NOTICE

Medicine is an ever-changing science. As new research and clinical experience broaden our knowledge, changes in treatment and drug therapy are required. The authors and the publisher of this work have checked with sources believed to be reliable in their efforts to provide information that is complete and generally in accord with the standards accepted at the time of publication. However, in view of the possibility of human error or changes in medical sciences, neither the authors nor the publisher nor any other party who has been involved in the preparation or publication of this work warrants that the information contained herein is in every respect accurate or complete, and they disclaim all responsibility for any errors or omissions or for the results obtained from use of the information contained in this work. Readers are encouraged to confirm the information contained herein with other sources. For example and in particular, readers are advised to check the product information sheet included in the package of each drug they plan to administer to be certain that the information contained in this work is accurate and that changes have not been made in the recommended dose or in the contraindications for administration. This recommendation is of particular importance in connection with new or infrequently used drugs.

Artificial Intelligence in Surgery

Artificial Intelligence in Surgery
Understanding the Role of AI in Surgical Practice

Editor

Daniel A. Hashimoto, MD, MS
Associate Director of Research
Surgical AI and Innovation Laboratory
Massachusetts General Hospital
Harvard Medical School
Boston, Massachusetts

Associate Editors

Ozanan R. Meireles, MD
Director
Surgical AI and Innovation Laboratory
Assistant Professor of Surgery
Harvard Medical School
Massachusetts General Hospital
Boston, Massachusetts

Guy Rosman, PhD
Associate Director of Engineering
Surgical AI and Innovation Laboratory
Massachusetts General Hospital
Boston, Massachusetts
Senior Research Scientist
Toyota Research Institute
Cambridge, Massachusetts

New York   Chicago   San Francisco   Athens   London   Madrid
Mexico City   Milan   New Delhi   Singapore   Sydney   Toronto

ISBN 978-1-260-45273-0
MHID 1-260-45273-5

This book was set in Times NR MT Std by KnowledgeWorks Global Ltd.
The editors were Andrew Moyer and Peter J. Boyle.
The production supervisor was Richard Ruzycka.
Project management was provided by Sarika Gupta, KnowledgeWorks Global Ltd.
The cover designer was W2 Design.

This book is printed on acid-free paper.

Cataloging-in-Publication Data is on file with the Library of Congress

McGraw Hill books are available at special quantity discounts to use as premiums and sales promotions or for use in corporate training programs. To contact a representative, please visit the Contact Us pages at www.mhprofessional.com.

For Naomi. Thank you for supporting my dreams and goals—
even when they seem unreasonable and unachievable.
And to my parents and siblings.
Thank you for instilling in me a love of science and discovery.

—Daniel Hashimoto

To my family, my parents and my brothers.
And a very special thank you to my mother, Professor Marta Melo, for teaching
me the value of academia and instigating my curiosity and for demonstrating
that one's legacy lives forever through their intellectual production.

—Ozanan Meireles

To my family—my parents, brother, sisters, wife, and children.
Thank you for your unconditional love and support
throughout the years and across the ocean.

—Guy Rosman

Contents

Chapter 1

A Brief History of Artificial Intelligence 1

Maria S. Alteiri, Cara B. Jones, and Guy Rosman

Chapter 2

Large Databases in Surgery 15

Sanford E. Roberts and Rachel R. Kelz

Chapter 3

Machine Learning For Medicine 37

Frank Rudzicz

Chapter 4

Neural Networks and Deep Learning 59

Deepak Alapatt, Pietro Mascagni, Vinkle Srivastav,
and Nicolas Padoy

Chapter 5

Natural Language Processing 85

Leo Anthony Celi, Daniel Gruhl, Euma Ishii,
Chaitanya Shivade, Joseph Terdiman, and Joy Tzung-yu Wu

Chapter 6

Computer Vision in Surgery:
Fundamental Principles and Applications 115

Daniel A. Hashimoto, Amin Madani,
Allison Navarrete-Welton, and Guy Rosman

Contributors

Deepak Alapatt, MSc
Research Engineer ICube
French National Centre for Scientific Research
Institute for Image-Guided Surgery
University of Strasbourg
Strasbourg, France
Chapter 4

Maria S. Alteiri, MD, MS
Assistant Professor
Department of Surgery
East Carolina University Brody School of Medicine
Greenville, North Carolina
Chapter 1

Joel W. Burdick, PhD
Richard L. and Dorothy M. Hayman Professor of Mechanical Engineering
and Bioengineering
Division of Engineering and Applied Sciences
California Institute of Technology
Pasadena, California
Chapter 12

Leo Anthony Celi, MD, MS, MPH
Principal Research Scientist
Institute for Medical Engineering and Science
Massachusetts Institute of Technology
Cambridge, Massachusetts
Associate Professor of Medicine
Division of Pulmonary, Critical Care, and Sleep Medicine
Beth Israel Deaconess Medical Center
Boston, Massachusetts
Chapter 5

Venkat Devarajan, PhD
Professor
Department of Electrical Engineering
University of Texas at Arlington
Arlington, Texas
Chapter 7

Megan B. Diamond, BA, MS
Program Manager
Harvard Global Health Institute
Cambridge, Massachusetts
Chapter 15

Majed W. El Hechi, MD
Post-Doctoral Research Fellow
Division of Trauma, Emergency Surgery & Surgical Critical Care
Boston, Massachusetts
Chapter 9

Yuman Fong, MD
Sangiacomo Chair and Chairman
Department of Surgery
City of Hope Medical Center
Duarte, California
California Institute of Technology
Pasadena, California
Chapter 12

Mitchell G. Goldenberg, MBBS, PhD
Clinician Investigator
International Centre for Surgical Safety
Li Ka Shing Knowledge Institute
St. Michael's Hospital, University of Toronto
Surgical Safety Technologies
Toronto, Ontario, Canada
Chapter 10

Teodor P. Grantcharov, MD, PhD
Professor of Surgery
International Centre for Surgical Safety
Li Ka Shing Knowledge Institute
St. Michael's Hospital, University of Toronto
Surgical Safety Technologies
Toronto, Ontario, Canada
Chapter 10

Daniel Gruhl, PhD
Distinguished Research Staff Member
International Business Machine Research–Almaden
San Jose, California
Chapter 5

Daniel A. Hashimoto, MD, MS
Associate Director of Research
Surgical AI and Innovation Laboratory
Massachusetts General Hospital
Harvard Medical School
Boston, Massachusetts
Chapters 6, 17, and 18

Euma Ishii, MD
Research Affiliate
Institute for Medical Engineering and Science
Massachusetts Institute of Technology
Cambridge, Massachusetts
MD-PhD Candidate
Tokyo Medical and Dental University
Tokyo, Japan
Chapter 5

Benjamin H. Jacobson, BA
Research Assistant
Harvard Global Health Institute
Cambridge, Massachusetts
Chapter 15

Cara B. Jones
Undergraduate Research Assistant
Columbia College
Columbia University
New York, New York
Chapter 1

Haytham Kaafarani, MD, MPH
Associate Professor of Surgery
Division of Trauma, Emergency Surgery and Surgical Critical Care
Massachusetts General Hospital
Harvard Medical School
Boston, Massachusetts
Chapter 9

Rachel R. Kelz, MD, MSCE, MBA
Professor of Surgery
Department of Surgery
Perelman School of Medicine at the University of Pennsylvania
Philadelphia, Pennsylvania
Chapter 2

Marc Levin, MD
Otolaryngology Resident
International Centre for Surgical Safety
Li Ka Shing Knowledge Institute
St. Michael's Hospital
University of Toronto
Toronto, Ontario, Canada
Chapter 10

Quanzheng Li, PhD
Associate Professor
Scientific Director
Center for Clinical Data Science
Massachusetts General Hospital
Harvard Medical School
Boston, Massachusetts
Chapter 11

Amin Madani, MD, PhD
Staff Surgeon
Division of General Surgery
University Health Network–Toronto General Hospital
Toronto, Ontario, Canada
Chapter 6

Anand Malpani, PhD
Assistant Research Scientist
Malone Center for Engineering in Healthcare
Johns Hopkins University
Baltimore, Maryland
Director of Data Science
Mimic Technologies Inc.
Seattle, Washington
Chapter 8

Pietro Mascagni, MD
PhD Candidate
ICube
French National Centre for Scientific Research
Institute for Image-Guided Surgery
University of Strasbourg
Strasbourg, France
Fondazione Policlinico Universitario Agostino Gemelli
Istituto di Ricovero e Cura a Carattere Scientifico
Rome, Italy
Chapter 4

Winta T. Mehtsun, MD, MPH
Complex Surgical Oncology Fellow
Harvard Global Health Institute
Cambridge, Massachusetts
Dana-Farber Cancer Institute
Brigham and Women's Hospital
Massachusetts General Hospital
Boston, Massachusetts
Chapter 15

Ozanan R. Meireles, MD
Director
Surgical AI and Innovation Laboratory
Assistant Professor of Surgery
Harvard Medical School
Massachusetts General Hospital
Boston, Massachusetts
Chapter 18

Daniel Naftalovich, BS
MD-PhD Student, Caltech-USC MD-PhD Program
Engineering and Applied Sciences
California Institute of Technology
Keck School of Medicine
University of Southern California
Pasadena, California
Chapter 12

Babak Namazi, PhD
Postdoctoral Research Fellow
Baylor University Medical Center
Dallas, Texas
Chapter 7

Allison Navarrete-Welton, AB
Research Assistant
Surgical AI and Innovation Laboratory
Massachusetts General Hospital
Boston, Massachusetts
Chapter 6

Samer A. Nour Eddine, MD
Cognitive Science and Psychology PhD Candidate
Department of Psychology
Tufts University
Medford, Massachusetts
Chapter 9

Nicolas Padoy, PhD
Professor of Computer Science
ICube
French National Centre for Scientific Research
Institute for Image-Guided Surgery
University of Strasbourg
Strasbourg, France
Chapter 4

Sanford E. Roberts, MD
General Surgery Resident
Department of Surgery
Perelman School of Medicine at the University of Pennsylvania
Philadelphia, Pennsylvania
Chapter 2

Guy Rosman, PhD
Associate Director of Engineering
Surgical AI and Innovation Laboratory
Massachusetts General Hospital
Boston, Massachusetts
Senior Research Scientist
Toyota Research Institute
Cambridge, Massachusetts
Chapters 1 and 6

Frank Rudzicz, PhD
Associate Professor of Computer Science
Department of Computer Science
International Centre for Surgical Safety
Li Ka Shing Knowledge Institute
St. Michael's Hospital
University of Toronto
Surgical Safety Technologies
Vector Institute for Artificial Intelligence
Toronto, Ontario, Canada
Chapters 3 and 14

Daniela Rus, PhD
Andrew (1956) and Erna Viterbi Professor of Electrical Engineering and Computer Science
Director
Computer Science and Artificial Intelligence Laboratory
Primary Investigator
Distributed Robotics Laboratory
Massachusetts Institute of Technology
Cambridge, Massachusetts
Chapter 18

Ganesh Sankaranarayanan, PhD
Assistant Director
Center for Evidence Based Simulation
Baylor University Medical Center
Clinical Associate Professor
Texas A&M College of Medicine
Dallas, Texas
Chapter 7

Raeid Saqur, MBA, MScAC
PhD Candidate
Department of Computer Science
University of Toronto
Toronto, Ontario, Canada
Princeton University
Princeton, New Jersey
Chapter 14

Chaitanya Shivade, PhD
Research Staff Member
International Business Machine Research–Almaden
San Jose, California
Chapter 5

Vinkle Srivastav, MS
PhD Candidate
ICube
French National Centre for Scientific Research
Institute for Image-Guided Surgery
University of Strasbourg
Strasbourg, France
Chapter 4

Camille Stewart, MD
Surgical Oncology Fellow
Department of Surgery
City of Hope Medical Center
Duarte, California
Chapter 12

Joseph Terdiman, MD, PhD
Research Staff Member
International Business Machine Research–Almaden
San Jose, California
Chapter 5

David Y. Ting, MD
Chief Medical Information Officer
Massachusetts General Physicians Organization
Assistant Professor
Harvard Medical School
Boston, Massachusetts
Chapter 13

Thomas Ward, MD
Surgical AI and Innovation Fellow
Surgical AI and Innovation Laboratory
Massachusetts General Hospital
Boston, Massachusetts
Chapter 16

Joy Tzung-yu Wu, MBChB, MPH
Research Staff Member
International Business Machine Research–Almaden
San Jose, California
Chapter 5

Preface

Artificial intelligence (AI) is a rapidly growing field that is touching or will touch nearly every element of modern life. One of the biggest areas of potential impact for AI is in health care, and there has been growing interest in understanding and evaluating how AI can affect different specialties across medicine. Although radiology and pathology have thus far been leading the charge in developing and adopting AI, other specialties are in hot pursuit. Surgery is one field with tremendous potential for disruption by AI. While there is no replacement for the formal study of a field through graduate education or research fellowships, we feel it is important for clinicians, educators, and researchers in surgery to gain an understanding of the fundamental topics, concepts, techniques, and considerations that go into research and development in AI in order to better understand its current abilities and future potential.

The overall objective of this book is to provide an *approachable* resource on AI to those in surgery who do not necessarily have a technical background in mathematics, engineering, or computer science. It will provide a foundation of knowledge on the history, principles, and main subfields of AI. It will then provide examples of current and near future use cases for AI in surgery and then transition to a discussion of the ethical implications of AI and its potential impact on health policy. Finally, it will provide those interested in AI research with an introduction to the practical aspects underlying research in the field to help readers develop a foundation in reading and interpreting existing work and to seek further education and training to grow as a surgical data scientist.

We are excited to be part of your journey in exploring the bright future of this field!

Daniel A. Hashimoto, MD, MS
Ozanan R. Meireles, MD
Guy Rosman, PhD

Acknowledgments

This textbook would not have been possible without the support of mentors, colleagues, and collaborators both at home in Boston and around the world. In particular, we thank Drs. Keith Lillemoe and David Rattner, who supported the vision of establishing a line of research at Massachusetts General Hospital (MGH) on the development of artificial intelligence for surgery; and Professor Daniela Rus of the Massachusetts Institute of Technology, who has contributed her genius, expertise, and experience toward developing and translating these technologies for the benefit of surgical patients. We also wish to thank the faculty, residents, and operating room staff at MGH, Newton Wellesley Hospital, and North Shore Medical Center who have supported the quest for a data-enabled future of surgery.

Now more than ever, science is a product of teamwork, and the Surgical AI and Innovation Laboratory at MGH has had success due to the contributions of a great team of fellows, students, and staff. We are grateful for the hard work and dedication of Dr. Thomas Ward, Dr. Yutong Ban, Dr. Mikhail Volkov, Caitlin Stafford, Allison Navarrete-Welton, Will Specht, and Gloria Indelicato.

We thank all the chapter authors and contributors to the textbook. Your expertise is invaluable to our community, and we appreciate you sharing it with us in an accessible manner. The advancement of surgical artificial intelligence is a global effort to improve access to and the quality of surgical care; such advances would not be possible without the collaborative efforts of surgeons, researchers, and patients around the world. A very special thanks to the McGraw Hill team, especially Andrew Moyer, Peter Boyle, and Leah Carton, for recognizing the importance of providing a source of fundamental knowledge of concepts in artificial intelligence to surgeons and surgical researchers.

Finally, we wish to thank all our colleagues and frontline workers around the world who have been engaged in the fight against the COVID-19 pandemic. Although work on this textbook began well before the start of the pandemic, we have all been affected—either through direct patient care, in our research efforts, or through personal experience with friends and family who were impacted by the virus. Thank you for your selfless dedication to the health and wellness of the world.

A BRIEF HISTORY OF ARTIFICIAL INTELLIGENCE 1

Maria S. Alteiri, Cara B. Jones, and Guy Rosman

HIGHLIGHTS

- Artificial intelligence is a field that has been influenced by mathematics, computer science, psychology, neurobiology, linguistics, economics, and others.
- The term *artificial intelligence* (AI) was officially coined in 1956 at the Dartmouth Summer Research Project meeting; however, the concept of AI can be traced to as far back as 700 BC, when tales of "mechanical" humans were incorporated into Greek mythology.
- Developments in AI often occurred in parallel with different research streams converging to lead to significant advances in the technology.

█ INTRODUCTION

Artificial intelligence (AI) has a variety of definitions depending on the context, basic theory, or era under consideration[1]; however, it can be understood broadly as the "the capability of a machine to imitate intelligent human behavior."[2] An intelligent machine that can understand and solve problems in a manner similar to, if not superior to, the human brain is perhaps the ultimate goal of AI. However, because this goal is undoubtedly ambitious, it remains far out of reach despite significant advances that have occurred in the field. AI is a broad and disparate discipline derived from a vast array of fields that have made many significant contributions to the development of AI throughout history. Disciplines such as biology, philosophy, and computer science, among others, have each played an important role in AI's development,

With contributions from Vinkle Srivastav, Nicolay Padoy, PhD, and Pietro Mascagni, MD, of University of Strasbourg.

sometimes working in parallel before intersecting at various points in time as technology and interests have converged.

Fundamental advances in philosophy and biology led to analogous advances in applied fields such as economics, engineering, and computer science. The interaction and cross-integration of these various disciplines and their visions promoted growth and stimulated creative thinking. Together, centuries of small discoveries in philosophy, mathematics, economics, linguistics, psychology, neurobiology, and computer science laid the foundation upon which the concept of AI was established. In our view, there were 3 notable pillars of progress that led to the advancement of AI as we know it today. The first is marked by the attempt to connect basic machinery to the philosophy of thinking—as seen in works spanning from Leonardo da Vinci to Alan Turing—and the rise of numerical reasoning and computing. The second pillar is the establishment of a basic understanding of logical reasoning coupled with attempts to define a reasoning machine. The third surrounds the development of techniques to answer the question of how one can quantify reasoning.

We see these pillars often occurring in parallel over time. Because the development of AI did not occur in discrete segments but rather as amorphous advances occurring together across history and different fields, it is quite difficult and arbitrary to divide the history of AI into specific time periods. Thus, although we provide some distinctions for relative time periods in this chapter, please note that these are not, by any means, "official" transitions or historical markers. The sections are meant to provide conceptual categorization for the reader.

Although an in-depth exploration of the history of AI is outside the scope of this chapter (and this book), it is important to understand the historical context that has led to the modern field of AI and its applications to surgery. This chapter provides a brief overview of and our perspective on some of the major events across various fields that have led up to the principles and applications of AI presented throughout this book.

▌ HISTORICAL FOUNDATIONS

Although *artificial intelligence* as a term was not coined until 1956,[1] it was a concept hundreds of years in the making. Having autonomous machines that mimic humans has been a property of human imagination for centuries. Hesiod described the ancient Greek myth of Hephaestus, a god of invention, who created a mechanical servant known as Talos. Talos was created from a life force called "ichor" to be a protector of Crete from invaders.[3] Ichor powered Talos's movements and thoughts and was the placeholder for the unobtainable, artificial production of a mind and, arguably, an early conceptualization of AI. Indeed, beyond mythology, the Greeks' contributions to philosophy, perhaps one of the most ancient disciplines, have been considered foundational for the social sciences as well. Their advances in philosophy laid the foundation for later advances in fields such as economics, mathematics, information science, and statistics.

For example, Aristotle described laws of thought, used to set parameters around the rational mind, that became the beginning of the field of logic—an outsize influence in learning and mathematics. In addition, around 250 BC, Ktesibios of Alexandria created the first self-controlling machine, a water-controlled clock that demonstrated self-regulating feedback. Although logic and clocks alone are certainly not AI, their development does highlight important historical and philosophical contributions that later enabled the development and enhancement of fields such as mathematics and engineering. Fast-forwarding to the 14th century, logical and mechanical advancements started to accelerate at a swift pace. Around 1500, Leonardo da Vinci described a design for a mechanical calculator, but it was not until 1623 that Wilhelm Schickard built the first known calculating machine—the Speeding Clock or Calculating Clock—that was able to add and subtract 6-digit numbers.

Although many historical advances in philosophy have occurred, those pertaining to logic, reason, and probability have had notable impacts on mathematics and AI. In 1662, Antoine Arnauld and Pierre Nicole published *The Logic or the Art of Thinking*, defining actions, judgments, and inferences through the rules of reason and creating a quantitative formula for deciding what action a person could or should take. This ultimately influenced Thomas Bayes, who further built upon ideas of probability in his work, "Essay Towards Solving a Problem in the Doctrine of Chances," published after his death in the *Philosophical Transactions of the Royal Society of London*. His findings and the description of Bayes's rule have become crucial to modern approaches in AI, particularly around the reasoning of uncertainty.[4] David Hume further described the principle of induction in his *A Treatise of Human Nature* as part of the empiricism movement. Hume explored the psychological part of human nature, hypothesizing that human knowledge was based on experience rather than reason alone.

By the 19th century, logic, philosophy, mathematics, and the first calculators had started paving the way for more complex machines and ushering in the second pillar of progress on the road to AI—the advancement of numerical reasoning and computing. In 1801, one of the first programmable machines, the Jacquard attachment or Jacquard mechanism, used interchangeable punch cards that individually indicated a systematic weaving pattern. It provided a stepping stone for the designs of the earliest computers with punch cards used in the 1830s in the design of Charles Babbage and Ada Byron's Analytical Engine.[5] The Analytical Engine was designed to be a programmable calculating machine that was steam-driven and controlled by a singular person. Although this machine was not built as a working model until 2002, it is often regarded as the first computer ever designed. It contained compartments that compare to modern computers' central processing unit, storage, memory, input, and output.

17TH CENTURY TO 20TH CENTURY ADVANCES: NEUROSCIENCE AND COMPUTING

Biology, and specifically neuroscience, has played an influential role in the advancement of AI. The intuitions behind artificial neural networks were profoundly inspired by those gained studying their biologic counterparts, as is often the case with technologic innovation. Scientific observations on the human brain date back to the start of the 20th century, when Santiago Ramón y Cajal and Camillo Golgi first hypothesized that neurons serve as the fundamental building block of the nervous system, a complex network that extends from the brain to the body periphery.

In 1873, Camillo Golgi observed neurons for the first time using a new staining technique now known as Golgi staining. Golgi staining is a process in which neurons are stained through the hardening of nervous tissue from the exposure to potassium bichromate and silver nitrate, thus giving a look into the subanatomy of the brain. He shared a Nobel Prize in 1906 with Santiago Ramón y Cajal, who had conducted similar work on the microscopic structure of the brain and illustrated the numerous cellular connections that formed what would later come to be known as neural networks.[6] Insights into the organization of neurons, as described later in this chapter, led to significant neuroscientific advances in the 1900s with subsequent impact on the development of several AI techniques.

The area of mathematics was advancing in parallel to advances in biology and neuroscience. In the early 20th century, a new approach to logic was described in Bertrand Russell and Alfred North Whitehead's *Principia Mathematica*. In *Principia Mathematica*, Russell and Whitehead defended logicism, the simplified idea that mathematics can be reduced to logic and is therefore an extension of it. These textbooks define mathematical principles (hence the name) from logical principles alone and became very influential in the 1910s to the 1950s. In the 1930s, Kurt Gödel proved his incompleteness theorems, which questioned the solvability of problems and demonstrated the inherent limitations of every formal axiomatic system capable of modeling basic arithmetic. Gödel, along with Russell and Whitehead, influenced Alan Turing and Alonzo Church (among others), leading to the notation of Turing machines, λ-calculus, the beginning of complexity theory, and a rigorous explanation of what functions are computable and with what computational effort.[7]

Such mathematical advances led to the design of one of the earliest operational computers in 1945 by Turing, known as the Automatic Computing Engine (ACE), which went on to serve as the model for the first personal computers.[8] However, Turing's work with ACE was overshadowed at the time by John von Neumann's Electronic Discrete Variable Automatic Computer (EDVAC) design. EDVAC became the first description of a stored-program computer design, where the program was stored in the same memory as the data on which it was working.[9] However, unlike EDVAC, which used binary, ACE used Turing's Abbreviated Instruction Code, which is now seen as an early programming language related to modern programming languages. ACE is also recognized as a general-purpose computer, able to perform multiple tasks without rewiring or programming.

Between 1939 and 1948, many different calculators and computers were rapidly produced. During that time, the complex number calculator was completed (1939) as the first remote access computer performing calculations from New York City to Dartmouth College.[10] A couple years later, in 1941, the first Bombe was completed, which was an electromechanical machine used in World War II to break the German Enigma codes.[11] The Atanasoff-Berry computer (ABC) was built as the first automatic electronic digital computer with the ability to compute complex calculations. The ABC adopted the use of a binary numbering system instead of base 10 numbering and contained memory for storing data.[12] Although this device was limited, it became the basis for the development of the Electronic Numerical Integrator and Computer (1946), commonly known as ENIAC, which was the first electronic computer, instead of a standard electromechanical machine.[13] This allowed the computations to be around 1000 times faster, computing more numbers than anything in history before it. Furthermore, around this time, Arthur Samuel created a computer algorithm that could allow a computer to play a game of checkers, perhaps the first example of a computer program with the ability to learn from its previous errors. Written for the IBM 701, it is the earliest example of nonnumerical computation and the first game-player program, demonstrating the computational ability to outperform the average person's learning patterns.[14]

In 1950, Alan Turing defined the Turing Test, which provided parameters to determine whether a computer program could think "original" thoughts. A computer was deemed successful if the test could not distinguish a computer from a human.[15] Turing provided what has become perhaps the most famous framework for evaluating a general AI and a goalpost for potential achievement in computing. In that same year, the National Physical Laboratory completed the Pilot ACE. Originally designed by Turing, the Pilot ACE became one of the first general-purpose computers to perform more than one specified task.[16] In that same year, Marvin Minsky and Dean Edmonds built the Stochastic Neural Analog Reinforcement Calculator (SNARC). Known as the first neural network computer, it used an automatic pilot mechanism to simulate a network of 40 neurons.[2]

In the midst of these advances in computing, scientists began to turn their attention to questions such as, "Can a machine solve a problem using machine intelligence?" The Dartmouth Summer Research Project on Artificial Intelligence (DSRPAI) attempted to answer this question and marked the founding of AI as an organized field. During this conference, a group of scientists proposed a 2-month summer research project known as the Stanford Artificial Intelligence Project with the shared vision of "a computer made to perform intelligent tasks," kicking off the current era of AI research as we largely know it today. Within this proposal, John McCarthy defined AI as "the basis of the conjecture that every aspect of learning or any other feature of intelligence can in principle be so precisely described that a machine can be made to simulate it."[17] The DSRPAI set off a cascade of foundational works in the field of AI.

Following the DSRPAI, during a September 1956 seminar at the Massachusetts Institute of Technology, 3 influential works were presented by George Miller, Noam Chomsky, Allen Newell, and Herbert Simon that covered the psychology of language, memory, and logical thinking. Miller discussed short-term memory in "The Magic Number Seven, Plus or Minus Two" paper, discussing cognitive limits. Chomsky published "Three Models for the Description of Language," which created a ranking of syntactic forms and became very influential in the development of natural language processing. Newell and Simon presented the Logic Theorist, perhaps the first "modern" AI program, which was able to prove the majority of the theorems of Russell and Whitehead's *Principia Mathematica*. It introduced several concepts that would be central to AI, such as reasoning to search, heuristics, and list processing.

In 1957, Chomsky, through his review of B.F. Skinner's *Verbal Behavior*, broke down the faults of behaviorist theory[18] and put forth a set of considerations in language that influenced much future work in computational linguistics and natural language processing. That same year, Richard Bellman formalized Markov decision processes and explored dynamic programming as a tool to solve them.

A year later, Herbert Simon and Allen Newell introduced the importance of heuristic problem solving in advanced computers. There was an unexplored management of present problems that Simon and Newell split into 2 categories: well-structured and ill-structured. Well-structured management problems are developed quantitatively and precisely and solved with known computational procedures. In contrast, ill-structured problems do not have tools that can solve them. They have variables that can be symbolic or verbal but not well represented quantitatively. They defined heuristic problem solving as the approach that allows humans to solve these ill-structured problems without mathematical tools and computational algorithms. The theory of heuristics, in contrast to traditional algorithmic problem solving, aims to understand the imperfect yet practical problem-solving processes in which humans often engage and to simulate such processes in computers.

As the underlying philosophy and mathematics of computational approaches to problem solving were worked out, programming languages and programs were developed to meet the needs of the scientific community. In 1960, LISP (list processing), a programming language, was developed. LISP was founded on the mathematical theory of recursive functions as applied to large data sets. This language was common for AI programming of the time and has been further modified over time. General Problem Solver (GPS) was subsequently created by Allen Newell and Herbert Simon to trace the reasoning of computer programs and compare it to human reasoning. Through observation and experimentation, a theory of mind was developed and replicated as a computer program. This further led to a connection between the manipulation of symbolistic data structures based on human or AI actions that created the physical symbol system in 1976.

In 1963, Lawrence Roberts published *Machine Perception of Three-Dimensional Solids*, which included an algorithm to render 3-dimensional objects from 2-dimensional photographs using rules of depth perception derived from edge information.[19] In Roberts's work, we again see the influence of neuroscience as Hubel and Wiesel's landmark work on edge perception by cats informed an understanding of biologic perception of edges that could be translated to computational work.

The DENDRAL project was initiated in 1965 and aimed to see if scientific discoveries were possible using a computer software system. DENDRAL's first application was in organic chemistry as one of the first expert systems. DENDRAL would use mass spectra information as input to identify the possible chemical structures that could be producing such data by relying on its knowledge of information such as atomic number and valence rules to quickly generate a list of possible chemical structures.[20]

Parallel to these developments in programming, a simplified mathematical formulation of the behavior of a neuron and the concept that synaptic (ie, Hebbian) plasticity contributes to learning paved the way for the development of computational neural networks.[21,22] As the theoretical understanding of the neuron was gaining traction in biology, computer scientists also started prototyping functional neurons on chips. In 1958, Frank Rosenblatt proposed the first computational model of a neuron known as the *perceptron*. The perceptron takes the weighted sum of inputs and outputs a "1" if the sum exceeds a given threshold, a process analogous to neurons firing an action potential if a certain threshold potential is reached.[23] Similar to biologic neural networks, the perceptron's internal parameters update much like neurons' connections strengthen or weaken with learning. The hierarchical processing of neural networks, an extremely relevant insight linking biologic and artificial neural networks, was a concept introduced by Hubel and Wiesel in 1962.[24] They observed that specific neurons in the primary visual cortex of cats responded based on the orientation of edges shown to them in images and hypothesized that neurons in early layers (ie, closer to the retina) extract low-level features such as edges, while downstream layers extract higher-level semantic information. As further described in Chapter 4 (Neural Networks and Deep Learning), their work played a key role in establishing the concept of hierarchical organization of neural networks.

Excitement regarding the potential of neural networks led to a flurry of activity in attempting to develop AI systems based on multilayer networks. Unfortunately, the computational power at the time was largely insufficient to tackle some of the more ambitious projects that were proposed. As failures mounted in the 1960s and 1970s, the first AI "winter" occurred—a period in which decreased enthusiasm from the scientific community led to decreased interest in AI, including a reduction in funding opportunities. The computational power for AI programs at the time was quite limited, particularly in the goal to produce several complex computations. Furthermore, the vast amount of information needed to build reasoning in an AI algorithm was unattainable at the time. Perhaps one of the most influential factors in bringing about the first AI winter was the Lighthill report of 1973. This report (officially named "Artificial Intelligence: A General Survey") critiqued the applicability of AI techniques to broader and more realistic problems and pointed to the paucity of discoveries that had been promised.[25] This pessimistic view of AI led to the decrease of government funding in the United States and Great Britain, dampening the earlier excitement for AI.[26]

Despite the AI winter, some research in AI persisted, particularly in medicine. In the 1970s, Edward Shortliffe, Ed Feigenbaum, and Bruce Buchanan created MYCIN, a system that demonstrated knowledge representation and inference in medical diagnosis and therapy using a 450-rule system. MYCIN was used to identify blood infections for treatment and was understood as the first expert system that used heuristic programming. Unlike DENDRAL, all the rules and calculation of the certainty of the given answer (certainty factors) were created from an extensive amount of literature and expert interviews instead of a general theoretical model. Overall, this program was comparable to experts and, in some applications, better than junior doctors. A notable feature of this program was the explainability of its results (ie, its ability to explain its diagnoses and conclusions).[27,28]

Jack Myers and Harry People developed INTERNIST, a knowledge-based medical diagnosis program created from the PDP-10 assembly language and LISP. Notably, all the knowledge from this program was reported to be from published literature as a standard source instead of the usual single-source domain expert. This database later led to Quick Medical Reference and the follow-up program INTERNIST-1.[29] That same year, Kunihiko Fukushima published an article on the unsupervised learning network known as neocognitron. This new algorithm was organized into 3 layers: the photoreceptor layer, S-cells layer, and C-cells layer, reflecting the Hubel and Wiesel model of the visual nervous system previously described.[30]

As LISP-based systems continued to improve, a resurging interest in LISP-based AI systems led to increased commercial investment in expert systems in the late 1970s and early 1980s, with both major companies (eg, Xerox, Texas Instruments) and start-ups releasing LISP machines for enterprise use. However, advances in personal computing workstations led to computers that became both more powerful and less expensive than AI-specific LISP machines. As businesses began to realize that specific AI hardware no longer held a computational advantage over more cost-effective computer workstations, interest in further development in the AI approaches of the time again began to wane in the early 1990s, leading to a second AI winter.

THE MODERN AI PERIOD

Although the AI winters may have temporarily dampened the momentum of AI, progress continued to be made in various elements of the field throughout both winters. From a theoretical perspective, Peter Cheeseman's *In Defense of Probability* defended the validity of using probability for uncertainty reasoning. Prior to his work, one of the dominant beliefs in the field was that probability was unable to accurately describe reasoning, and Cheeseman's text paved the way for the ideas captured by Judea Pearl in *Probabilistic Reasoning in Intelligent Systems*. This textbook is a landmark in the transition from the symbolic AI approaches of the 1960s and 1970s toward uses of Bayesian inference approaches that treat learning as a probabilistic inference from observations, formalizing uncertainty reasoning and causal reasoning.

The late 1980s saw the development of the Soar project, a cognitive architecture and a theory—based on works by Allen Newell, John Laird, Paul Rosenbloom, and others—composed of hypotheses that ultimately support 3 levels of processing: (1) bottom-up, parallel automatic processing; (2) deliberative processing of knowledge from the first level to select an action; and (3) complex processing of uncertainty.[31,32] Soar presented an agent architecture using explanation-based learning, which takes previously applied computations and, through observations, derives generalized rules that can be applied to future computations. It has had numerous applications ranging from natural language understanding to robotics to gaming and mobile AI.

As AI moved out of its second winter, there was a shift to machine learning using data-based information rather than knowledge-based information. The traditional rule-based systems generated from knowledge-based information used expert knowledge from a targeted area, where a set of facts was used to create rules from expert knowledge. However, these rules could become complex and unwieldy, leading to overly complex, expensive computation. As will be discussed in greater detail in Chapters 3 and 4, data-based systems offer more flexibility because they only use the outcomes of experts and without necessarily needing to learn or address their process of decision making. The algorithm, using probability, can begin to learn its own parameters from input variables to optimize output. Such an approach underlies much of the current work in deep learning.

Deep learning, a subfield of AI that has become incredibly popular today, has now grown to outsize influence in the AI world (Chapter 4 covers deep learning as applied to surgery in detail). The development of deep learning spans back decades, having been developed (at first slowly and then quite rapidly) in parallel since the first computational descriptions of the neuron. To consider some of the more recent work in deep learning, in 1989, Yann LeCun published work on connectivity systems, emphasizing the ability to learn from examples and the generalization of performance, concluding that a multilayer constrained network performed well when organized in a hierarchical structure that minimized the number of free parameters. His example included the application of this approach to image recognition (specifically digit recognition), and this efficient use of invariance in a neural network model would influence subsequent developments in deep learning.[33] Building off that work, Yann LeCun, Yoshua Bengio, and colleagues demonstrated that their multilayer convolutional neural network (CNN) known as LeNet could accurately recognize handwritten digits, the "Hello world!" of AI.[34] Still, at the time, neural networks were trained and tested on small data sets and had limited computing power, limiting their applicability outside of controlled environments.

By the mid-2000s, however, computing power and access to large data sets had begun to improve significantly. Neural networks quickly became the focus of the most recent decade of AI research and advancement, especially after Alex Krizhevsky, Geoff Hinton, and colleagues debuted a CNN called AlexNet in 2012 and trained it on a large-scale image classification data set, ImageNet,[35] using graphics processing units (GPUs). AlexNet represented a pivotal point in neural network research because it was able to show how deep learning could beat carefully crafted systems.[35] Since then, research on neural networks has flourished, leading to improved performance and new applications. For instance, neural networks such as Deeplab[36] or Mask R-CNN[37] can localize different objects in images. Generative adversarial nets (GAN) are a framework invented in 2014 that represents a modern view of machine learning through the joining of the probabilistic reasoning community and neural networks (see Chapter 4).

Applications of neural networks and deep learning gained momentum in the medical field with applications ranging from predicting outcomes using electronic health records[38] to medical imaging analysis[39] and surgical data science.[40] For example, variants of UNet[41] have been used to highlight anatomic structures down to the pixel level, and EndoNet,[42] an extension of AlexNet, has been used to analyze surgical workflow in endoscopic videos. Several chapters of this textbook will provide additional examples of neural networks and deep learning in medicine and, of course, surgery.

The modern period of AI is not limited to deep learning, however. As understanding of algorithms continues to grow and computational power becomes more accessible, interesting work exploring causality, explainability, and transparency and modeling of uncertainty are moving to the forefront of AI research. As narrow or specific AI (ie, AI that is adept at solving certain, defined problems) continues to be perfected, interest has grown in developing a framework of general AI (ie, AI that is able to tackle a wide range of tasks or problems). In other words, there has been a push toward developing truly intelligent machines that can more closely approximate natural intelligence, with the ability to generalize.[43]

▌CONCLUSION

An overview of the roots of AI as a field provides necessary context in appreciating the complex web of influences that has led to the current state of the art. Surgery is a recent application for a field that has been decades in the making. Both fields, however, have benefited from the influence of similar fields, such as biology, philosophy, mathematics, and computer sciences. The remainder of this textbook will provide surgeons, surgical researchers, medical students, and other interested individuals who do not necessarily have a mathematical or computational background with the foundation necessary to begin to appreciate advances that are being made in surgical AI.

▌REFERENCES

1. Definition of artificial intelligence. Merriam-Webster.com. Accessed August 26, 2020. https://www.merriam-webster.com/dictionary/artificial+intelligence.
2. Russell S, Norvig P. *Artificial Intelligence: A Modern Approach*. Global Edition. Pearson; 2016.
3. Graves R. *The Greek Myths*. Penguin UK; 1990.
4. Bayes T. An essay towards solving a problem in the doctrine of chances. 1763. *MD Comput*. 1991;8:157-171.
5. Bromley AG. Charles Babbage's analytical engine, 1838. *IEEE Ann Hist Comput*. 1998;20:29-45.
6. Kandel E. *Principles of Neural Science*. 5th ed. McGraw-Hill Professional; 2013.
7. Baaz M, Papadimitriou CH, Putnam HW, Scott DS, Harper CL Jr. *Kurt Gödel and the Foundations of Mathematics: Horizons of Truth*. Cambridge University Press; 2011.
8. Turing AM. Proposed electronic calculator (1945). In: Copeland J, ed. *Alan Turing's Automatic Computing Engine*. Oxford University Press; 2005:369-454.
9. Von Neumann J. First draft of a report on the EDVAC. Moore School of Electrical Engineering, University of Pennsylvania; 1945. doi:10.5479/sil.538961.39088011475779
10. Ritchie D. *The Computer Pioneers: The Making of the Modern Computer*. Simon & Schuster; 1986.
11. Welchman G. *The Hut Six Story: Breaking the Enigma Codes*. McGraw-Hill New York; 1982.
12. Chang C. John Vincent Atanasoff and the birth of electronic digital computing: Atanasoff-Berry Computer. Accessed August 26, 2020. http://jva.cs.iastate.edu/operation.php.

13. Weik MH. The ENIAC story. 1961. Accessed August 26, 2020. https://ftp.arl. army.mil/~mike/comphist/eniac-story.html.

14. Samuel AL. Some studies in machine learning using the game of checkers. *IBM J Res Dev.* 1959;3:210-229.

15. Turing AMI. Computing machinery and intelligence. *Mind.* 1950;LIX:433-460.

16. Vowels RA. The Pilot ACE: from concept to reality. In: Copeland J, ed. *Alan Turing's Automatic Computing Engine.* Oxford University Press; 2005:223-259.

17. McCarthy J, Minsky ML, Shannon CE, Rochester N, Dartmouth College. A proposal for the Dartmouth summer research project on artificial intelligence. August 31, 1955. Accessed August 26, 2020. http://www-formal.stanford.edu/jmc/history/dartmouth/dartmouth.html.

18. Chomsky N. A review of B. F. Skinner's verbal behavior. *Readings in Philosophy and Psychology.* 2013;1:48-64.

19. Roberts LG. Machine perception of three-dimensional solids. Dissertation. 1980. Accessed August 26, 2020. https://dspace.mit.edu/handle/1721.1/11589.

20. Buchanan BG, Feigenbaum EA. DENDRAL and meta-DENDRAL: their applications dimension. *Artif Intell.* 1978;11:5-24.

21. McCulloch WS, Pitts W. A logical calculus of the ideas immanent in nervous activity. 1943. *Bull Math Biol.* 1990;52:99-115; discussion 73-97.

22. Hebb DO. *The Organization of Behavior: A Neuropsychological Theory.* Psychology Press; 2002.

23. Rosenblatt F. The perceptron: a probabilistic model for information storage and organization in the brain. *Psychol Rev.* 1958;65:386-408.

24. Hubel DH, Wiesel TN. Receptive fields, binocular interaction and functional architecture in the cat's visual cortex. *J Physiol.* 1962;160:106-154.

25. Lighthill Report. Artificial intelligence: a general survey. Accessed August 26, 2020. http://www.chilton-computing.org.uk/inf/literature/reports/lighthill_report/p001.htm.

26. National Research Council, Computer Science and Telecommunications Board and Committee on Innovations in Computing and Communications. Lessons from history. In: *Funding a Revolution: Government Support for Computing Research.* National Academies Press; 1999:136-156.

27. Shortliffe EH, Davis R, Axline SG, et al. Computer-based consultations in clinical therapeutics: explanation and rule acquisition capabilities of the MYCIN system. *Comput Biomed Res.* 1975;8:303-320.

28. Buchanan BB, Buchanan BG, Shortliffe EH, Heuristic S. *Rule-Based Expert Systems: The MYCIN Experiments of the Stanford Heuristic Programming Project.* Addison Wesley Publishing Company; 1984.

29. Myers JD. The background of INTERNIST-1 and QMR. In: *A History of Medical Informatics.* Association for Computing Machinery; 1990:427-433.

30. Fukushima K. Neocognitron: a self-organizing neural network model for a mechanism of pattern recognition unaffected by shift in position. *Biol Cybernet.* 1980;36:193-202.

31. Newell A. *Unified Theories of Cognition.* Harvard University Press; 1994.

32. Laird JE, Newell A, Rosenbloom PS. SOAR: an architecture for general intelligence. *Artif Intell.* 1987;33:1-64.

33. LeCun Y. Generalization and network design strategies. In: Pfeifer R, Schreter Z, Fogelman F, Steels L, eds. *Connectionism in Perspective*. Elsevier; 1989:143-155.

34. Lecun Y, Bottou L, Bengio Y, Haffner P. Gradient-based learning applied to document recognition. *Proc IEEE*. 1998;86:2278-2324.

35. Krizhevsky A, Sutskever I, Hinton GE. ImageNet classification with deep convolutional neural networks. *Commun ACM*. 2017;60:84-90.

36. Chen L-C, Barron JT, Papandreou G, Murphy K, Yuille AL. Semantic image segmentation with task-specific edge detection using CNNs and a discriminatively trained domain transform. Presented at the 2016 IEEE Conference on Computer Vision and Pattern Recognition. Accessed August 26, 2020. https://arxiv.org/abs/1511.03328.

37. Kaiming H, Georgia G, Piotr D, Ross G. Mask R-CNN. 2017. Accessed August 26, 2020. http://paperpile.com/b/1Gzjbj/ah6h.

38. Shickel B, Tighe PJ, Bihorac A, Rashidi P. Deep EHR: a survey of recent advances in deep learning techniques for electronic health record (EHR) analysis. *IEEE J Biomed Health Inform*. 2018;22:1589-1604.

39. Schaffter T, Buist DSM, Lee CI, et al. Evaluation of combined artificial intelligence and radiologist assessment to interpret screening mammograms. *JAMA Netw Open*. 2020;3(3):e200265.

40. Maier-Hein L, Vedula SS, Speidel S, et al. Surgical data science for next-generation interventions. *Nat Biomed Eng*. 2017;1:691-696.

41. Ronneberger O, Fischer P, Brox T. U-Net: convolutional networks for biomedical image segmentation. In: *Medical Image Computing and Computer-Assisted Intervention—MICCAI 2015*. Springer International Publishing; 2015:234-241.

42. Twinanda AP, Shehata S, Mutter D, et al. EndoNet: a deep architecture for recognition tasks on laparoscopic videos. *IEEE Trans Med Imaging*. 2017;36:86-97.

43. Pennachin C, Goertzel B. Contemporary approaches to artificial general intelligence. In: Goertzel B, Pennachin C, eds. *Artificial General Intelligence: Cognitive Technologies*. Springer; 2007:1-30.

LARGE DATABASES IN SURGERY 2

Sanford E. Roberts and Rachel R. Kelz

HIGHLIGHTS

- An understanding of the information input and export processes is critical to the appropriate use of large data sets. As some would say, garbage in equals garbage out.
- Proper study design and knowledge of programming and statistics are imperative to the safe use of big data in health care.
- Many data sets and registries exist. The selection of the proper data source for a specific question or problem is necessary to achieve success.
- Collaborative practice including multidisciplinary teams of clinicians, statisticians, medical anthropologists, and programmers, among others, is encouraged when working with big data.
- Artificial intelligence has the capacity to change the way humans see and use data. Ethics panels and review boards must remain in place to safeguard the public and investigators.

▌ INTRODUCTION

The 21st century has seen the rise of "big data" in many different industries, including biology and medicine. The use of large data sets in academia has enhanced researchers' ability to tackle large-scale issues and identify broader patterns. Furthermore, enhanced computing power and sophisticated programming have unlocked the world of artificial intelligence. When combined, big data and artificial intelligence will improve our ability to study health care and to deliver personalized medicine. The applications for big data in surgery are similar to those in health care and health at large, and they are limitless (Figure 2-1). Because the development and deployment of artificial intelligence are highly dependent on the proper utilization of data, it is important for surgical researchers and

	Diagnostics	Data mining and analysis for early detection of disease and warning of impending deterioration
	Prevention	Predictive analytics to avoid unnecessary treatment and adverse events and to improve surgical technique
	Precision	Data analysis of genetic, lifestyle, and historical encounter repositories to personalize care recommendations
	Standardization	Identification of best practices to improve quality and efficiency and reduce cost and waste
	Care organization and delivery	Utilize encounter data to direct provider and hospital selection for patients and resource allocation across facilities
	Research	Harness the information contained in aggregated databases to advance surgical practice and design new approaches to care
	Education and training	Capture the wisdom and knowledge of experts to enhance the process of education and accelerate the pace of training
	Certification, privileging, and credentialing	Automated collection and analysis of data on surgeon and hospital performance to inform maintenance of certification programs, and privileging and credentialing of providers within practice settings

Figure 2-1 • Applications of big data in surgery.

clinicians to first understand what types of data currently exist in database form as well as the strengths and weaknesses of specific databases.

▌ BIG DATA

To date, there has been no formal definition of *big data*. A well-formed and unambiguous understanding of the term big data is important for a shared understanding of the term. Widely used features to describe big data are the 3 V's: volume, variety, and velocity.[1] Succinctly, volume refers to the size of the data, velocity refers to the frequency of update, and variety refers to the diversity of the data. The ambiguity of these terms reflects the challenges posed by the use of big data in general (Figure 2-2).

Volume, variety, and velocity are in no way completely descriptive of large data sets, but they do illustrate some important features. A threshold for what volume constitutes big data is not consistently given. Some studies cite terabytes, petabytes, or exabytes as thresholds; others simply state that size is relative and intentionally do not define it.[2] Velocity refers to the high frequency (sometimes near real time) with which data are generated,

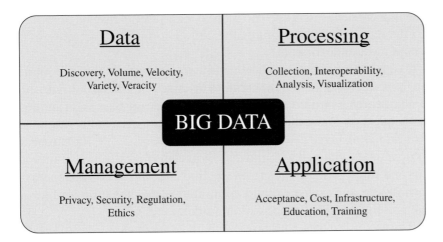

Figure 2-2 • The challenges of harnessing the power of big data.

delivered, and processed.[3] Variety is often achieved via the aggregation of widely disparate data from independent sources. Each of these dimensions of big data poses its own unique challenges to use of big data.

Data sets designed to integrate patient and provider data from various sources such as clinical, administrative, and regulatory repositories hold significant value to public health both indirectly via research and directly via the resultant knowledge, tools, and practices applied to patient care. There are many examples of how data sets and registries have been used to define clinically significant practice patterns and treatment strategies. These data sources have proven useful in answering important clinical questions and confirming conclusions derived from smaller studies, such as the benefit of anatomic resection for early-stage disease,[4] the impact of adjuvant therapy on survival,[5] and the association of patient-specific metrics on outcomes.[6] Large data sets have also been used to track changes in utilization, identify practice patterns over time, uncover disparities in care, and describe outcomes associated with rare events that would otherwise be difficult to study with smaller samples. This is just to name a few of the countless ways large data sets can be used. These data sets take many forms, with claims databases, discharge data sets, and registries being among the most common.

More recently, with continuous streams of data from infusion pumps and monitors, the rise in popularity of opt-in genomics companies, and the transition from paper medical records to electronic medical record systems, there has been an exponential growth of health-related data.[7] These data can take many forms such as numerical, text, coded, graphical, images, physiologic measures, or audio.[8] The volume of unstructured data presents a challenge to those who wish to make useful insights or inquiries into the data and often requires the conversion or restructuring of the data into workable formats.[9]

Acquisition of raw data has historically often been the rate-limiting step for researchers. Before the creation of large centralized data sets, individual researchers would have to dedicate significant time and funding to data acquisition. Now that large amounts of data are readily available, a new field has emerged centered on outcomes research.[10-12] Researchers in this domain are charged with the task of asking clinically important questions and interpreting trends from existing data in the correct context.[13] Study design and statistical and computational innovation and knowledge present great challenges within outcomes research.

The use of big data within research and patient care faces many challenges related to data processing. The collection of the data can be labor intensive, and duplication of efforts is common and wasteful. In addition, new tools and services for data discovery, integration, interoperability, analysis, and visualization are required to make sense of large amounts of data.[2] Researchers and statisticians must develop innovative ways to eliminate noise and erroneous data (ie, data cleaning) so that data may be interpreted in a meaningful way. Currently, there is a relative dearth of human experts who possess both the clinical and analytic knowledge necessary to harness large clinical databases.[14]

The effective use of big data in surgery will necessitate the development of teams to oversee the management and application of its use. Governance will be required for regulation and resolution of ethical issues that arise in the process of integrating and using big data in surgery (see Chapter 14). These teams will need to provide data security to ensure the protection of data privacy.

At present, big data and the associated tools are often met with awe and skepticism. As such, as with all new knowledge, implementation and dissemination of big data tools will require culture change. Education and training will be important to the optimal utilization of the vast amount of information emerging in surgery.

Investment in infrastructure for data, data processing, management, and applications will avoid unnecessary waste in the future. Unlike other capital campaigns raised to invest in bricks and mortar, the investment in data infrastructure must be designed to handle the costs of human capital such as clinical scientists and computer scientists who can provide the fluid and adaptable recommendations needed to handle the rapidly expanding field. In addition, teams of coders and database managers will be needed. Thus, the infrastructure for big data will require spending on storage, data, and human capital. While many large databases are now publicly available, they are not free. Most data sets and registries require either a purchasing or membership fee from individuals and institutions who wish to use them. In addition, the storage space to house the data and the hardware and software necessary to secure and use the data can be costly and are needed in perpetuity.

The costs associated with the use of big data will lessen as competition in the market grows; however, overall spending is likely to continue to increase as the products of big data become more valuable. Although public access to the data sources is unlikely due to the sensitive nature of the information, publicly available code sharing in an open source context, such as that made available by Healthcare Cost and Utilization Project,[15] is feasible. As code sharing and automation become more common, access and collaboration will improve. Over time, increased availability of common applications will facilitate use of big data in surgery.

Today, large databases are providing surgical researchers, and health care researchers in general, with a tremendous amount of new opportunity and challenges. Currently, most surgical databases are classified by the source of their raw data. Some of these sources include insurance claims (eg, those made available by the Centers for Medicare and Medicaid Services [CMS]), registry data, survey data, and electronic medical record data. Each of these sources of data carries its own unique set of opportunities and challenges and, like all data, must be interpreted in the correct context. Throughout the rest of this chapter, we will provide examples of several of the large data sets commonly used in surgical research. In each section, we will note the unique features and advantages and disadvantages of the data source. We will include examples of projects published using each type of repository.

COMMONLY USED DATA SETS IN HEALTH CARE

Claims Data Sets

Medicare Files

Medicare is the federal health insurance program for individuals in the United States who are aged 65 years or older, select individuals with disabilities aged less than 65 years, and individuals with end-stage renal disease. In 2015, more than 55 million beneficiaries were covered by Medicare. Given the aging population in the United States, Medicare data will certainly be an important source of data for health researchers moving forward.

The CMS is a federal agency that collects data for every person and provider using Medicare health insurance. The CMS makes a uniform national claims database available for research purposes and offers researchers and other health care professionals a broad range of quantitative information on Medicare programs, such as information on Medicare and Medicaid spending, enrollment, claims data, and a broad range of consumer research.

The CMS produces annual standard analytic files (SAFs) for researchers containing final (adjudicated) action claims for Parts A and B services and Part D prescription drugs, which reflect care received in the hospital, physician offices, skilled nursing facilities, and hospice settings through December 31 of the latest available calendar year. These claims capture inpatient and outpatient diagnoses, procedures, devices, and medication information in the form of alphanumeric codes, dates of service, charged amounts and paid claims, and a limited number of provider characteristics, such as provider number and geographic information (state, county, and zip code) for facilities as well as national physician number and clinical specialty for physicians. SAFs also contain information on beneficiary enrollment and demographic data, including race, ethnicity, and date of death.[16]

The CMS files have several strengths that are common to claims data sets. The database contains longitudinal data on health care services. Withdrawal from Medicare is very rare; typically, patients are followed from enrollment until death. Medicare data reflect near-complete capture of health care services across all settings of care. Therefore, the data can be used to answer a wide range of health care–related questions, including understanding the epidemiology of a disease; quantifying the costs related to health care interventions; describing treatment utilization patterns and the delivery of health care services; comparing the effectiveness, safety, and costs of interventions; and studying the effects of policy changes on prescribing patterns and clinical outcomes. In doing so, broad changes in clinical practice patterns can be traced, evidence useful for developing and evaluating adherence to clinical practice guidelines can be generated, and the effects of CMS payment policy decisions can be evaluated.[16]

Although the Medicare data have many strengths, there are some limitations to consider. These limitations also are common across claims data sets. Information on behavioral characteristics, such as diet, exercise, and alcohol and tobacco use; biochemical laboratory data; imaging data (eg, computed tomography scans, magnetic resonance imaging); and other disease severity indicators, is not available. As in other claims databases, diseases are defined by the presence of a diagnostic code, which can be prone to misclassification, and severity of disease may also not be captured. In addition, Medicare data, like other claims data, are not collected for the purpose of research. Claims are for reimbursement and are thus subject to possible financial influence and misclassification.

Classic examples of surgical outcomes studies using Medicare claims exist across the decades. Medicare claims linked to Surveillance, Epidemiology, and End Results (SEER) data were used to document the volume-outcome relationship in surgery.[17] Medicare claims linked to chart abstraction were examined to confirm that patients who have one complication are at risk for additional complications and death.[18] Medicare claims alone have been used to develop new measures of hospital quality such as failure to rescue.[19] More recently, Medicare claims linked to information on surgeon training have been used to assess the performance of the system of graduate medical education in surgery.[20] These are just a few examples of the broad contributions to science that have been made possible by the use of Medicare claims.

Discharge Data Sets

Over the past 40 years, hospital discharge data have become a mainstay data source for health services research. Nearly all states have data organizations collecting administrative data (ie, discharge records) for all nonfederal hospitalizations in their state. The discharge data often represent a subset of the data submitted to insurance payers by hospitals and providers for payment of claims. In health care, most of the charges for patient care are paid by an insurance carrier. The "bills" are referred to as claims, which are often filed by the provider on behalf of the recipient of the services, the patients. Data are often collected in multiple contexts, including inpatient, emergency department (ED), observation visits, ambulatory surgery, and other outpatient visits. These data sets often include records for all payers and the uninsured.

Generally, hospitals are required to submit all the data elements the state data organization requests, but in certain states, some data elements are voluntary to submit (eg, race/ethnicity).[21] Originally, the standards for data collection varied significantly. However, in the early 1990s, most states transitioned to uniform bill (UB). The UB, created by the National Uniform Billing Committee (NUBC), was developed to maintain a single billing format and to standardize data used by institutional, private, and public providers and payers for health care claims. This also had a secondary benefit of ensuring uniformity for the data when used for research purposes. When purchased directly through state agencies such as the state-specific departments of health, the data sets often have additional features such as the inclusion of hospital identifiers that permit linkage to other data sources, such as the American Hospital Association data set or the Hospital Compare Data, to expand the possible areas of investigation.

Statewide discharge data have some limitations that affect their usefulness and accuracy in analysis. Several of the described limitations include issues with quality of data elements, missing data elements, and excluded populations.[22] A data quality problem arises with the accuracy of some International Classification of Diseases (ICD)-9-CM/ICD-10-CM coded diagnoses and procedures, because these can be subject to miscoding and omission of comorbidities. Quality of information in the medical record, coder training, experiences, quality control, and coding errors have all been described as potential issues that affect the quality of this type of data. Incentives to maximize reimbursement may also bias data. Finally, discharge data sets typically use the same administrative data collected for filing claims, although they often lack the identifiers needed to connect multiple encounters for individual patients. As such, in discharge databases, a single patient may be included many times without the ability to differentiate them across encounters.

Missing data elements also provide a challenge to discharge/claims data. For example, the statewide discharge data may include hospital charges but not include the hospital's costs to provide the services or the reimbursed amounts from payments by health plans or patient copays.[23] Many data sets also do not include any patient identifiers, which makes linkage to outside data sets challenging. Similarly, physician identifiers are not collected in all states, limiting analysis on physician practice patterns or outcomes. Federal hospitals are also not included in the data sets.

Researchers can attempt to attenuate some of these limitations through statistical approaches, data manipulation, or linkage to other data sources. For example, researchers have linked discharge data to hospital cost reports to estimate the costs to hospitals to produce their care[24] or price of the stay.[25]

Health care discharge data have been useful in the study of public safety, injury surveillance and prevention, public health, disease surveillance, disease registries, health planning, community assessments, public reporting for purchasing and comparative reports, quality assessment, performance improvement, commercial applications, and health services and policy research.[22]

Healthcare Cost and Utilization Project

The Healthcare Cost and Utilization Project (HCUP) is a group of discharge databases developed through a federal-state-industry partnership sponsored by the Agency for Healthcare Research and Quality (AHRQ). Beginning in the early 1990s, HCUP began a voluntary collaboration with statewide data organizations and private data organizations (called HCUP partners) to leverage their data collection efforts to build uniformly formatted national and state hospital encounter-level data sets for research.[26]

HCUP is the largest collection of all-payer, encounter-level hospital data in the United States. HCUP data are useful for researchers who wish to explore health care use, access, outcomes, and costs related to hospital inpatient stays, ambulatory surgery and services, ED visits, and readmissions. The data set is updated and released annually. The data sets in aggregate contain data from more than 7 million hospital stays annually. New databases are created annually and maintained by the AHRQ through a federal-state-industry partnership. Data are typically made available 1 to 2 years after the dates of service.

Costs of purchasing the data sets are relatively inexpensive, ranging from $350 to $500 depending on the year of availability and state. Additional supplementary data files and equipment and tools needed to successfully use the data sets include a DVD drive, a minimum of 15 gigabytes of space available on a hard drive for each year of data, a third-party file compression utility, and statistical analysis software.

The HCUP data sets are designed to protect the privacy of contributing hospitals by hiding and removing data that may reveal hospital identification and location. However, this strategy also creates barriers for researchers to answer and study many important questions. The lack of lower-level identifiers also makes it difficult to link HCUP data to other data sets, such as pollution data on the city and state level.[27]

Currently, 49 partners (48 states and the District of Columbia) provide HCUP with statewide inpatient data, 35 partners provide ambulatory surgery and services data, and 39 partners provide ED data. The inpatient data represent more than 97% of inpatient discharges from community hospitals.

HCUP divides its data into smaller more specific data sets based on certain categories. These subdivisions can be useful to researchers who wish to query a narrower field of data. Following is a brief summary of the HCUP databases and their data sources:

- The National Inpatient Sample (NIS) is the largest publicly available all-payer inpatient database in the United States. Released annually, the NIS approximates 20% of the discharges from all US community hospitals.
- The Kids' Inpatient Database (KID) is the largest publicly available, all-payer, national pediatric database in the United States. It was designed to facilitate study of hospital services, outcomes, and charges for children and adolescents. It contains a sample of 2 to 3 million hospital pediatric discharges per year.[28]

- The Nationwide Emergency Department Sample (NEDS) is a database that yields national estimates of ED visits. Released annually, the NEDS database enables researchers to study a broad range of conditions and procedures related to ED use. It includes approximately 31 million records each year for patients who were either treated in the ED and released or treated in the ED and admitted to the same hospital.[29]
- The Nationwide Readmissions Database (NRD) supports analyses of repeat hospital visits in a year, addressing the need for nationally representative information on hospital readmissions for all ages and payers, including the uninsured. The NRD is released annually.[30]
- The State Inpatient Databases (SID) is a collection of hospital inpatient discharge information. The SID can be used to investigate questions that are unique to one state or to compare data from 2 or more states.[31]
- The State Ambulatory Surgery and Services Databases (SASD) include encounter-level data for ambulatory surgery and other outpatient services from hospital-owned facilities. Some states provide data for ambulatory surgery and outpatient services from non–hospital-owned facilities.[32]
- The State Emergency Department Databases (SEDD) contain discharge information on all ED visits that do not result in a hospital admission.[33]

HCUP databases have been used for a variety of different research projects within the field of surgery. The HCUP data set is large, with over 100 variables, creating the opportunity for researchers to ask a huge variety of research questions. Studies that have used the HCUP data sets have investigated emerging treatments, surgery rates and surgical complications, predictors of outcomes, and population-based mortality risk factors.

Survey-Based Data Sets

American Medical Association Physician Masterfile

The American Medical Association (AMA) Physician Masterfile is a database of current and historical information on all physicians, medical residents, and students in the United States, including those with MD and DO degrees. Information contained in the AMA Masterfile includes physician contact information (including name and professional mailing address) and basic professional information (including date of birth, sex, year of graduation, medical school, training history, specialty, hospital affiliations, and type of practice). Historical data can also be accessed.

The Masterfile contains current and historical data on approximately 940,000 living and deceased residents and physicians in the United States and on 77,000 students in schools of medicine and osteopathy. It includes data on 243,000 foreign medical graduates who live in the United States and have met basic credentialing requirements. Data have been collected since 1906.

AMA Masterfile data are typically used to identify random samples of US physicians or trainees for surveys or to determine the distribution of physicians across specialties or geographic regions. This data set provides basic demographic information about physicians as well as contact information. It is primarily useful for 2 main purposes: (1) identifying a population-based cohort of physicians for surveys and (2) obtaining physician characteristics for other studies (eg, studies using claims data for which unique physician identification numbers are available).

It has also been used to examine trends in physician specialty over time; however, one of the major limitations of the AMA Masterfile database is that it provides few opportunities for using it as a stand-alone database for research given its limited scope of data.

The pricing structure is contingent on the number of records plus service and handling charges; price also varies between data licensees even for the same request. As a rough example, the price to obtain contact information on a random sample of 2000 general internists is approximately $400. In addition, a written agreement, regardless of requesting party, content, or media, is required.[34]

American Hospital Association Data Set

American Hospital Association produces an annual survey database. These data represent information that is directly provided by nearly 6300 hospitals and more than 400 health care systems. The data set covers an array of variables including demographics, operations, service line, staffing, executive information, expenses, physician organization structures, beds, utilization, and more. Although this data set does not include specific patient information as might be contained in other data sets, it may be used in conjunction with outside data such as the discharge data sets previously described. Historical data sets are available for many of these tools.[34]

Dartmouth Atlas Project

Wennberg and Gittelsohn published a study on small area variation in 1973, which subsequently led to the creation of the Dartmouth Atlas of

Health Care (also known as the Dartmouth Atlas Project).[35] Since then, the Dartmouth Atlas Project has documented variations in how medical resources are distributed and used in the United States. The broad project uses Medicare and Medicaid data to provide information and analysis about regional patters in health care spending and utilization. The Dartmouth Atlas Project uses a methodology, commonly known as small area analysis, that is population based. The focus of small area analysis is on the experience of the population living in a defined geographic area or the population that uses a specific hospital. Studies are often performed using supplemental information from other sources such as the US Census, the American Hospital Association, the AMA, and the National Center for Health Statistics.

The Dartmouth Atlas Project offers access to many sources of data at the level of zip codes. This can be linked to other data sets, with permission, to allow population-based studies incorporating information on social determinants of health and other important parameters that are often missing from claims and discharge data sets, which contain information at the individual level.[36]

Clinical Registries

Clinical registry data are generally considered to be a more valid and reliable data source for quality measurement than administrative claims because data are collected prospectively and specifically for the purpose of research and quality improvement.[37] Registry data have notable advantages over claims data because the data elements are designed specifically to capture information for clinical care rather than for billing purposes.

National Surgical Quality Improvement Program

The National Surgical Quality Improvement Program (NSQIP), which was started in the Department of Veterans Affairs in 1994 and expanded into the private sector in 2004 through the efforts of the American College of Surgeons (ACS), is the first national, validated, outcome-based, risk-adjusted, peer-controlled program for the measurement and enhancement of the quality of surgical care.[38]

Each hospital assigns a trained surgical clinical reviewer (SCR) to collect preoperative through 30-day postoperative data on randomly assigned patients. The number and types of variables collected will differ from hospital to hospital, depending on the hospital's size, patient population, and quality improvement focus. The ACS provides SCR training, ongoing education opportunities, and auditing to ensure data reliability.

Data are entered online in a Health Insurance Portability and Account-ability Act (HIPAA)-compliant, secure, web-based platform that can be accessed 24 hours a day. A surgeon champion assigned by each hospital leads and oversees program implementation and quality initiatives.

Blinded, risk-adjusted information is shared with all hospitals, allow-ing them to nationally benchmark their complication rates and surgical outcomes. Many complications occur after the patient leaves the hospi-tal, often leading to costly readmissions. For example, in the case of col-ectomies, one of the most common procedures performed in hospitals, one-half of cardiac arrests and two-thirds of infections occur after the patient leaves the hospital.[39] Therefore, ACS NSQIP tracks patients for 30 days after their operation. ACS also provides monthly conference calls, best practice guidelines, and many other resources to help hospitals target problem areas and improve surgical outcomes.

ACS NSQIP is risk adjusted, based on models in use for more than 20 years. This allows for better comparative analysis between differ-ent patient populations and hospitals. Hospitals caring for higher acu-ity pathology or sicker patient populations will no longer be dinged for having comparatively worse outcomes than hospitals caring for healthier groups. Similarly, ACS NSQIP allows a hospital that takes on more com-plex surgical cases to meaningfully calibrate its results against one that performs more straightforward procedures. ACS NSQIP accounts for the complexity of operations performed, allowing for more accurate national benchmarking.[40]

Data abstracted from the medical record and hospitals by ACS NSQIP trained and tested clinical personnel are audited to ensure stan-dardized data collection. This provides a high standard of data quality to registry users. In a study comparing ACS NSQIP data to administrative and claims data collected by the University Health System Consortium (UHC) program,[41] ACS NSQIP identified 61% more complications than UHC. This sort of discrepancy has been replicated in numerous con-texts in the literature.[42] A deidentified participant use file is available for research efforts for participating members.

Unfortunately, participation in clinical registries can be burdensome to hospitals, especially smaller ones. A clinical registry necessitates employ-ing a data abstractor, and mining clinical data from medical records is labor intensive. Some of this labor may become automated with innova-tion in electronic medical records; however, currently, human labor is the only option for many hospitals. In this regard, administrative claims data may be advantageous for certain outcomes because they are routinely in large aggregated databases and can be used without incurring extra costs to hospitals.[43]

Metabolic and Bariatric Surgery Accreditation and Quality Improvement Program

The Metabolic and Bariatric Surgery Accreditation and Quality Improvement Program (MBSAQIP) database was created in 2012 by the ACS and the American Society for Metabolic and Bariatric Surgery. The MBSAQIP database participant user data files have been available for analysis since 2015 and include HIPAA-compliant patient-level data on more than 150,000 metabolic and bariatric cases performed between January 1 and December 31, 2015, at 742 centers across the United States and Canada. The MBSAQIP is a rigorous data set that captures 100% of all bariatric cases at each participating institution, has clear definitions of data parameters, and has the data collected by a clinical reviewer. A deidentified participant use file is available for research efforts for participating members.[44]

Trauma Quality Improvement Program

The Trauma Quality Improvement Program (TQIP) is a program provided by the ACS to improve the quality of care in trauma centers in the United States. The program began as a pilot in 2008 and opened for formal enrollment in 2010. TQIP accomplishes its work by collecting data from more than 800 trauma centers, with the goal of providing direct feedback about performance and quality. The data are also entered into a large clinical data repository.[45] The program provides a measure of external reference by using risk-adjusted benchmarking to accurately provide national comparisons. Data are only available for participant sites.[46]

Society of Thoracic Surgeons Database

The Society of Thoracic Surgeons (STS) national database was established in 1989 as a quality improvement initiative for cardiothoracic surgery. The database is divided into 4 components: adult cardiac surgery, general thoracic surgery, congenital heart surgery, and mechanical circulatory support via the Intermacs database.[47]

There are several examples of how STS data have greatly impacted clinical practice. During the field's early stages, clinicians and researchers questioned whether minimally invasive lung resection would yield oncologic equivalence when compared to open operations, including the thoroughness of lymph node dissection and the accuracy of pathologic staging.[48,49] Initially founded in single-institution data, the advantages of minimally invasive resection were not fully realized until the outcomes associated with large data were available to support a shift in practice.

In the absence of large randomized trials, 3 studies derived from the STS General Thoracic Surgery Database demonstrated that minimally invasive resection by video-assisted thoracoscopic surgery (VATS) yielded comparable outcomes to open resection with regard to postoperative complication risk, the completeness of lymph node dissection, and long-term survival.[50]

Vascular Quality Initiative

The Vascular Quality Initiative (VQI) is a set of 12 registries that contain demographic, clinical, procedural, and outcomes data from more than 500,000 vascular procedures performed nationwide and in Canada. Each entry contains information from the patient's initial hospitalization and 1 year of follow-up data. The high rate of long-term follow-up is a somewhat unique part of the VQI. Achieving patient contact a year after the initial procedure is resource intensive but offers hospitals and researchers a robust data source. Each participating center receives biannual reports of their performance.[51]

Electronic Health Records

Physicians everywhere in the United States interact with electronic medical records (EMRs) daily. Some studies have demonstrated a 2:1 ratio of EMR work to direct patient care in some situations. Given this significant time investment into the EMR, it is postulated that the EMR could be used as a tool for data collection and quality assurance. Medical records are created for the purpose of clinical work and billing and thus are not optimized for data acquisition. The majority of clinical data in EMRs is in free-text format. This type of data has high volatility and changes rapidly as disease state evolves. Manual data extraction is tedious, costly, time consuming, and an error-prone process when there are often missing elements of data. Some studies have trialed using progress note templates with key research elements that could be extracted automatically by automated programs. This has resulted in high rate of data retrieval and accuracy. The disadvantages of this approach are that it requires prospective planning to create the progress note templates and clinicians must be educated on the proper use of these data entry forms.

Raw EMR data are disorganized and full of uncodified variables. Working directly with EMR data for statistical analysis is a challenge in and of itself. Intimate knowledge of the data structure of the EMR is necessary for even the simplest of queries. Extracting EMR data is a difficult, time-consuming, and often pragmatic process. In addition, EMR-derived data may not be comprehensive enough for research unless multiple sources capturing several workflows are queried.

The Medical Information Mart for Intensive Care (MIMIC) database from the Massachusetts Institute of Technology Laboratory for Computational Physiology is a deidentified health database derived from intensive care admissions at a large academic health center and includes structured data that have been curated from that hospital's EMR specifically for the purposes of critical care research. This data set has been used in many of the machine learning studies that have been published in the critical care field.

Natural language processing is an exciting field in computer science that may one day help computers interpret free-text clinical information found in the EMR (see Chapters 5 and 14); however, the technology is still under development.

Other Databases and Resources

The data sets noted in this chapter (Table 2-1) represent some of the most common big data repositories currently used in health care delivery.

Table 2-1   COMMONLY USED DATA SETS AND LINKS TO PURCHASE PROCEDURES AND RELATED RESOURCES

Data Sets	Link to Access Purchase Procedures and Related Resources for Data Sets
Claims Data Sets	
Medicare files	https://www.cms.gov/newsroom/data https://www.resdac.org/cms-data/files/medpar
Healthcare Cost Institute (HCCI)	https://www.healthcostinstitute.org/research/research-resources
TRICARE	https://health.mil/Military-Health-Topics/Privacy-and-Civil-Liberties/Submit-a-Data-Sharing-Application?page=2#pagingAnchor
Discharge Data Sets	
State specific[a]	
New York State database	https://www.health.ny.gov/statistics/sparcs/access/
Pennsylvania State database	http://www.phc4.org/services/datarequests/data.htm

(continued)

Table 2-1	COMMONLY USED DATA SETS AND LINKS TO PURCHASE PROCEDURES AND RELATED RESOURCES (CONTINUED)
Data Sets	**Link to Access Purchase Procedures and Related Resources for Data Sets**
National data and state specific	
AHRQ HCUP data sets	https://www.hcup-us.ahrq.gov/databases.jsp
Military Health System Data Repository	https://www.health.mil/Military-Health-Topics/Technology/Clinical-Support/Military-Health-System-Data-Repository
Registry Databases	
NSQIP Participant Use Data File	https://www.facs.org/quality-programs/acs-nsqip/participant-use
MBSAQIP Participant Use Data File	https://www.facs.org/quality-programs/mbsaqip/participant-use
National Cancer Database	https://www.facs.org/quality-programs/cancer/ncdb
National Trauma Data Bank	https://www.facs.org/quality-programs/trauma/tqp/center-programs/ntdb/about
United Network for Organ Sharing	https://unos.org/data/data-collection/
Survey Data Sets	
American Medical Association Masterfile	https://www.ama-assn.org/practice-management/masterfile/data-services-publications
American Hospital Association	https://www.aha.org/data-insights/aha-data-products
Dartmouth Atlas Project	https://www.dartmouthatlas.org/data/

All websites were accessed on June 24, 2019.

[a]A few state-specific discharge data sets are included to provide examples of the types of organizations that collect and distribute these data. There are many more such data sets available for use in research and quality and safety work.

Many other important disease-specific data sets exist, such as the National Trauma Database,[52] the National Cancer Database,[53] and the United Network for Organ Sharing database.[54] In addition, access to data from state medical boards, specialty boards, and licensing agencies can be obtained with special authorization for defined studies. Opt-in genomics companies (eg, 23 and Me, Ancestry.com) are also becoming a large source of raw genetic information. Furthermore, the National Institutes of Health is currently engaged in a historic effort to gather a wide array of health information including genetic, environmental, and lifestyle factors from over 1 million patients.

In essence, if there is an important reason to conduct a study or a method to advance population health and data are required, creativity will often prevail, and data can be made available. As an investigator, look for existing sources and consider contacting agencies and principal investigators of prior cross-sectional surveys and clinical trials to reuse existing information. Frequently, the limitations of big data use begin where the human mind can no longer see.

CONCLUSION

Big data present researchers with unique opportunities but also unique challenges. Those who intend to compare or interpret the data must often spend a significant amount of time transforming the data into usable formats. Furthermore, the responsible use of the data requires clear and concise definitions of terms, knowledge on the accuracy of the input and export of the data, and transparency of the coding algorithms to ensure reliability and reproducibility.

The collection of data from multiple sources permits the investigation of issues that cross disciplinary lines and allows inquiries into a broad array of issues to advance care. Resultant higher-order outcome studies can be performed with large patient cohorts and adjustment for confounders that is often not achievable with single- or multi-institutional data. Furthermore, as data sets can often be linked to examine the totality of care within regions, states, and nations or across all settings for individuals, with appropriate study design, this information can be used to minimize the risk of selection bias and allow for adequately powered analyses. With the appropriate use of artificial intelligence, these data can also be used to diagnose disease,[55,56] warn providers of the risk of a poor outcome[57] (in real time), and aid clinicians in the treatment of disease to improve the odds of success.[58] Although still in its infancy, the use of big data in medicine, coupled with developments in computing power and artificial intelligence, holds the promise of an acceleration in the pace of advancement of knowledge. Hopefully, the human mind will be able to keep pace and learn to apply this new information to improve health.

REFERENCES

1. Berger ML, Doban V. Big data, advanced analytics and the future of comparative effectiveness research. *J Comp Eff Res*. 2014;3(2):167-176.
2. van Horn JD, Toga AW. Human neuroimaging as a "Big Data" science. *Brain Imaging Behav*. 2014;8(2):323-331.

3. Jee K, Kim GH. Potentiality of big data in the medical sector: focus on how to reshape the healthcare system. *Healthc Inform Res*. 2013;19(2):79-85.

4. Altekruse SF, McGlynn KA, Reichman ME. Hepatocellular carcinoma incidence, mortality, and survival trends in the United States from 1975 to 2005. *J Clin Oncol*. 2009;27(9):1485-1491.

5. Aro K, Ho AS, Luu M, et al. Survival impact of adjuvant therapy in salivary gland cancers following resection and neck dissection. *Otolaryngol Head Neck Surg*. 2019;160(6):1048-1057.

6. Pusic AL, Klassen AF, Scott AM, Klok JA, Cordeiro PG, Cano SJ. Development of a new patient-reported outcome measure for breast surgery: the BREAST-Q. *Plast Reconstr Surg*. 2009;124(2):345-353.

7. Sessler DI. Big Data—and its contributions to peri-operative medicine. *Anaesthesia*. 2014;69(2):100-105.

8. Baro E, Degoul S, Beuscart R, Chazard E. Toward a literature-driven definition of big data in healthcare. *Biomed Res Int*. 2015;2015:639021.

9. Matheson GO, Klügl M, Engebretsen L, et al. Prevention and management of noncommunicable disease: the IOC consensus statement, Lausanne 2013. *Clin J Sport Med*. 2013;23(6):419-429.

10. DeMaria EJ, Pate V, Warthen M, Winegar DA. Baseline data from American Society for Metabolic and Bariatric Surgery-designated bariatric surgery centers of excellence using the bariatric outcomes longitudinal database. *Surg Obes Relat Dis*. 2010;6(4):347-355.

11. Hogue CW, Barzilai B, Pieper KS, et al. Sex differences in neurological outcomes and mortality after cardiac surgery: a Society of Thoracic Surgery national database report. *Circulation*. 2001;103(17):2133-2137.

12. Gandhi GY, Nuttall GA, Abel MD, et al. Intraoperative hyperglycemia and perioperative outcomes in cardiac surgery patients. *Mayo Clin Proc*. 2005;80(7):862-866.

13. Ward JC. Oncology reimbursement in the era of personalized medicine and big data. *J Oncol Pract*. 2014;10(2):83-86.

14. Mavandadi S, Dimitrov S, Feng S, et al. Crowd-sourced BioGames: managing the big data problem for next-generation lab-on-a-chip platforms. *Lab Chip*. 2012;12(20):4102-4106.

15. Healthcare Cost and Utilization Project. Agency for Healthcare Research and Quality. Accessed on May 22, 2019. https://hcup-us.ahrq.gov/tools_software.jsp.

16. Mues KE, Liede A, Liu J, et al. Use of the Medicare database in epidemiologic and health services research: a valuable source of real-world evidence on the older and disabled populations in the US. *Clin Epidemiol*. 2017;9:267-277.

17. Begg CB, Cramer LD, Hoskins WJ, Brennan MF. Impact of hospital volume on operative mortality for major cancer surgery. *J Am Med Assoc*. 1998;280(20):1747-1751.

18. Silber JH, Rosenbaum PR, Trudeau ME, et al. Changes in prognosis after the first postoperative complication. *Med Care*. 2005;43(2):122-131.

19. Silber JH, Romano PS, Rosen AK, Wang Y, Even-Shoshan O, Volpp KG. Failure-to-rescue comparing definitions to measure quality of care. *Med Care*. 2007;45(10):918-925.

20. Kelz RR, Niknam BA, Sellers MM, et al. Duty hour reform and the outcomes of patients treated by new surgeons. *Ann Surg.* 2019;271(4):599-605.

21. Andrews RM. Statewide hospital discharge data: collection, use, limitations, and improvements. *Health Serv Res.* 201;50(suppl 1):1273-1299.

22. Schoenman JA, Sutton JP, Elixhauser A, Love D. Understanding and enhancing the value of hospital discharge data. *Med Care Res Rev.* 2007;64(4):449-468.

23. Riley GF. Administrative and claims records as sources of health care cost data. *Med Care.* 2009;47(7 suppl 1):S51-S55.

24. Friedman B, de La Mare J, Andrews R, McKenzie DH. Practical options for estimating cost of hospital inpatient stays. *J Health Care Finance.* 2002;29(1): 1-13.

25. Levit KR, Friedman B, Wong HS. Estimating inpatient hospital prices from state administrative data and hospital financial reports. *Health Serv Res.* 2013;48(5):1779-1797.

26. Lupo P, Neale A, Bowman MA. Agency for Healthcare Research and Quality (AHRQ) webinar features 3 journal of American Board of Family Medicine practice-based research (PBR) articles. *J Am Board Fam Med.* 2015;28(4):438.

27. Overview of the National (Nationwide) Inpatient Sample (NIS) Healthcare Cost and Utilization Project. Accessed May 22, 2019. https://www.hcup-us.ahrq.gov/ nisoverview.jsp.

28. Overview of the Kids' Inpatient Database (KID). Healthcare Cost and Utilization Project. Accessed May 22, 2019. https://www.hcup-us.ahrq.gov/kidoverview.jsp.

29. Overview of the Nationwide Emergency Department Sample (NEDS). Healthcare Cost and Utilization Project. Accessed May 22, 2019. https://www.hcup-us. ahrq.gov/nedsoverview.jsp.

30. Overview of the Nationwide Readmissions Database (NRD). Healthcare Cost and Utilization Project. Accessed May 22, 2019. https://www.hcup-us.ahrq.gov/ nrdoverview.jsp.

31. Overview of the State Inpatient Databases (SID). Healthcare Cost and Utilization Project. Accessed May 22, 2019. https://www.hcup-us.ahrq.gov/sidoverview.jsp.

32. SASD Database Documentation. Healthcare Cost and Utilization Project. Accessed May 22, 2019. https://www.hcup-us.ahrq.gov/db/state/sasddb-documentation.jsp.

33. Overview of the State Emergency Department Databases (SEDD). Healthcare Cost and Utilization Project. Accessed May 22, 2019. https://www.hcup-us.ahrq. gov/seddoverview.jsp.

34. AMA Physician Masterfile. American Medical Association. Accessed May 22, 2019. https://www.ama-assn.org/practice-management/masterfile/ama-physician-masterfile.

35. Wennberg J, Gittelsohn A. Small area variations in health care delivery. *Science.* 1973;182(4117):1102-1108.

36. AHA data products. American Hospital Association. Accessed May 22, 2019. https://www.aha.org/data-insights/aha-data-products.

37. Lawson EH, Louie R, Zingmond DS, et al. A comparison of clinical registry versus administrative claims data for reporting of 30-day surgical complications. *Ann Surg.* 2012;256(6):973-981.

38. Khuri SF, Daley J, Henderson W, et al. The Department of Veterans Affairs' NSQIP: the first national, validated, outcome-based, risk-adjusted, and peer-controlled program for the measurement and enhancement of the quality of surgical care. *Ann Surg*. 1998;228(4):491-507.

39. Wick EC, Shore AD, Hirose K, et al. Readmission rates and cost following colorectal surgery. *Dis Colon Rectum*. 2011;54(12):1475-1479.

40. ACS National Surgical Quality Improvement Program. American College of Surgeons. Accessed May 22, 2019. https://www.facs.org/quality-programs/acs-nsqip.

41. Steinberg SM, Popa MR, Michalek JA, Bethel MJ, Ellison EC. Comparison of risk adjustment methodologies in surgical quality improvement. *Surgery*. 2008;144(4):662-667.

42. Dixon JL, Papaconstantinou HT, Hodges B, et al. Redundancy and variability in quality and outcome reporting for cardiac and thoracic surgery. *Proc (Bayl Univ Med Cent)*. 2015;28(1):14-17.

43. Lawson EH, Louie R, Zingmond DS, et al. Using both clinical registry and administrative claims data to measure risk-adjusted surgical outcomes. *Ann Surg*. 2016;263(1):50-57.

44. Metabolic and Bariatric Surgery Accreditation and Quality Improvement Program. American College of Surgeons. Accessed on May 22, 2019. https://www.facs.org/quality-programs/mbsaqip/about.

45. Hemmila MR, Cain-Nielsen AH, Jakubus JL, Mikhail JN, Dimick JB. Association of hospital participation in a regional trauma quality improvement collaborative with patient outcomes. *JAMA Surg*. 2018;153(8):747-756.

46. Trauma Quality Improvement Program. American College of Surgeons. Accessed on May 22, 2019. https://www.facs.org/quality-programs/trauma/tqp/center-programs/tqip.

47. STS National Database. Society of Thoracic Surgeons. Accessed on May 22, 2019. https://www.sts.org/registries-research-center/sts-national-database.

48. Medbery RL, Gillespie TW, Liu Y, et al. Nodal upstaging is more common with thoracotomy than with VATS during lobectomy for early-stage lung cancer: an analysis from the national cancer data base. *J Thorac Oncol*. 2016;11(2):222-233.

49. Licht PB, Jørgensen OD, Ladegaard L, Jakobsen E. A national study of nodal upstaging after thoracoscopic versus open lobectomy for clinical stage I lung cancer. *Ann Thorac Surg*. 2013;96(3):943-949.

50. Resio BJ, Dhanasopon AP, Blasberg JD. Big data, big contributions: outcomes research in thoracic surgery. *J Thorac Dis*. 2019;11(suppl 4):S566-S573.

51. Vascular Quality Initiative. Accessed on May 22, 2019. https://www.vqi.org/.

52. About National Trauma Data Bank American College of Surgeons. Accessed on June 25, 2019. https://www.facs.org/quality-programs/trauma/tqp/center-programs/ntdb/about.

53. National Cancer Database. American College of Surgeons. Accessed on June 25, 2019. https://www.facs.org/quality-programs/cancer/ncdb.

54. Data collection. United Network for Organ Sharing. Accessed on June 25, 2019. https://unos.org/data/data-collection/.

55. Ardila D, Kiraly AP, Bharadwaj S, et al. End-to-end lung cancer screening with three-dimensional deep learning on low-dose chest computed tomography. *Nat Med.* 2019;25(6):954-961.
56. Hu L, Bell D, Antani S, et al. An observational study of deep learning and automated evaluation of cervical images for cancer screening. *J Natl Cancer Inst.* 2019;111(9):923-932.
57. Amorim FF, Santana ANC. Automated early warning system for septic shock: the new way to achieve intensive care unit quality improvement? *Ann Transl Med.* 2017;5(1):17.
58. Hashimoto DA, Rosman G, Rus D, Meireles OR. Artificial intelligence in surgery: promises and perils. *Ann Surg.* 2018;268(1):70-76.

MACHINE LEARNING FOR MEDICINE 3

Frank Rudzicz

HIGHLIGHTS

- Machine learning is a deeply statistical science, built largely out statistics and algebra, neither "logistic regression on steroids" nor a panacea for all data-derived difficulties - it's just another tool whose utility, like others, greatly depends on how it's used.
- Although the learning algorithms themselves are of course important, the relevance of high-quality, representative, and voluminous data cannot be understated.
- Machine learning is increasingly being used in surgical settings. This chapter focuses on more traditional aspects of machine learning.

INTRODUCTION

Machine learning is neither "logistic regression on steroids" nor a panacea for all data-derived difficulties; it is just another tool whose utility, like others, greatly depends on how it is used. As it and other technologies have graduated into public discourse, experts in domains other than computer science are now trying to work out what all the fuss is about, and it may be difficult to separate the expectation from the truth.

Artificial intelligence (AI) is often used as if it is synonymous with machine learning (ML), and vice versa, which is not accurate—at least not yet. Although the specific definitions for these terms are constantly in flux, the consensus is that AI involves any sufficiently complex software that mimics human behavior on some task, which could reasonably include a circuitous flow chart designed by a committee, with branches marked "if" and "otherwise" that one may follow downward toward the output, mechanistically. Thus, AI includes software that may be explicitly instructed by human experts on how to mimic their domain expertise, whereas ML—a *subset* of AI—foregoes humans altogether, to the extent possible, and learns from experience (ie, from *data*). The nature of this learning is also typically quite limited to a very specific (or domain-specific) task. In surgery, we might have a piece of ML that can predict the presence of a hypoxemic event, for example, but might have nothing to say about the severity of that event or about sepsis, anaphylaxis, or bleeding, unless the data allowed for those aspects to be learned.

The field of ML has been steadily moving from expert-defined deterministic rules to data-defined statistical patterns, although domain experts still serve their purpose in increasingly niche areas. The various subfields of AI, including computer vision (CV) and natural language processing (NLP), have tended to incorporate considerable domain expertise (eg, in understanding and interpreting issues of syntax or lexicography in language, in the latter), but modern ML has slowly eroded the necessity for such prior knowledge. One reason for this gradual shift, which may have begun as a mere trickle as far back as the 1980s, is the tidal wave of data now being recorded, including in health care. The average clinic or small hospital may have on the order of a petabyte (1024 terabytes) of patient data or more, approximately 80% of which is *unstructured* (eg, computed tomography [CT] scans, textual clinical notes), which ML excels at organizing. As data become more plentiful, the cost of collecting data becomes cheaper, which only amplifies the deluge. In fact, we may soon find ourselves entirely overwhelmed by its sheer volume. Fortunately for us, in the mountainous pile of hay that is modern big data, the needle can still be quickly located, if we have the right metal detector.

▌ TRADITIONAL MACHINE LEARNING

ML is a deeply statistical science and one built largely out of the bricks of linear and nonlinear algebra. Even a cursory summary of the relevant first principles is beyond our scope here, but in practice, it is crucial to be familiar with vectors, matrices, and their various forms of algebraic manipulation (eg, multiplication, pseudo-inverses, and decompositions), as well as with probability and information theory (including various distributional forms and entropy). These building blocks construct a tool that is useful where there is no human expertise, where humans cannot explain their expertise fully (as in automatic speech recognition), or when explaining human expertise is too expensive (hence the shift from paying experts to encode their knowledge in deterministic, and perhaps brittle, systems).

In 1997, Tom M. Mitchell provided a definition for ML that has not really been supplanted:

> A computer program is said to learn from experience E with respect to some class of tasks T and performance measure P, if its performance at tasks in T, as measured by P, improves with experience E.

In most cases, experience E is synonymous with data D, which itself is of course tightly correlated to the task T. For example, a program with the task T = *detect left ventricular hypertrophy* would more likely be associated with data D = *echocardiographic views* than with D = *blood work*.

Implicit here is a distinction as to the *type* of task being undertaken. Perhaps the de facto task *type* for ML has been **classification** in which a data sample x is assigned to a category or class y (from among k available categories) according to a learned function f or, more formally, $y = f(x)$ where $f{:}R^n \to \{1, \ldots, k\}$ translates real-valued vectors of length n into one of k classes. In perhaps the simplest case, which we call the *binary task*, $k = 2$, as in when the outcome is either positive or negative. There are several subareas of AI whose tasks have variously appropriated different approaches from ML. For example, early approaches to NLP involved explicit grammatical rules provided by linguists, whereas now those rules can be automatically induced, with probabilities, from data. How ML goes about the task of classification is varied; it can partition a map of all possible data points with boundaries between classes, or it can simply assign likelihoods or scores to the available classes, for example. The most common alternative task type for ML is **regression**, in which the output is not a discrete nominal category but instead a value on a continuum (which itself may be composed of real-valued numbers [eg, the estimated size of a tumor] or integer-valued numbers [eg, scores on a Likert-type scale]). Despite its name, logistic regression may more rightly be considered a nominal classifier. There are, as one would expect, various peculiar variants of these types, and we will soon see examples from *deep learning*, a relatively new form of ML, in which other forms of output and tasks have become possible.

Data

Although the learning algorithms themselves are of course important, the relevance of high-quality, representative, and voluminous data cannot be understated. Data provide the statistical power for ML. Regardless of the elegance of an engine, it cannot take you across the country without fuel.

First, the data collected must be **representative**. That is, we should aim for our data to be as free of sampling bias as possible. For instance, the distribution of categories or covariates in the data should be identical to their distribution in the real world, to the extent possible. In health care, this may primarily relate to demographic covariates; a well-known ML approach to distinguishing malignant skin lesions from benign ones using CV techniques on a small sample size[1] did not account for skin color in the analysis or data collection.[2] A data set recorded in a large urban center may similarly not generalize to rural populations, or a system trained with postoperative clinical data alone may not serve well to predict outcomes given only preoperative data. There may be special considerations to this point. To some extent, models trained on historical data may encapsulate biases from the past that the developers wish removed, such as demographic biases toward recidivism or gender biases in models of language[3]; if the system is meant to enable decision support prospectively, techniques to mitigate bias should be undertaken.

The mere size of the data is also often a primary factor. There is a reason big data has taken off, while neither medium data nor teensy data has really caught on. Although it may seem blatantly obvious, the more data we can collect—and the more varied it is—the sharper and more accurate representations we can achieve of the underlying process. However, acquiring large amounts of data is easier said than done. At the scale of a population, we will often either require something like (1) a randomized controlled trial, which can be prohibitively costly in time and other resources to run (at least, for 2 innovative programmers in their garage), or (2) some secondary use of retrospective data, as in the sharing of "anonymized" electronic medical records. Beyond the cost of actually anonymizing the data, even with the current best practices, there is the risk of reidentification either directly through errors in those practices* or through the use of auxiliary data sources.[4] As the open world of ML research increasingly bears down on the walls of patient data, new discussions (or at least reinvigorations of old discussions) concerning patient privacy will need to take place.[5]

Training and Testing Data

A model trained in the lab will only be as useful as its generalizability to real-world, previously unseen scenarios. Therefore, given some large set of data D, the common practice is to partition those data into subsets—typically a training set and a test set—which are respectively used to produce the model itself and to estimate its performance on unseen data. A standard split will have 80% to 90% of the data used for training and the remaining 10% to 20% used for evaluation, once the data have been sufficiently randomized to reduce the risk of covariate influence, although this approach is also subject to some risk, which can be mitigated, as described later. A fundamental scientific priority is to ensure that no data in the test set have also occurred in the training set; otherwise, we are essentially allowing our ML model to cheat by seeing the answers to a test before the exam.

---

*A 99.7% success rate in anonymization sounds impressive, until we realize that 0.3% of, say, 750,000 records is still 22,500 people with their records entirely exposed.

Further to the earlier distinction, often some proportion of the training set (usually approximately 10%) is used as a validation set. Because many ML models learn their internal parameters iteratively—that is, by repeatedly updating a model—we are interested in identifying a good time to stop that iteration. Essentially, the validation set is treated similarly to the testing set in that we are only interested in how the model performs on it; the distinction is that we can track the improvements to performance on the validation set over the iterations of training and stop when the improvement has dropped below some (possibly predefined) threshold.

When several ML models are compared, the data used to train those models or, separately, evaluate those models should be identical. These data should be ecologically valid, statistically consistent, or otherwise similar to data expected to be observed in deployment. It would not make sense to train ML for CV on simulated laparoscopic videos and expect it to be useful in vivo directly without some modification.

Running Appropriate Experiments

In a classification experiment, each element of a set of test data will be provided to the learned model, and the outcome will be evaluated according to some criterion. For example, *accuracy* may be computed as the proportion of correctly classified data points to the total number of data points in a testing set [or $= (TP + TN)/(TP + TN + FP + FN)$ in a binary task, where TP is true positive, TN, true negative, FP, false positive, and FN, false negative]. Just as Mitchell's invocation of experience E (or data D) is tightly coupled with the task in the definition of ML, so is the performance measure P. Naturally, it would not make sense to compute accuracy for a regression task or a root mean squared error for a nominal classification task. In health care in particular, we may also take special consideration to value certain outcomes more highly than others. For example, a false positive on a screening test that only leads to more assessment may carry a certain financial burden for the government or institution (or for the patient, depending on the jurisdiction), but a false negative that leads to a disease going unrecognized and therefore untreated may carry a more significant burden (again, depending on the jurisdiction) of the loss of life or well-being.

In the frantic race to outcompete alternative algorithms in the dogged pursuits of efficiency and accuracy, there is a glaring risk that the bare methodologic concepts of science may be misapplied or even ignored when comparing our systems. The mythical label *state-of-the-art* is often applied to one approach or another, as if a medal won through an unambiguous contest, which becomes suspect when one considers the supposed rules of the contest. Typically, state-of-the-art may only apply on a certain (sometimes small) data set, on a certain (sometimes esoteric) task that by no means is guaranteed to generalize to yours, and given only a particular set of initial conditions.

When describing the performance P of one or more models, the following aspects must be carefully controlled and reported[6]:

Implementation. The computer language (eg, R or Python), the library or framework (ie, a collection of tools to build a model, such as PyTorch or TensorFlow), and other considerations (eg, whether an algorithm requires massively parallel processing using modern graphics processing units to be tractable or whether there is some arbitrary stop learning condition in the code) can affect outcomes and must be made explicit.

Hyperparameters. The numeric hand-tunable configurations of an ML algorithm, such as a learning rate (the amount to change the components of a model iteration to iteration) or the number of artificial neurons in a neural network, are called *hyperparameters*, and their manual settings can have a profound effect on downstream tasks. If they are optimized, the hyperparameters of the comparative ML models should also be optimized, except when the hyperparameters themselves are being compared.

Preprocessing. Data are often scrubbed of elements that may confound the training process or that are superfluous and therefore distracting to the learning algorithm. Modification of the data before training is called *preprocessing*. For example, we may remove stop words, such as prepositions, from a data set of text messages between nurses and attending physicians in an intensive care unit (ICU) if our goal is to train an NLP model to detect urgency (a subtype of sentiment) from those texts, because prepositions and adverbs rarely carry any affect. However, the same preprocessing step would not be appropriate when more specific semantics are required (eg, indicating whether a reanastomosis was *above* or *below* a prior anastomosis).

Appropriate measures. There is a tendency to report accuracy or area under the precision-recall (or other operator characteristic) curves in nominal classification; however, this is not always correct. For example, systems that predict cause of death according to international standards for disease coding should not merely report accuracy, but should also include the cause-specific mortality fraction, which is the fraction of in-hospital deaths for a given cause normalized over all causes[7]; it is a measure of predictive quality at the population level.

Clearly, the particular measure used can be highly context dependent and may result in very different outcomes for different samples.

Beyond the standard controls in the prior list, we must also be sensitive to other details in our experimental processes that may affect the observed behaviors of a model. Human examiners may have an inherent or subconscious bias or conflict of interest in favor of a model that they themselves devised, so it can be difficult to notice when their thumb is on the scale, so to speak. Inadvertently or not, experiments may be set up so that information can leak from the training set to the test set in such a way so that no latent information exists across sets, other than directly obtained from observation variables. This can occur when latent information is highly correlated to labels, annotation, or other supervised information. For example, a system may be designed to classify between CT scans with and without the presence of cancer and may have multiple data points recorded, for example, at different tomographic slices. Some visual features, such as the size or shape of tissue contours, may help to identify pathology cross-sectionally, but they can also be used to identify patients themselves. Because each patient may be associated with a label for his or her diagnosis, even if individual samples are partitioned across training and test sets, it would be inappropriate if an individual patient is represented in both training and test sets. This is because any model could learn the identity of a patient from the training data and apply the known label to test data, tainting the results. Leave-one-out cross-validation is one mitigation strategy.

Other considerations may also taint an experiment. A *channel effect* occurs when a model may learn characteristics of the manner in which data were recorded, in addition to the nature of the data themselves. For example, a system may be designed to classify patients into their required levels of care upon presenting at an emergency department. However, if all (or most) patients with complex cancers travel to seek treatment in urban centers, then a classifier may learn to associate those cancers with certain regions. For example, Caruana et al[8] trained a model to predict which patients presenting with pneumonia would die upon being admitted to a hospital, but this model learned to associate the presence of asthma with a *lower* risk of death, which confounded the investigators. Later, it was found that the particular hospital where these data were recorded has a procedure in place to shunt patients with asthma and symptoms of pneumonia directly to the ICU, which in fact improved their outcomes given the higher levels of care. This kind of channel effect, and others, can be caused by the mechanism used to obtain the data, any preprocessing that occurred on one or more subsets of the data, the identity of the individuals obtaining the data, or environmental changes in which data were recorded. If these effects cannot be controlled, they would ideally be accounted for as covariates during statistical significance testing. The typical scientific and engineering issues of repeatability (related to the variation that occurs despite efforts to keep conditions constant) and reproducibility (related to the variation that occurs given different conditions or evaluators) are, of course, present here, too.

Supervised and Unsupervised Learning

We often consider it to be ideal when a set of data D has been appropriately labeled (ie, annotated) with some outcome measure that we mean to predict or infer. This is the case of **supervised learning**, in which human labelers may apply their insights or expertise to provide the targets of a presumed function over the features of the data.

However, not only is this becoming more difficult to assume (the pace of data acquisition far exceeds the pace of proper labeling), but a lot can be accomplished with *unlabeled* data. **Unsupervised learning** involves automatically recognizing patterns emergent from the data, such as latent or hidden structures therein, without any guidance whatsoever. In deep learning, this can take the form of probability distributions over features or aspects of the data, which can be used directly for some future estimation or for synthesis of artificial data. Clustering algorithms and Gaussian mixture modeling are common examples of unsupervised learning.

Bias, Variance, Overfitting, and Underfitting

Bias and variance are twin descriptive statistics of ML output that can affect our interpretation of ML performance. Bias is the difference between the average model prediction and the correct value. If a model is highly biased, it may result in a simple model, but one bearing little resemblance to training data (and therefore little resemblance to an accurate model). Variance is the spread of predictions for a given data type; it may be highly sensitive to the training data but will therefore not generalize well to new data. Formally, if we mean to predict some outcome Y of some true process, we can model it as $Y = f(X) + e$, where e is an error term with mean 0. This process will produce some artifact model $\hat{f}(X)$ that is not fully accurate.

In this second formulation, the first term is the squared bias, the second is the variance of the predictions, and the third (σ_e^2) is an irreducible error term (caused by error in the data itself, perhaps). Figure 3-1 shows

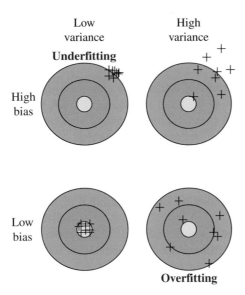

Figure 3-1 • The trade-off between bias and variance in machine learning (ML) model output. The center of each bull's eye represents the true target, and the X marks indicate the actual predictions made by an ML model.

the relationship between variance and bias, with regard to the true output. If a model is too simple *relative to the data*, we risk **underfitting** to those data, or having a model whose output shows high bias and low variance; a linear approximation to nonlinear data may fall into this trap. Conversely, an overly complex model that is able to very tightly fit to its training data will risk **overfitting** to those data; it will have low bias but high variance and will similarly not generalize well to unseen data. There is no de facto preference between under- and overfit models, but in health care, we may generally prefer low bias and control for variance using various **regularization** techniques, such as the L1 norm (lasso regression) or the L2 norm (ridge regression).

Feature Engineering

One hallmark of older approaches to AI remains the presence of *feature engineering*, which involves small functions or pieces of code that transform the raw input into certain intermediate representations. For example, a time series from an electrocardiogram may consist of raw voltages over time, but a Fourier transform will serve to extract spectral information from those signals, thereby obtaining the features of *frequency* that are more directly applicable to analysis. Not only does this aid in the interpretation of results, through the principle of decomposability,[9] but these intermediate representations often simplify the learning process by purposefully extracting information that is expected to be most relevant to a task. While still potentially useful in a variety of settings (including when data are scarce), the advent of deep learning has, to some extent, replaced the need for intermediate feature engineering, as the methods themselves can learn to identify features of the original, raw output that are most discriminative of some downstream task or most representative of some underlying structure in the data.

In cases where the number of extracted features outweighs the number of data samples in a training set, various methods may be applied to reduce the number of the former, which can help avoid overfitting. Feature selection chooses a subset from an available set of features that are most useful to the task, whereas dimensionality reduction (eg, principal components or factor analysis) projects these features into some latent space, which is defined by hidden dimensions in the data, as in principal components analysis. ML methods themselves can be used as advanced feature selectors; for example, Alonzo-Atienza et al[10] used an ML technique called *support vector machines*, discussed later, to identify the most useful features for the early detection of ventricular fibrillation.

Generative Models

A generative model is one in which synthetic examples may be automatically produced by sampling from the model. At its most primitive, the set of generative models may be represented by a simple statistical distribution; the normal (or Gaussian) distribution is controlled by only 2 parameters—mean μ and standard deviation σ—yet sampling uniformly across the independent variable (or domain) x gives synthetic sample outputs $(= e^{-\frac{(x-\mu)^2}{2\sigma^2}} / \sqrt{2\pi\sigma^2}$), which will mimic the behavior of whatever data were used to train the distribution in the first place. Generative models can be useful in synthesizing data that are realistic (at least to the capabilities of the model), but as a consequence of their typical incorporation of the observation space's prior probabilities, they are usually less accurate in classification tasks than discriminative methods. Of course, a lot depends on the *choice* of model. Two generative models are discussed in the following sections.

Naïve Bayes

Thomas Bayes was an 18th-century English statistician whose works provide a sort of backbone to much of the work we now do in ML. Broadly,

Bayesian probability conceives of probability not as frequency of some phenomenon occurring, but rather as an expectation related to our own knowledge—to what extent we can be certain of something. In this way, the classic *Bayes theorem* emerges where, for a class c (ie, the target or outcome) and for predictor x (ie, attributes or features), we can rewrite the probability of c given x as

$$P(c \mid x) = \frac{P(x \mid c)P(c)}{P(x)}$$

This simple reformulation typically allows us to make use of (or ignore) probabilities we can more easily obtain or that are not useful. Specifically (and ironically), we can take the frequentist approach to estimate $P(c)$ as just the proportion of instances in which we have observed outcome c over all instances, and estimate $P(x \mid c)$ as the distribution of x in the subset of all data where the outcome is specifically c (which is relatively easy to compute). Moreover, if our goal is merely to find the class c that maximizes $P(c \mid x)$, given x, then Bayes theorem allows us to ignore the prior probability of the input features (which are useless, because we have already observed the specific input) by simply computing the probabilities in the numerator. Importantly, however, Bayes theorem assumes independence among the predictors, which, to put it in a word, may be naïve in real-world tasks.

However, if the assumption of independence holds (or can be safely assumed to hold), naïve Bayes is relatively quick to make inferences in practice, particularly performant on large data sets (often being just as good as more complicated approaches), and performs especially well if the input is categorical or nominal, rather than continuous or numeric. In the latter case, the normal distribution is normally (pun intended) assumed, which is another, sometimes unreasonable, assumption. Furthermore, if a class has not been observed in training, Bayes will assume it to be impossible and give it a zero probability. Therefore, in practice, one should consider adding "smoothing" methods that redistribute probability mass to unseen events, and one should also consider selecting only one from among sets of correlated input features, so that the assumptions in the model can hold.

Hidden Markov Models

We are often concerned with observations that change over time. This can include high-frequency measures, such as heart rate or intubated breathing rate, as well as long-term measures, such as the sequence of progress notes.

Consider the situation where we wish to estimate the risk of sepsis s over time given some observable indicators x. We can represent the sequence of each of these variables by subscripts, so $x_{0:t}$ represents the sequence of indicators from the baseline at time 0 up until some given time t. Modeling these sequences of indicators and risks together is $P(x_{0:t}, s_{0:t})$, which can be decomposed to $P(s_{0:t})P(x_{0:t} | s_{0:t})$ by the chain rule. However, each of these 2 factors will also factor out over time in long chains of probabilities that become so specific to our previous experience that they simply cannot generalize to new data. That is why we apply the *Markov assumption*, that the observation at time t depends not on the *entire* history of observations that preceded it but is approximately estimated by only the recent past. If we assume that the risk of sepsis at time i depends only on the immediately preceding risk, s_{i-1}, then $P(S_{0:t}) \approx \Pi_{i=0}^{t} P(S_i | S_{i-1})$; furthermore, if we assume that the observations at time i depend only on the risk at time i, then $P(x_{0:t} | S_{0:t}) \approx \Pi_{i=0}^{t} P(x_i | S_i)$. Graphically, this sequence looks like the following:

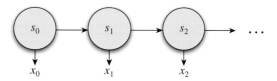

Here, each circle represents a variable, and each arrow represents a particular conditional probability—the first downward arrow represents $P(x_0 | s_0)$ and the first rightward arrow represents $P(s_1 | s_0)$. These simple probabilities are easy to compute, which is a result of the first core aspect of *hidden Markov models* (HMMs)—the Markov assumption. The second core aspect is also in the title—hidden.

Typically, we do not have direct access to measures that we would like to estimate, such as sepsis risk. Instead, these variables are *hidden*—unknown. If our aforementioned probabilities are already established, we can infer s_t at each point in time using the Viterbi algorithm,[11] which uses dynamic programming to efficiently find the state sequence $s_{0:t}$ that maximizes the probability $P(x_{0:t}, s_{0:t})$, given the observations $x_0.t$. If our aforementioned probabilities are *not* already established, then we have to learn them from data. But how can we learn probabilities about the states s if we can never actually measure s?

In a concept to which we will return briefly when discussing neural networks, internal model representations are rarely as explicit as the earlier example. If we cannot actually measure the state, but we know some conditioning state exists, we can let the data infer the presence of such a state automatically. This is similar, in some sense, to the notion of *clustering*, in which some hidden structure emerges naturally from the data, or to the notion of *principal components analysis (PCA)*, in which some hidden dimensions emerge as capturing much of the variance in the data. This brings us to the notion of the **latent space**—a hidden world of structure and dimension but one that we cannot observe.

In HMMs, we assume there to be some conditioning state but, like the dimensions in a PCA analysis, we cannot necessarily give it a name. We infer its presence and behavior by an iterative method called the *expectation-maximization (EM) algorithm*. Here, we take a preexisting model of our probabilities (the arrows in the graph above) to estimate what the states $s_{0:t}$ *should* be, and then given that expectation (step 1), we recompute those probabilities using the traditional *maximum likelihood estimate* (step 2, ie, the frequentist approach of merely counting instances of a thing, over all observed instances in the data set). The challenge here, of course, is that we cannot count the number of times we are in some particular state if we cannot know when we are actually in one state or another at a particular time; the solution is to compute these probabilities in a soft manner, weighing all possible instances. Given that the recomputation of the probabilities will probably give better estimates of the training data than their previous version, iterating between the expectation steps and the maximization steps will give us better and better models until some stopping condition.

In HMMs, the hidden variable is the time-varying state s, which has a direct effect on our observations (eg, symptoms); however, the EM algorithm generalizes to other generative models, including mixtures of Gaussians, where the hidden variable is the identity of a Gaussian distribution that produced an observation (where any observation may actually be the soft combination of multiple Gaussians). The details of HMMs and the EM algorithm are beyond the scope of this chapter but are beautiful and open our interpretation of phenomena to unknowable, hidden aspects that behave not unlike Schrödinger's cat—we must consider all possible states of the hidden phenomena (even states that are not so definable as alive or dead). We will return to this unintuitive but powerful concept in our discussion of neural networks.

Discriminative Models

A discriminative model more directly solves the classification task by explicitly learning parameters to minimize error. For example, consider the probability distribution $P(O,K)$, which computes the joint probability of an observation O and class K occurring together. Some generative models may learn this distribution to decide whether some particular class

$K = k_1$ gives higher probability than some other class $K = k_2$. Indeed, a model that describes the data is what we tend to expect in the traditional sciences. However, this results in wasted effort; if we expand this distribution, $P(O,K) = P(O)P(K|O)$, we see that the probability of the observation $P(O)$ is useless to our classification decision, when all we really want is $P(K|O)$, and our learning should be focused there.

But focusing on the conditional distribution is not enough. In ML, we are dealt all manner of tasks to solve, and we should effectively pass our goals along to the algorithms themselves. In optimization, we talk about a **loss function** or a **cost function**, which maps observations or outcomes onto a real number that we want to minimize; for example, if our model predicts $f(x)$ given input x, but the actual target output is y, then a loss could be the squared difference between the two, scaled by some constant hyperparameter c: $c(y - f(x))^2$ (this is actually called the quadratic loss). Naturally, we want to minimize the loss. There are, of course, other loss functions; we can talk about minimizing regret (however precisely defined) or some expected loss. Somewhat more generally, we can talk about **objective functions**, which are either loss functions we want to minimize or their inverse (or some other desirable outcome) that we want to maximize. Defining our objective functions precisely and appropriately to the task is important to think about, although frankly, in most ML tasks, we simply wish to minimize the error. We discuss 2 approaches to minimizing error in the following sections.

Support Vector Machine

The support vector machine (SVM) is similar to logistic regression in that we assume a linear function $w^\mathrm{T}x + b$, where w and b must be tuned to data, except the output is only nominal—positive when that function is positive and negative otherwise (ie, the SVM does not estimate probabilities). The parameters w and b are typically tuned so that the boundary they produce between the 2 classes is positioned as far away from either class as possible (Figure 3-2). More specifically, we define the *margin* as the empty space extending orthogonally from this boundary toward the closest data points from each class (called *support vectors*). Intuitively, the larger this margin, the more confident we can be in the position of our boundary, since we have cautiously reduced the chances that future, so-far-unseen examples of our classes would naturally pop up on the wrong side of this boundary (eg, if the boundary was too close to the data from one class, if we keep sampling from that class, we expect new samples to fall on the other side of the boundary).

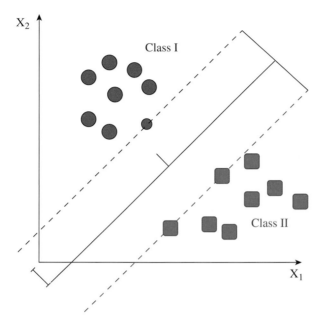

Figure 3-2 • Support vector machine (SVM) between class I and class II, showing the maximum margin between these 2 classes, given 1 support vector in the former and 2 in the latter.

SVMs seem to be restricted to problems where we only have 2 classes or 2 problems where we can draw a clean, straight boundary between the classes, but both of these restrictions have been surmounted by extensions of the core concept. First, SVMs generalize to situations where we have an arbitrary number of classes k—all we need to do is learn a collection of binary classifiers. For example, if we wish to classify between low, moderate, or high risk of transfusion, we can first classify between high risk and not high risk with one binary SVM and then iterate to a second binary SVM that classifies not high risk cases into low- or moderate-risk instances.

One of the key innovations associated with SVMs is the **kernel trick**, which is the ability to project data into other spaces by replacing dot products between weights and inputs with arbitrary functions. That is, we can replace the contributions of our inputs x with some function $\phi(x)$, and we can replace the dot product in $w^T x + b$ with a function $k(x, x^{(i)}) = \phi(x) \cdot \phi(x^{(i)})$, called the kernel function, where $x^{(i)}$ is an example from the training data. This allows us to learn models that are no longer linear, as in the introduction earlier, but nevertheless converge to good solutions during optimization. For example, a common kernel is the Gaussian kernel, also called the radial basis function kernel, $k(u, v) = N(u - v; \mu = 0,$

$\Sigma = \sigma^2 I$), for mean μ and variance Σ, which allows us to perform dot products over infinite-dimensional spaces.

▌DEEP NEURAL NETWORKS

Deep learning is dealt with in greater detail in Chapter 4 of this book; however, a brief overview of the connections between the concepts introduced earlier and neural networks can help one better understand the intersectionality of these techniques.

Recurrent Neural Networks

HMMs introduced us to the idea of learning about temporal dynamics in data, using simple Bayesian statistics and a few (perhaps overbearing) assumptions about statistical independence. However, their simplicity places certain limitations on us that we may want to avoid, such as potential nonlinear relationships between input variables that we wish to preserve. A recurrent neural network (RNN) is simply a type of neural network that projects hidden layers or outputs computed at one point in time t, in a sequence, to be used in subsequent points in time (usually $t + 1$). Graphically, this looks like:

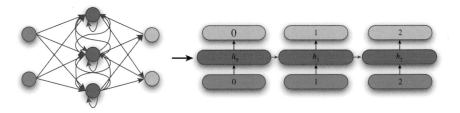

Where x_t, h_t, and y_t are the input, hidden, and output layers of neurons at time t. Moreover, the hidden layer can be computed as $ht = g(W_I[x;h_{t-1}] + c)$ for some activation function g and constant bias term c, and the output can be computed as $y_t = W_O h_t + b$ for some bias term b. Note that we have some freedom to choose the activation g, but typical choices are:

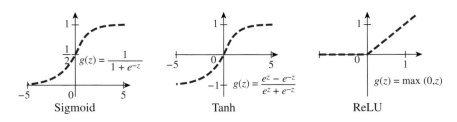

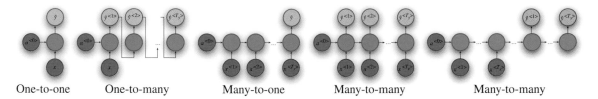

Figure 3-3 • Five variants of recurrent neural network (RNN). An input sequence x can be associated with either a single output or a sequence of outputs y, and those outputs can all be generated once all inputs have been read, or synchronously—one output with each input.

A core concept here is that the hidden layer h_t is constantly updated with information from the past. If the input sequence x_t is a series of tumor markers such as carcinoembryonic antigen over time, the hidden layer essentially encodes information about the latent disease trajectory. Like the HMM, the actual representation of this layer may not be explicitly nameable using typical methods. There are also, as is almost always the case in ML, various alternatives to the underlying model. As shown later, RNNs can have one output at each input, one output at the end of a sequence of inputs, or an arbitrary number of outputs after an arbitrary number of inputs (Figure 3-3). This last type of RNN has its own name—2 actually—a sequence-to-sequence model or, alternatively, an encoder-decoder network (since it first encodes information and then decodes it). The choice of architecture depends, as always, on the task.

Unlike SVMs or traditional feedforward neural networks, RNNs can process input sequences of any length, without having to resort to hacks like padding inputs to be of some arbitrarily constant length. However, like HMMs, RNNs soon forget information as new information is written to the hidden layer. This catastrophic forgetting is also somewhat related to the problem of vanishing or exploding gradients. Because the loss function needs to be propagated backward through time, the gradients often become iteratively smaller (ie, the error signal becomes weaker as it is passed backward through the network, like light becoming dimmer as it penetrates deeper into the sea), limiting the influence of the loss and therefore also of the ability of the network to learn. An innovation to accommodate this phenomenon is to add a "highway" through time, called a *cell state*, in which useful information is explicitly written, overwritten, and saved.

The classic use of the cell state is within the long short-term memory (LSTM) network that uses 4 gates. Each gate is a smooth function between 0 and 1 that either lets information pass through or filters it out. The first is the forget gate, which decides what information should be removed from the cell state; the second decides what information from the hidden and input layers should be stored; the third actually adds that information to the cell state; and the fourth updates the hidden state. This can be a lot to learn, and even somewhat redundant, so more modern approaches forego the cell state and the multiple steps altogether and instead make precise and deliberate changes to the hidden state in a gated recurrent unit.

Convolutional Neural Networks

When the dimensions of data can be strictly ordered, not just as points in time, but according to any continuum, then convolutional neural networks (CNNs) may be useful. In the most basic case, we have 2-dimensional images in which the dimensions are the dimensions of the image (ie, pixels ordered along the height and width). Fundamentally, a convolution is an operation on 2 functions (f and g) that produces a third expressing how the first modifies the second, that is, $\int_{t=-\infty}^{\infty} f(\tau)g(t-\tau)\,d\tau$. The profundity of this operator is beyond the scope of this chapter. Suffice it to say that, for practical purposes, this can be viewed as taking a small lens (called a filter whose own height and width is a tunable hyperparameter) over a small region of the image and then scanning it across the dimensions of the image and applying a pooling operation to obtain a single value representing the respective region. This is visualized in Figure 3-4.

Figure 3-4 represents one layer of a deep CNN (or ConvNet). We can imagine multiple such operations processed one after the other, so that a very large 2-dimensional image is "boiled down" to smaller and smaller pseudo-images, representing more and more abstract representations of the input image. Crucially, a CNN is focused on local variation, which is why it is crucial that the dimensions over which the convolution is performed are well ordered. This focus allows us to make the neural network sparser (ie, it permits us to ignore some possible connections in the goal of efficiency). This is visualized in the 2 alternative connective layers in

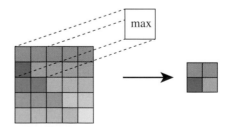

Figure 3-4 • Here, the filter is of size 2×2 pixels, its stride is 2 pixels, and the operation is max pooling.

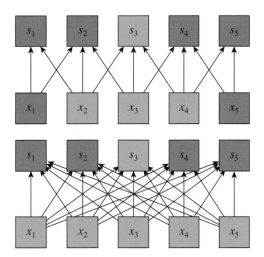

Figure 3-5 • The top layer is sparsely connected in that unit s_3 only takes input from a relatively small region in the top example but from all possible inputs in the bottom example. (Reproduced from Goodfellow I, Bengio Y, Courville A. Convolutional networks, in *Deep Learning*. Accessed October 5, 2020. https://www.deeplearningbook .org/contents/convnets.html.)

Figure 3-5. Local assumptions were also applied to HMMs, in time, and allow us to learn more effectively or to generalize better.

The common wisdom is that layers closer to the input will encapsulate relatively surface-level phenomena (eg, word choice in progress notes or edges in images), and deeper layers closer to the output will encapsulate information relevant to the task (eg, semantic information relevant to risk or regions resembling tumors).

▌ FUTURE TENSE

From Basement to Bedside

To some extent, AI and ML have been less visible in surgery than in other specialties during this recent technologic expansion. Indeed, surgery was not among the specialties explored by Topol[12] in his recent survey of AI in medicine, which included radiology, pathology, dermatology, ophthalmology, gastroenterology, and cardiology. Furthermore, although AI is often associated with robotics, the current status quo in surgical robotics has been more about highly complex engineering challenges than about ML.

However, this is changing, and ML is increasingly being used in surgical settings. Several studies have explored the use of CV, typically through

CNNs, to identify tools and estimate surgical skill.[13] By automatically identifying and tracking tools in video, we can effectively assess for surgical quality through the analysis of tool usage patterns, movement, and economy of motion. More classic approaches, including basic control and CV, have even recently begun to augment[14] or even supersede human performance on very specific skilled tasks, such as suturing, in highly controlled settings. The days are, as they say, still early.

▌ CONCLUSION

On its own, ML is neither a harbinger nor an emancipator, as it is alternatively portrayed in the common discussion. As with many things, the truth may fall somewhere in between. Certainly, to the extent that ML is embodied within statistical *models*, it can be neither intrinsically dangerous nor safe—that depends on the context *around* the model, including the task, the data, the empirical training procedure, and the eventual use. It is not the model that counts, but how we use it. We have discussed a few concepts, at a high level, that should be part of any evaluation of ML models.

In addition to the practical considerations described earlier for ML in general, deep learning presents its own unique challenges. For one, its complexity leads to computational requirements that cannot be ignored. It simply will not be reasonable to use a deep CNN on a volume of data large enough to account for the necessary variation *without* a high-performance computer, for example.

It is also important to note that discussions of ML are often conjugated in the future tense. Our community has made fantastic progress over the decades, and especially recently, but the fact remains that the *promise* of AI is exactly that—a pledge of some future potential. Despite the great impacts that have already been made, we still expect the future impacts of ML to be even more profound. As we move into the future, we have several preparatory steps we can take in the present.

First, we need to continue to build a welcoming and vibrant cross-disciplinary community in ML and health care. This will require health care workers, technologists, and social scientists to work devotedly together on common challenges. At an abstract level, those in health care tell us what to solve, the technologists tell us how to solve it, and the social scientists tell us why we should care about the solution. At a more realistic level, progress will depend on the diverse perspectives of all stakeholders, and to build those solutions, we will require a common language. This has not always been easy. For one, the vocabularies can be quite divergent (eg, active learning means different things in different contexts). Second, the "grammar" of the scientific process has also been different across disciplines; whereas clinicians will often approach a problem top-down with a null hypothesis H_0 that can be tested given a sample size emergent from a power analysis, ML engineers have sometimes taken a more, let us say, "discovery-based" approach from the data upward. A common question that clinicians ask of computer scientists is "How much data will you need?" to which a reasonable response would be "everything you can give me."

A second step we can take toward the future of ML in health care—and we can never emphasize this enough—is for us to realize that we do not know what we do not know. André Gide advised us to "believe those who are seeking the truth; doubt those who find it." Socrates, supposedly, emphasized that the one thing he knew was that he knew nothing. Amid the popular, frothing-at-the-mouth, and frenzied discussion of the promises and perils of ML, we need to remember the purpose to which we are applying these modern tools and that, after Marshall McLuhan, when we shape these tools we must consider how these tools shape us.

REFERENCES

1. Esteva A, Kuprel B, Novoa RA, et al. Dermatologist-level classification of skin cancer with deep neural networks. *Nature*. 2017;542(7639):115-118.
2. Adamson AS, Smith A. Machine learning and health care disparities in dermatology. *JAMA Dermatol*. 2018;154(11):1247-1248.
3. Bolukbasi T, Chang K, Zou J, Saligrama V, Kalai A. Man is to computer programmer as woman is to homemaker? Debiasing word embeddings. Accessed September 30, 2020. https://arxiv.org/abs/1607.06520.
4. Na L, Yang C, Lo CC, Zhao F, Fukuoka Y, Aswani A. Feasibility of reidentifying individuals in large national physical activity data sets from which protected health information has been removed with use of machine learning. *JAMA Netw Open*. 2018;1(8):e186040.
5. Culnane C, Rubinstein BIP, Teague V. Health data in an open world. Accessed September 30, 2020. http://arxiv.org/abs/1712.05627.
6. Rudzicz F, Paprica PA, Janczarski M. Towards international standards for evaluating machine learning. Accessed September 30, 2020. http://ceur-ws.org/Vol-2301/paper_10.pdf.
7. Jeblee S, Gomes M, Jha P, Rudzicz F, Hirst G. Automatically determining cause of death from verbal autopsy narratives. *BMC Med Inform Decis Mak*. 2019;19(1):127.
8. Caruana R, Lou Y, Gehrke J, Koch P, Strum M, Elhadad N. Intelligible models for healthcare. Accessed September 30, 2020. http://people.dbmi.columbia.edu/noemie/papers/15kdd.pdf.

9. Lipton ZC. The mythos of model interpretability. Accessed September 30, 2020. https://arxiv.org/abs/1606.03490.

10. Alonso-Atienza F, Rojo-Álvarez JL, Rosado-Muñoz A, Vinagre JJ, García-Alberola A, Camps-Valls G. Feature selection using support vector machines and bootstrap methods for ventricular fibrillation detection. *Exp Syst Appl.* 2012;39:1956-1967.

11. Forney GD. The Viterbi algorithm. *Proc IEEE.* 1973;61(3):268-278.

12. Topol E. High-performance medicine: the convergence of human and artificial intelligence. *Nat Med.* 2019;(25):44-56.

13. Jin A, Yeung S, Jopling J, et al. Tool detection and operative skill assessment in surgical videos using region-based convolutional neural networks. *IEEE.* 2018:691-699.

14. Leonard S, Wu KL, Kim Y, Krieger A, Kim PCW. Smart tissue anastomosis robot (STAR): a vision-guided robotics system for laparoscopic suturing. *IEEE Trans Biomed Eng.* 2014;61(4):1305-1317.

NEURAL NETWORKS AND DEEP LEARNING 4

Deepak Alapatt*, Pietro Mascagni*, Vinkle Srivastav, and Nicolas Padoy

HIGHLIGHTS

- The growing availability of digital data and computational power enables the training of deep neural networks useful for real-world applications.
- Deep neural networks are typically composed of multiple convolutional layers used to efficiently extract information from high-dimensional inputs, pooling layers to reduce dimensions, and fully connected layers to aggregate neuron activations into output values.
- Neural networks learn to approximate a function by forward propagating the input layer by layer, calculating a loss comparing the current output to the ground truth, and then updating the network's weights and biases through backpropagation.
- Deep architectures are selected based on the nature of the input and desired output data to perform tasks such as classification, detection, semantic segmentation, and temporal recognition.
- Deep-learning strategies to guarantee the security of sensitive medical data, train networks using less supervision, increase model explainability, and deliver real-time predictions in the operating room are being developed to generate value in surgery.

▮ INTRODUCTION

Instead of trying to produce a programme to simulate the adult mind, why not rather try to produce one which simulates the child's? If this were then subjected to an appropriate course of education one would obtain the adult brain.

Alan Turing, 1950, "Computing Machinery and Intelligence"

The question of whether machines could be capable of thinking and learning like humans has always allured mankind. As briefly discussed in

*Deepak Alapatt and Pietro Mascagni share co-first authorship.

Chapter 1, ancient mythology dating back more than 2500 years ago already made references to modern concepts such as self-moving objects, robots, and what we now refer to as artificial intelligence (AI). The recent surge in deep learning is contributing to turning these antic fantasies into today's reality. Deep-learning breakthroughs in fields ranging from image and speech recognition to game playing have been widely covered by the press, generating enthusiasm in the general public as well as among businesses and funding agencies. Replicating biologic neurons on silica chips is by no means a novel idea; however, the incredible amount of digital data we now ubiquitously generate—together with the growing availability and decreasing cost of computational power—makes training deep neural networks practical. Furthermore, open source programming frameworks have lowered the barrier to entry, allowing quick prototyping for real-world applications.

Deep-learning models are already in use for applications such as automatic recommendations of media content and smart assistants in our homes and self-driving cars. Health care is a very active field of research for AI given its social and economic relevance. In this sector, surgery is a particularly interesting and challenging subfield because it is a high-stakes discipline where multiple people interact, make quick decisions based on a large amount of sparse information, and act to alter a patient's anatomy. Despite clear opportunities and widespread hype, deep learning has yet to impact surgical patients. Thus, it is the ideal moment for surgeons to understand the intuitions behind neural networks, become familiar with deep-learning concepts and tasks, grasp what implementing a deep-learning model in surgery means, and finally appreciate the specific challenges and limitations to address for deep learning and AI to benefit patients and surgical practices.

ARTIFICIAL AND CONVOLUTIONAL NEURAL NETWORKS

A function in mathematics is a relation that assigns one or more unique output values to any given input. It may be trivial to define a function to detect atypical values in routine blood tests; however, defining a function to detect abnormalities in radiologic scans may not be as straightforward a task due to the varied appearance of both normal and abnormal scans. Neural networks offer a means to approximate an unknown function when the output values for a large number of sufficiently informative inputs are known but the relationships between them cannot be deduced easily using conventional approaches. This is why neural networks, also known as universal function approximators, are an extremely useful tool for a variety of applications.

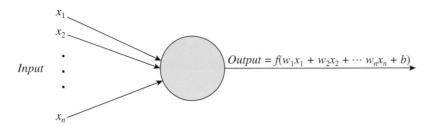

Figure 4-1 • Artificial neuron.

Artificial Neuron and Neural Networks

The fundamental building block of neural networks is the *artificial neuron* (Figure 4-1) or node (hereinafter referred to as neuron), which is used to map a multidimensional input $(x_1, x_2, \cdots, x_n)$ to a single output value.

The 3 main components of the neuron are a set of weights $(w_1, w_2, \ldots, w_n)$, a bias (b), and an *activation function* (f). The weights and biases of the neuron are numeric values or *parameters* that can be used to represent any linear combination of the inputs in the form:

$$w_1x_1 + w_2x_2 + \cdots + w_nx_n + b. \qquad \text{(Eq 4-1)}$$

The activation function f then transforms the sum of weighted inputs by applying nonlinearity to the output of that neuron. This operation is performed because these neurons are used to learn real-world representations, which are seldom linear. Some useful activation functions are described in Table 4-1. The choice of activation functions is based on a number of factors such as speed of computation, the purpose of the neuron, and the nature of the data it operates on. Some of the activation functions mentioned earlier can be used to "squeeze" the output of the neuron to a fixed range. For instance, *sigmoid* transforms the input function to an output between 0 and 1 (Table 4-1). This type of activation function is known as a *saturating function* and may be useful if the expected output of the neuron is within a fixed and known range of values, for example, to represent the probability of an event occurring where the only plausible values would be between 0 and 1. Rectified linear unit (or ReLU) is another commonly used choice of activation function because it is computationally inexpensive to calculate.

A *neural network* is a collection of interconnected neurons. Each neuron takes a set of inputs, processes them, and sends a signal (a numerical one in this case) that in turn serves as an input to other neurons. In this section, we will introduce the key concepts involved in designing and implementing a neural network.

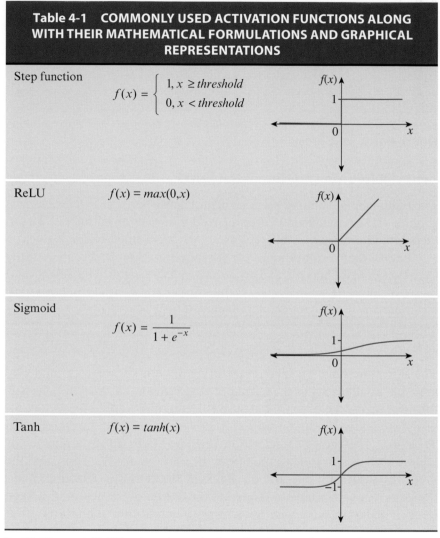

Table 4-1 COMMONLY USED ACTIVATION FUNCTIONS ALONG WITH THEIR MATHEMATICAL FORMULATIONS AND GRAPHICAL REPRESENTATIONS		
Step function	$f(x) = \begin{cases} 1, x \geq threshold \\ 0, x < threshold \end{cases}$	
ReLU	$f(x) = max(0,x)$	
Sigmoid	$f(x) = \dfrac{1}{1 + e^{-x}}$	
Tanh	$f(x) = tanh(x)$	

Rectified linear unit (ReLU) and step show a simple nonlinearity at $x = 0$, whereas sigmoid and tanh represent more complex nonlinear functions.

In Figure 4-2, each of the different colors represents one layer of the neural network, and each of the individual circles represents a neuron in that layer. The network consists of an input layer, one or more hidden layers that are used to extract meaningful information from the input, and finally an output layer that aggregates this information into a desired form. If the input layer is, for example, a computed tomography (CT) scan slice showing a tumor, then the output could represent the probability

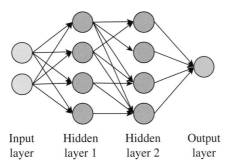

Input   Hidden   Hidden   Output
layer   layer 1   layer 2   layer

Figure 4-2 • Example of a neural network.

of malignancy. When there are multiple hidden layers between the input and output layers, the network is said to be a *deep neural network*, and training such a network to perform a task is referred to as *deep learning*. Lower layers can be thought to extract simple information, such as edges for images, and higher layers build on that information to develop an understanding of more complex concepts, such as parts and then more complex shapes.[1]

Let us now look at how neurons function together in a layer beginning with the simplest kind, the *fully connected layer*. A fully connected layer is basically a collection of neurons each connected to every neuron of the previous layer. Every neuron of the fully connected layer thus receives n input values (i_1, i_2, ... , i_n), where n is equal to the number of neurons in the previous layer, and the output of that neuron is given by:

$$w_1 i_1 + w_2 i_2 + \cdots + w_n i_n + b. \qquad \text{(Eq 4-2)}$$

In fact, the output of an entire fully connected layer containing m neurons can be calculated using a single matrix multiplication:

$$
\begin{bmatrix} o_1 \\ o_2 \\ \cdots \\ o_m \end{bmatrix}
=
\begin{bmatrix} w_{11} & w_{12} & \cdots & w_{1n} \\ w_{21} & w_{22} & \cdots & w_{2n} \\ \cdots & \cdots & \cdots & \cdots \\ w_{m1} & w_{m2} & \cdots & w_{mn} \end{bmatrix}
\begin{bmatrix} i_1 \\ i_2 \\ \cdots \\ i_n \end{bmatrix}
+
\begin{bmatrix} b_1 \\ b_2 \\ \cdots \\ b_m \end{bmatrix}. \qquad \text{(Eq 4-3)}
$$

Here o_i, (w_{i1}, w_{i2}, ..., w_{in}), and b_i correspond to the output, weights, and bias of the ith neuron in the layer, respectively. A nonlinear activation function can then be applied on each of these outputs before passing it as the input to the next layer, if any.

Taking the previous example, suppose the CT scan slice showing a tumor is provided as input to a neural network that uses 2 or more fully

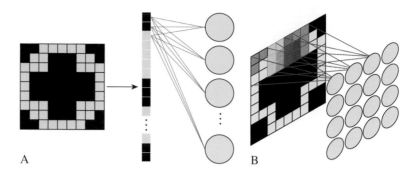

Figure 4-3 • Depiction of neurons and their inputs for (**A**) a fully connected layer and (**B**) a convolutional layer.

connected layers that outputs the probability of malignancy. The slice is first converted into a machine-interpretable format as a 2-dimensional (2D) matrix of numeric values representing the brightness of each pixel in the scan slice. In order to be fed to the first fully connected layer of the network, this 2D matrix has to first be transformed into a 1-dimensional (1D) *vector* (Figure 4-3A) in order to perform the matrix multiplication described in Equation 4-3. Then the network is trained to find appropriate values for the parameters (ie, the weights and biases of all the neurons in the network). Finally, the result is computed from different pathways of neurons that extract the visual cues representative of malignancy in the input.

Using only fully connected layers in a network presents 2 potential issues that can make the process of finding the right parameter values difficult. The first issue is that such a layer does not leverage the information provided by the order in which pixels appear in the original image. For instance, even neighboring pixels in the original 2D image can appear far apart in the transformed 1D vector used as input, as seen in Figure 4-3A. The other issue is that fully connected layers require a large number of parameters to operate on high-dimensional inputs, often in the range of millions for a single layer to operate directly on a high-quality image. One way to address both of these issues is to use a 2D layout of neurons that each only operates on a smaller region of the input and that share the same parameter values in order to identify the same visual cues at different positions (Figure 4-3B). Mathematics conveniently packages this solution in the form of the *convolutional layer*, wherein a smaller set of weights and a bias can be "slid" across different parts of the input.

Figure 4-4 shows a depiction of how the convolution operation works on an input of size 5 × 5. A small matrix of 3 × 3 weight values (known as a *filter*) and 1 bias value is applied on 3 × 3 patches of the input column

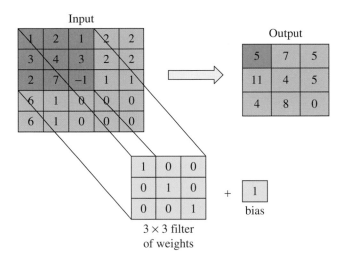

Figure 4-4 • Visualization of a 3 × 3 convolutional filter operating on a 5 × 5-sized input producing an output of size 3 × 3.

by column and row by row. Because convolution uses the same parameters at different positions, this operation is much more memory efficient than the fully connected layer. In fact, in the given example, the convolutional layer only stores 9 weights plus 1 bias per neuron, whereas a fully connected layer would have required the storage of 25 weights plus 1 bias per neuron to operate on the same input. Because each convolutional operation generates a 2D output, using stacks of such filters would generate a 3-dimensional (3D) output. When working with 3D features as inputs to convolutional layers, each convolution filter must also be 3D in order to apply it on 3D patches when moving across the length and breadth of the input. The *stride* of the convolution is the amount the filter is shifted at every step as it is moved over the input. Note that the size of the output is less than the input and decreases even further when using a larger stride value when shifting the filter. It may also be useful to add a border of 0 values around the input to conserve the size of the output. This is known as *zero padding*.

Another layer fundamental to modern neural networks is the *pooling layer*, which can be used to reduce the size of the inputs through mathematical operations, such as averaging and maximum, applied in a similar "sliding" fashion. Figure 4-5 shows an example of the output of a pooling layer using the maximum and average functions.

Neural networks that use the convolutional layer are often referred to as *convolutional neural networks*. Typical network designs involve many convolutional layers, each followed by activation functions and pooling operations and finally a fully connected layer to produce the final output.

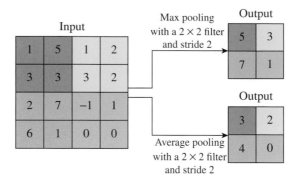

Figure 4-5 • Visualization of pooling with 2 × 2 filters and stride 2 using maximum (top) and average (bottom) pooling.

For a binary classification task like the previously discussed case of tumor classification, we can use a fully connected layer comprising 1 neuron with a sigmoid activation to generate a valid probability of malignancy. Suppose now that we want to classify the same tumor as one of several considered histologic classes using a larger fully connected layer that outputs the probability of each class. In this case, using sigmoid activations could potentially classify the tumor as all of the classes at the same time or as none of them by returning only 1s or 0s, respectively. Here, it would be more appropriate to have an activation function that converts the output into a vector of probabilities that sum to 1. It follows that when one class is classified as more likely, the probability of the other classes decreases. The *softmax* activation allows us to satisfy this constraint by converting the outputs of a layer $(o_1, o_2, \ldots, o_n)$ into a valid probability distribution $(p_1, p_2, \ldots, p_n)$ using the following formula:

$$p_i = \frac{e^{o_i}}{\sum_{j=1}^{n} e^{o_j}}. \qquad \text{(Eq 4-4)}$$

Taking the exponential of the class output ensures that every output is positive, and the division by the sum of the exponential of every class guarantees that all the outputs sum to 1.

Figure 4-6 shows a simple design for a neural network based on AlexNet[2] that can be used to identify which surgical tools are present in an image. The H × W × C notation has been used to express the size of the output of each layer in the network, where H, W, and C are the height, width, and depth of the matrix, respectively. Each of the C slices of size H × W of this matrix is referred to as a *channel*.

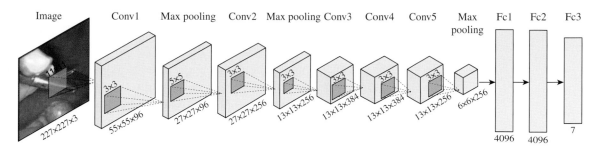

Figure 4-6 • Network architecture used to generate the probability that a tool is visible in an input image.

Every pixel of the input endoscopic image can be expressed as a combination of 3 fundamental colors (red, green, and blue). So, if the input image contains 227 × 227 pixels, it can be expressed by a matrix of 227 × 227 × 3 numeric values (one channel corresponding to each fundamental color). Note that convolutional layers are used to increase the number of channels (by using more filters) as we go deeper into the network, allowing us to extract richer semantic information as the network derives more abstract features. In contrast, the spatial size (height and width) is reduced using max pooling as we go deeper in order to reduce the number of values that must be stored and to simultaneously compress spatial information. Assuming that 7 different tools can possibly appear in any given endoscopic image, 3 fully connected layers are then used at the end of the network to aggregate these high-level representations into 7 values representing the probability that each of those tools is visible in the input.

Training Neural Networks

The first step to training neural networks, as with most machine learning models, is dividing the data into training and test data sets. The training data set is a subset of the data from which the network learns, and once the network is trained, the test data set is used to evaluate the network's ability to generalize to "unseen" data. Additionally, a third subset known as the validation data set can be defined to test different values of manually chosen parameters, known as *hyperparameters*, that affect the training process. The validation data set is also commonly used in the training process to assess whether the model is able to properly generalize to new data. For supervised learning, it is also important to define or annotate the expected output or the *ground truth* for each data point in the data set so that the network can learn a function that approximates the ground truth output for each respective input data point.

Unfortunately, neural networks do not come off-the-shelf with the "right" parameter values to approximate an appropriate function for every given task. Once the structure or the *architecture* of a neural network is defined in terms of the order and types of layers to be used, the network must be trained to learn effective values for its parameters to perform its intended task. This process usually begins by setting or *initializing* the parameters with random values and then defining a *loss* or *objective function L*, which represents how far the prediction is from its ground truth value. For a *binary classification* problem like the benign versus malignant tumor case discussed previously, if the network outputs value between 0 and 1 representing the probability that a given CT scan contains a malignant tumor, a simple loss could be the *mean absolute error* from its ground truth, where the ground truth is defined as 1 if the tumor is malignant and 0 otherwise. Minimizing this loss through iterative updates in the parameters of the network leads, by definition, to better values of these parameters for the classification task. This process is known as *optimization*.

Suppose the loss function *L* is calculated based on one parameter *w*. A sample visualization of the values of *L* (blue line) over the entire parameters space (ie, all possible parameter choices) is shown in Figure 4-7.

The gradient $\frac{\partial L}{\partial w}$ of the loss function with respect to the parameter *w* informs us on the direction to change *w* to cause the largest increase in *L*. In this example where we have only one parameter, a positive value of $\frac{\partial L}{\partial w}$ implies that increasing *w* will lead to the largest increase in *L*, and a negative value of $\frac{\partial L}{\partial w}$ tells us that decreasing *w* would have the same effect. Logically, the negative of the gradient leads to the largest decrease in that function's value. So, for every iteration τ of the optimization process, we can calculate a better value for *w* at the next iteration $\tau + 1$ that corresponds to a lower loss. This method of minimizing the loss by following

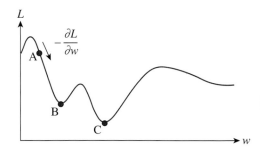

Figure 4-7 • Visualization of an example loss curve. "B" represents a local minimum, whereas "C" represents the global minimum.

the negative direction of the gradient is an optimization technique known as *gradient descent*:

$$w^{\tau+1} = w^{\tau} - \lambda \frac{\partial L}{\partial w}. \qquad \text{(Eq 4-5)}$$

In Equation 4-5, the gradient informs us on which direction to change *w*, and the *learning rate* λ (where $\lambda > 0$) is a manually chosen hyper-parameter that determines how big of a step we take in that direction. If our initial random choice of *w* was at point A (Figure 4-7), a low value of λ may cause the network to converge to the value of *w* at point B because it is in the direction of steepest descent for all small enough changes in *w*. B is known as a *local minimum* of the loss curve because the value of *L* at B is less than the value of *L* at all points within some fixed distance around B. Similarly, point C is known as the *global minimum* of the curve because it corresponds to the lowest value of *L* over the entire parameter space and so should also correspond to the target value for *w* that we are trying to learn. Choosing a larger learning rate can help us step over the local mini-mum but could also potentially cause the network to step over point C and oscillate around it. Thus, a careful choice of learning rate can be a crucial factor in minimizing the loss. Finding the right value often involves some trial and error or, alternatively, using methods such as ADAM,[3] RMSProp,[4] and ADAGRAD[5] that adaptively tune the learn-ing rate during training. This learning process can be extended to any loss function irrespective of the number of parameters involved.

It is important to note that the loss and gradient mentioned in the previous paragraph are calculated for the entirety of the training data set, often comprising thousands to millions of data points. However, load-ing that much data all together into the computer's memory to perform complex calculations may not always be feasible, especially when work-ing with image data. Using *mini-batch gradient descent*, we overcome this issue by calculating the gradients and performing parameter updates on smaller subsets (known as *batches*) of the training data set. When using batches containing only 1 training example each, this process is referred to as *stochastic gradient descent*. The number of times the entire training data set passes through the network during training is denoted by the number of *epochs*. Recent advances in graphics processing unit (GPU) technology, which parallelizes operations, have also made it faster to per-form the matrix operations involved in this process on batches compared to providing the same number of training examples sequentially to the network.

To summarize the training procedure, for a given input, we sequentially go layer by layer forward through the network until we eventually calculate the network's output. This phase of the process is aptly referred to as *forward propagation* because information flows forward through the layers of the network. Using this output, we calculate a loss representing the error in that output and then go layer by layer backward through the network to calculate the gradient of the loss with respect to the parameters of each layer and make updates to the weights in order to decrease the loss. This is known as *backpropagation*. This entire process is repeated iteratively until a stopping criterion is met such as when our loss for the validation data set stops decreasing or after a fixed number of iterations.

Techniques for Deep Learning

Training neural networks is not a trivial exercise. Over the years, several structural tricks that have emerged as standard practices in deep learning have allowed for the training of deeper networks on smaller data sets, transforming the field into a real game-changer across various domains. We will briefly describe here a few of these techniques to improve the learning process and increase a network's ability to generalize to new data.

Preprocessing

Preprocessing, or suitably altering the data set before passing it to the network, can greatly improve the learning process in terms of stability, preventing overfitting, and time to converge to a good minimum corresponding to a sufficiently low loss. Data normalization is a commonly used preprocessing strategy where the input data are scaled down to a smaller range of values such as between 0 and 1. One normalization method is to *standardize* the input to be zero-centered with unit standard deviation over the training data set. If μ and σ are the mean and standard deviation, respectively, of the inputs for all the training data, each individual input x can be standardized using:

$$\underline{x} = \frac{x - \mu}{\sigma}.$$
(Eq 4-6)

Data Augmentation

When working with small data sets, the size of the training subset can usually be inflated by adding additional data generated using modifications of the available training data set. This is done to increase the diversity of training examples available without having to actually collect, clean, and label more data. For example, when working with an image data set, using additional data generated through small and random rotations and translations of the original data set during training may make the model more robust to varying positions and orientations of objects in images.

Regularization

Large neural networks learning from small data sets tend to *overfit* to the training set and perform poorly on the test set. *Regularization* is the process of providing additional constraints to reduce overfitting. The most widely used regularization technique is *L2 regularization*, wherein an extra component for every weight parameter of the network is added to the loss function to prevent the network from learning arbitrarily large values.

$$L_{total} = L_{task} + \lambda_r \sum_{i=1}^{n} \|w_i\|^2, \qquad \text{(Eq 4-7)}$$

where n is the total number of weights in the network and the *regularization strength* λ_r is a manually set hyperparameter that needs to be carefully chosen. This effectively prevents the network from learning overly complex functions that fit perfectly to the training data but do not generalize well to new data. Regularizing the bias parameters usually has much less of an impact toward preventing overfitting compared to weight regularization and so is not as common.

Dropout

One technique that relates to regularization is *dropout*.[7] As neural networks are trained, the contribution of certain pathways of neurons in the network may gradually become more and more irrelevant or crucial toward making correct predictions on the training data set. Excluding random subsets of neurons from training at every iteration could force these neurons to learn representations less reliant on specific pathways. This effectively forces the network to learn smaller weights corresponding to multiple paths rather than large weights along specific ones. Thus, this technique, known as dropout, can provide a similar regularizing effect as L2 regularization.

Batch Normalization

Another technique that has become standard practice in deep networks training is batch normalization—an intermediate layer that attempts to normalize the inputs of each layer during each training batch. This prevents numerical problems during the update of the network weights and is available in most network training frameworks.

Transfer Learning

A strategy to pretrain a neural network on an alternate but similar task and/or data set and then optimize or fine-tune a subset of the network's parameters on the target data set is known as *transfer learning*. In practice, it may be very difficult to learn optimal parameter values from scratch (ie, randomly initializing parameters values), especially when working with large networks and small data sets. Sometimes, in order to reduce the number of parameters that have to be learned, only the last layers are fine-tuned on the data set of interest. In such cases, parameter values for the lower layers are not retrained because they are thought to correspond to more generic features like edges, which apply to varying data sets. This approach is commonly used in surgical research where networks that have been pretrained on the ImageNet database are subsequently fine-tuned on a more specific surgical data set such as the Computational Analysis and Modeling of Medical Activities research group's Cholec80 data set of laparoscopic cholecystectomy or the Massachusetts General Hospital Surgical Artificial Intelligence and Innovation Laboratory's SleeveNet database of laparoscopic sleeve gastrectomy (CAMMA, MGH SAIL).

Deep-Learning Tasks

A good starting point when deciding network architectures to solve a problem may be to look for networks that solve similar tasks and adapt them to the specific needs and data if necessary. This section will briefly describe some broad types of problems that deep learning is particularly efficient at solving and some of the involved network architectures. Most deep-learning tasks fit into 1 of 3 categories based on the type of output expected from the network: classification, detection, and semantic segmentation. We would like to stress that these categories are neither exhaustive nor unrelated.

Classification

Classification refers to the task of categorizing a given input into 2 or more possible classes (Figure 4-8A). For example, a classification network could be used to identify a lesion on a dermatoscopic image as benign or malignant or to classify an electrocardiogram (ECG) segment as normal or as showing an arrythmia. Note that lower dimensional convolutional

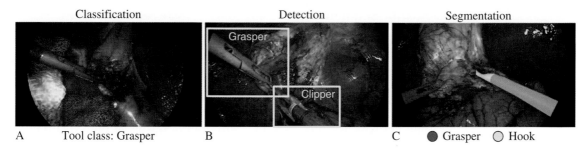

Classification   Detection   Segmentation

A   Tool class: Grasper   B   C   ● Grasper ○ Hook

Figure 4-8 • Visualization of network outputs for (**A**) tool classification, (**B**) tool detection, and (**C**) tool segmentation performed on images extracted from a laparoscopic cholecystectomy video.

filters are used when operating on lower dimensional inputs such as ECG segments, which consist of voltage values. Some network architectures frequently used for deep-learning tasks involving classification are ResNet[9] and VGGNet[10] (Figure 4-9). Most classification architectures involve a convolutional network ending with a fully connected layer with 1 neuron for every considered class. These neurons are generally used to output the probability of the input belonging to each class.

Detection

Detection, like classification, involves identifying the category of an object of interest in the input but additionally localizing its position spatially, as illustrated in Figure 4-8B. For image data, the position of a target object could be described by coordinates of the corners of a bounding box around the object predicted by the network. For every object of interest in the input, ground truth annotations (in a supervised setting) describe both the class of the object and sufficient information to completely describe the position of the object. An example of where neural networks have been used to achieve strong performance in a detection task is the identification and localization of tools in endoscopic images.[11]

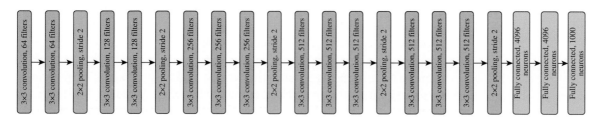

Figure 4-9 • Visualization of the VGGNet architecture used for classification. Here, *3 × 3 convolution, 64* implies that 64 3 × 3 convolutional filters are used to operate on that layer's input; the fully connected layers have 4096 outputs or neurons. Each time the spatial size is halved using a pooling layer, a convolutional layer is used to double the number of channels.

Semantic Segmentation

Semantic segmentation is the task of classifying every pixel of an image into a particular category (Figure 4-8C). As an example, segmentation of the cerebrovascular network in a magnetic resonance angiography[12] could be a useful tool for clinicians and radiologists to interpret those images because of the large interpatient variability of anatomy in such scans. Some network architectures that are commonly used by the computer vision community to solve segmentation problems are Deeplabv3+[13] and HRNet.[14] UNet[15] is another popular architecture that has shown promising results for semantic segmentation on medical images.

Unlike object detection and classification, semantic segmentation involves generating a much larger output representing predictions corresponding to every pixel of the input. Maintaining the input feature size at all layers of a very deep neural network is computationally intensive in terms of both speed and memory. To solve this issue, segmentation networks such as Deeplabv3+ and UNet use an encoder-decoder framework. These networks first use an encoder path to extract rich semantic information at reduced dimensions and then a decoder path to recover sharp boundaries while restoring the original dimensionality. An example of a naive decoder would be a simple resizing operation.

Synthetic Data Generation

Synthetic data generation is the task of creating new data mimicking the characteristics of a given training data set. Given the dearth of large and well-labeled medical data sets, data generation approaches can be used to synthesize additional training examples. For instance, such artificially augmented data sets have been successfully used to improve performance for lesion classification.[16] Additionally, these approaches have been proposed to create photo-realistic surgical simulations to aid trainees.[17] They have also been used to modify radiologic scans, with one paper[18] demonstrating a vulnerability of hospitals to CT scan attacks where such networks are used to inject or remove evidence of cancer, potentially leading to misdiagnosis.

One commonly used framework for data generation is the *generative adversarial network* (GAN), as depicted in Figure 4-10. In this framework, a model is trained to synthesize images resembling examples from a given training data set using 2 neural networks. The first network, or generator, tries to synthesize an output resembling the training data, while a second network, or discriminator, competes to identify whether the generated example was a fake. During training, as the discriminator gets better at discerning fake examples, the generator becomes more efficient at generating realistic fakes.

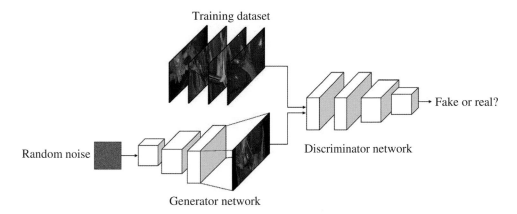

Figure 4-10 • An example of a generative adversarial network (GAN) being used to generate realistic laparoscopic images.

Another useful approach for generative modelling is to use *autoencoder* networks that first encode an input into a latent representation of lower dimensionality and then decode that representation to reconstruct the original image. Due to the dimensionality reduction in the first stage, these representations learn to encode only the most relevant features of the input needed for its reconstruction and to ignore noise. If encodings from real images are replaced by realistic guesses of latent representations, the decoding stage of the network can then be used to generate new examples. *Variational autoencoders* (VAE) leverage this property by constraining the network, through an additional loss term, to learn representations for different inputs that are sufficiently close numerically while still remaining distinct. This effectively forces the latent representations to represent common features whose variations are sufficiently descriptive to reconstruct realistic variations of the original input. An added benefit is that these representations are often easier to interpret. For example, when training a VAE to generate laparoscopic images, the variables that constitute the latent representation could correspond to size, orientation and position of different anatomical structures in the image.

Recognition With Temporal Models

Imagine trying to identify the type of surgical procedure being performed from just a single still endoscopic image versus having a sequence of frames or a video. For tasks involving sequential or time-series data, it may be useful and sometimes necessary to add a component to the network architecture that "remembers" information derived from previous inputs in the sequence. *Recurrent neural networks* (RNNs) add this concept of memory

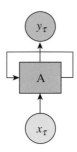

Figure 4-11 • Recurrent neural network receiving an input at time step τ and generating an output.

to the network by adding a loop between layers that allows information to persist in the network from previous steps in the sequence through a *hidden state* (Figure 4-11).

At every step τ, the RNN receives both the input x_τ for that time step as well as a learned hidden state h from step $\tau - 1$. An unrolled depiction of the RNN is shown in Figure 4-12. An initial assumption must be made for what will be passed to the network as the hidden state for the first step $\tau = 1$.

When backpropagation is performed on such a network, the gradients are calculated on the unrolled version of the RNN. This is known as *backpropagation through time (BPTT)*. Without going too deep into the mathematics of the gradient computation, this could lead to a numerical instability in the gradients that causes it to grow or shrink to arbitrarily large or small values, respectively. This predicament is known as the *vanishing or exploding gradients* problem and could severely hinder the learning process. Another major issue introduced by this kind of network is that a sequence of irrelevant data caused by some event such as an obstructed camera view may cause useless information to be propagated through the hidden state even though relevant inputs were available to

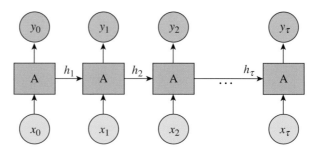

Figure 4-12 • Unrolled depiction of a recurrent neural network receiving inputs at different time steps.

the network at earlier steps. Two variants of RNNs that address these problems are the long short-term memory (LSTM)[19] model and the gated recurrent unit (GRU).[20] These models introduce separate neurons that control what information is stored and discarded for each step in the sequence of inputs. This helps filter out irrelevant information and emphasize important information.

Often, convolutional neural networks are first used to extract meaningful features that are then fed as input to an RNN that models temporal relationships between these features at different steps in the sequence. Some surgical applications where LSTM-based deep-learning models have demonstrated great success are surgical skill evaluation[21] and surgical activity recognition.[22]

DEEP LEARNING IN SURGERY

At this point, the reader should be familiar with the terminology necessary to read and think about deep learning. Here, we examine the implementation of a deep-learning pipeline to guide the reader through the application of concepts introduced earlier. These concepts can further be put in practice in the hands-on lab provided with the chapter, available at https://github.com/CAMMA-public/ai4surgery. Surgical phase and tool detection models,[23] 2 early examples of deep learning for surgical applications, will serve as examples. Detecting workflow and tool usage (Figure 4-13) is a necessary step to understand the surgical context, an essential milestone toward smart support or autonomous assistance systems.[24,25]

Data and Annotation

Choosing appropriate input data for a model to learn a given task is of fundamental importance. In most cases, a simple and effective way to check whether data are sufficiently informative is to ask an expert to look at the data and perform the same task for which the model will be trained. In our examples, given an endoscopic picture, one can easily say whether a tool is present but cannot easily infer the phase of a procedure from it. Videos are more suitable than pictures for tasks such as workflow (ie, phases and activity) detection for which knowing the temporal context intuitively helps. Unfortunately, there is no straightforward way to estimate how much data is needed other than gauging the variability in input data and evaluating model performance with data sets of different sizes. In classification tasks such as tool or phase detection, estimating interclass and

Preparation	Calot triangle dissection	Clipping and cutting	Gallbladder dissection	Gallbladder packaging	Cleaning and coagulation	Gallbladder extraction

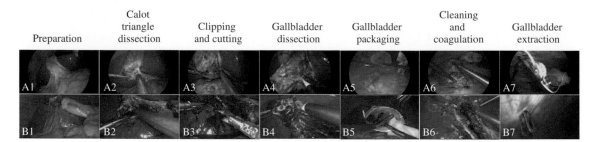

Figure 4-13 • Endoscopic images from 2 laparoscopic cholecystectomy procedures (**A** and **B**) representing the 7 phases defined in the Cholec80 data set.[23] The images contain the surgical tools typically used during cholecystectomy. Images taken from procedure A have a black frame around the endoscopic scene, whereas the others have none, showing the need for the preprocessing of endoscopic images.

intraclass similarities or variability can help understand the complexity of the problem. For instance, distinguishing a surgical hook from a scissors is clearly easier than differentiating a crocodile grasper from a Maryland grasper. Because the 2 types of graspers (ie, the 2 classes) are similar, an observer (or an algorithm) would need more experience (ie, more data) to learn to differentiate between them. In the case of surgical workflow analysis, the initial phase of a cholecystectomy could either be very short and straightforward or require extensive adhesiolysis. In other words, the same phase of a procedure can look very different (ie, there is a large intraclass variability), so to learn how to correctly classify surgical phases, this variability needs to be well represented in the data set. Informativeness of input data and interclass and intraclass variability also influence the consistency of annotations, a fundamental factor influencing model performance. In supervised learning, models are trained to approximate a function to go from the input data to the annotated information. It follows that if annotations are not consistent the model will compute a loss on incongruent data, deteriorating performance. In our example, persons with no medical education could correctly annotate tool presence or absence in images. The same cannot be said for annotating surgical phases because those require surgical understanding and a shared definition of what exactly describes and delineates phases.

Implementation

Here, we briefly present how to implement deep learning on surgical images. More details on data acquisition, storage, and annotation of surgical videos can be found in Chapter 16. First, data are analyzed and preprocessed. For phase and tool detection, preprocessing may include resizing, cropping (Figure 4-12), and padding input images and/or excluding data annotated with inconsistent labels. Then, the database is split into training, validation, and test sets. It is good scientific practice to keep these sets as independent from each other as possible because the network may develop biases (not to be confused with the network parameter) based on visual patterns not relevant to the network's task. Furthermore, when reporting results of deep-learning experiments, it is important to carefully describe the data set, its splits, and applied preprocessing because this may affect interpretation of outcomes.

At this point, one or more deep-learning architectures showing good performance on similar tasks or data are identified. Classifiers such as ResNet, VGGNet, or NASNet may work for phase and tool detection in images. However, as seen earlier, the temporal information captured by the video can be extremely relevant, at least for phase detection. Adding an RNN such as LSTM to model the temporal relationships could thus boost performance.

Before starting the learning process, the model parameters need to be initialized. Weights and biases can be initialized randomly or, in transfer learning, taken from the same model pretrained on a large data set. The latter is often the case in surgical data science given the limited size of annotated data sets. At this point, we are ready to start training the model.

In the case of a classification task such as phase and tool detection, the initialized model will output class scores reflecting the computed probability of each surgical tool or phase being represented in the input. Various loss functions can then be computed to quantify the error between class probabilities and ground truth. For instance, building on the surgical intuition that certain tools are more frequently used in certain surgical phases, as one can appreciate in Figure 4-12, a model for tool detection can compute a loss on the probability of tool and phase co-occurrence.[26] Once a suitable loss function is defined, gradients are calculated and neuron parameters are updated. This process is repeated for a number of iterations, usually until results plateau or after a predefined number of iterations. Before testing on unseen data, hyperparameters such as learning rate and batch size are tuned on the validation data set.

The model is then finally run on the test data set, and results are reported according to performance metrics chosen based on the nature of the task and the composition of the data set. These results are usually compared against one or more baselines. When aiming at improving performance of an already tackled problem like phase and tool detection, a good baseline for comparison is usually obtained by reimplementing related state-of-the-art architectures on the data of interest. However, when tackling a completely novel problem, the baseline is often represented by the results of a naive or random model—the equivalent of flipping a coin for a binary classification task. In addition, the contribution of each part of the proposed model to the outcome can be examined through an *ablation study* consisting of sequentially removing components of the model to see how performance changes. Finally, performance of deep-learning models should be examined in light of the intended clinical use. For instance, not detecting a grasper in an endoscopic image will have little to no impact, whereas a false negative in a screening mammography can have dramatic consequences; thus, metrics must be chosen that reflect these clinical priorities.

❚ CONCLUSION AND PERSPECTIVES

Even though biologically inspired artificial neural networks have been around for a while, deep networks for real-world applications have only recently appeared. This poses new fascinating questions to researchers and stakeholders, especially when looking at applications in highly regulated fields such as medicine and surgery. We will now briefly discuss some of the questions researchers are trying to address to translate the potential of neural networks to surgery.

Data privacy, security, and ownership are issues common to most data-driven approaches, especially when treating highly sensitive health data. It is beyond the scope of the present chapter to describe all possible methods to guarantee data privacy and security; however, it is important to know that deep learning can help in this regard. For instance, face detection models have been used to automatically hide identity of people recorded in the operating room,[27] and models capable of analyzing data acquired in an identity-preserving format, such as recording at extremely low resolutions[28] or with depth and thermal sensors,[29] have shown promising results. In addition, distributed learning approaches could allow training and validating algorithms on varied data generated in multiple institutions without the need to centralize and, hence, move and share, any data.

On top of the mentioned issues with clinical data, annotating raw data with surgical knowledge requires rare and expensive physician time. Hence, an important bottleneck slowing the development of deep-learning models in surgery is the scarcity of well-annotated data sets. Successes with deep networks in other domains are in great part fueled by big data sets such as ImageNet, a data set containing about 14 million images annotated with more than 20,000 classes of objects.[30] In surgery, we are far from having such a vast and well-annotated database; hence, methods able to learn on less data and with less supervision are the focus of many research groups. For instance, methods for tool detection,[31] tracking,[11] segmentation,[32] and phase detection[33] requiring very few annotations have been proposed.

Furthermore, understanding how and why a model returns a certain prediction is a priority, especially in the medical field, due to medicolegal considerations. Unfortunately, deep-learning approaches have been criticized as being black boxes because their internal logic is hard to explain. However, recent works such on *saliency maps*[34] and *class activation maps*,[35] methods that determine which parts of the input affect the output, have shown progress in improving the interpretability of deep-learning models. For example, Al Hajj et al[36] found that their deep model was "focusing" on the deformation of the anterior segment of the eye to infer whether surgical tools were in contact with the eye in cataract procedures.

Finally, to impact surgical care, models will have to communicate or be integrated within operating rooms. Real-time operating room–embedded vision applications could be possible with lightweight and efficient architectures such as mobile-net[37] and efficient-net[38] that use a computationally superior variant of convolution operation known as *depthwise separable convolution*. Another strategy to improve a model's run time is to use the *mixed-precision operation*. The latest versions of NVIDIA GPUs, for example, the NVIDIA-V100, include *tensor cores* that can perform a combination of low- and high-precision operations (ie, approximate numbers to different exactness levels). Mixed-precision computations are much more efficient than high-precision computation but are often considered much less accurate. This is disputed by recent studies[39] showing that, using better training techniques, mixed-precision computation can achieve performance comparable to high-precision computations.

In conclusion, despite the novelty of deep-learning applications in surgery and the numerous open challenges to address, the ability of neural networks and deep learning to extract meaningful information from the vast amount of raw data we continuously generate is likely to redefine surgical practices. It is now the ideal moment to join the discussion, team up with stakeholders, and help shape the impact of deep learning on patients and surgical practices.

▌HANDS-ON DEEP LEARNING LAB

A hands-on practical on deep learning for surgical data is available online as companion to this chapter. The interested reader can directly experiment with the methods presented in this chapter by following this link: https://github.com/CAMMA-public/ai4surgery.

❚ REFERENCES

1. Honglak L, Grosse R, Ranganath R, Ng AY. Convolutional deep belief networks for scalable unsupervised learning of hierarchical representations. *Proceedings of the 26th Annual International Conference on Machine Learning* 2009;609-616. Accessed September 30, 2020. https://web.eecs.umich.edu/~honglak/icml09-ConvolutionalDeepBeliefNetworks.pdf.

2. Krizhevsky A, Sutskever I, Hinton GE. Imagenet classification with deep convolutional neural networks. Accessed September 30, 2020. https://papers.nips.cc/paper/4824-imagenet-classification-with-deep-convolutional-neural-networks.pdf.

3. Kingma DP, Ba J. Adam: a method for stochastic optimization. Accessed September 30, 2020. https://arxiv.org/abs/1412.6980.

4. Hinton G. Neural networks for machine learning. Lecture 6a: overview of mini-batch gradient descent. Accessed September 30, 2020. http://www.cs.toronto.edu/~tijmen/csc321/slides/lecture_slides_lec6.pdf.

5. Duchi J, Hazan E, Singer Y. Adaptive subgradient methods for online learning and stochastic optimization. *J Mach Learn Res.* 2011;12:2121-2159.

6. Goodfellow I, Bengio Y, Courville A. *Deep Learning*: MIT Press; 2016.

7. Srivastava N, Hinton G, Krizhevsky A, et al. Dropout: a simple way to prevent neural networks from overfitting. *J Mach Learn Res.* 2014;15(1):1929-1958.

8. Baldi P. Autoencoders, unsupervised learning, and deep architectures. Accessed September 30, 2020. http://proceedings.mlr.press/v27/baldi12a/baldi12a.pdf.

9. He K, Zhang X, Ren S, Sun J. Deep residual learning for image recognition. Accessed September 30, 2020. https://www.cv-foundation.org/openaccess/content_cvpr_2016/papers/He_Deep_Residual_Learning_CVPR_2016_paper.pdf.

10. Simonyan K, Zisserman A. Very deep convolutional networks for large-scale image recognition. Accessed September 30, 2020. https://arxiv.org/abs/1409.1556.

11. Nwoye CI, Mutter D, Marescaux J, Padoy N. Weakly supervised convolutional LSTM approach for tool tracking in laparoscopic videos. *Int J Comput Assist Radiol Surg.* 2019;14(6):1059-1067.

12. Sanches P, Meyer C, Vigon V, Naegel B. Cerebrovascular network segmentation of MRA images with deep learning. Accessed September 30, 2020. https://deepai.org/publication/cerebrovascular-network-segmentation-on-mra-images-with-deep-learning.

13. Chen L-C, Zhu Y, Papandreou G, Schroff F, Adam H. Encoder-decoder with atrous separable convolution for semantic image segmentation. Accessed September 30, 2020. https://arxiv.org/abs/1802.02611.

14. Sun K, Zhao Y, Jiang B, et al. High-resolution representations for labeling pixels and regions. Accessed September 30, 2020. https://arxiv.org/abs/1904.04514.

15. Ronneberger O, Fischer P, Brox T. U-net: convolutional networks for biomedical image segmentation. Accessed September 30, 2020. https://arxiv.org/abs/1505.04597.

16. Frid-Adar M, Diamant I, Klang E, Amitai M, Goldberger J, Greenspan H. GAN-based synthetic medical image augmentation for increased CNN performance in liver lesion classification. *Neurocomputing.* 2018;321:321-331.

17. Engelhardt S, De Simone R, Full PM, Karck M, Wolf I. Improving surgical training phantoms by hyperrealism: deep unpaired image-to-image translation from real surgeries. Accessed September 30, 2020. https://arxiv.org/abs/1806.03627.

18. Mirsky Y, Mahler T, Shelef I, Elovici Y. CT-GAN: malicious tampering of 3D medical imagery using deep learning. Accessed September 30, 2020. https://arxiv.org/pdf/1901.03597.pdf.

19. Gers FA, Schmidhuber J, Cummins F. Learning to forget: continual prediction with LSTM. *Neural Comput*. 2000;12:2451-2471.

20. Cho K, Van Merriënboer B, Gulcehre C, et al. Learning phrase representations using RNN encoder-decoder for statistical machine translation. Accessed September 30, 2020. https://arxiv.org/abs/1406.1078.

21. Jin A, Yeung S, Jopling J, et al. Tool detection and operative skill assessment in surgical videos using region-based convolutional neural networks. Accessed September 30, 2020. https://ieeexplore.ieee.org/document/8354185.

22. Zia A, Hung A, Essa I, Jarc A. Surgical activity recognition in robot-assisted radical prostatectomy using deep learning. Accessed September 30, 2020. https://deepai.org/publication/surgical-activity-recognition-in-robot-assisted-radical-prostatectomy-using-deep-learning.

23. Twinanda AP, Shehata S, Mutter D, Marescaux J, De Mathelin M, Padoy N. Endonet: a deep architecture for recognition tasks on laparoscopic videos. *IEEE Trans Med Imaging*. 2016;36:86-97.

24. Padoy N. Machine and deep learning for workflow recognition during surgery. *Minim Invasive Ther Allied Technol*. 2019;28(2):82-90.

25. Vercauteren T, Unberath M, Padoy N, Navab N. CAI4CAI: the rise of contextual artificial intelligence in computer-assisted interventions. *Proc IEEE*. 2019;108:198-214.

26. Mondal SS, Sathish R, Sheet D. Multitask learning of temporal connectionism in convolutional networks using a joint distribution loss function to simultaneously identify tools and phase in surgical videos. Accessed September 30, 2020. https://arxiv.org/pdf/1905.08315.pdf.

27. Issenhuth T, Srivastav V, Gangi A, Padoy N. Face detection in the operating room: Comparison of state-of-the-art methods and a self-supervised approach. *Int J Comput Assist Radiol Surg*. 2019;14(6):1049-1058.

28. Srivastav V, Gangi A, Padoy N. Human pose estimation on privacy-preserving low-resolution depth images. Accessed September 30, 2020. https://arxiv.org/abs/2007.08340.

29. Yeung S, Downing NL, Fei-Fei L, Milstein A. Bedside computer vision-moving artificial intelligence from driver assistance to patient safety. *N Engl J Med*. 2018;378:1271.

30. Deng J, Dong W, Socher R, Li LJ, Li K, Fei-Fei L. Imagenet: a large-scale hierarchical image database. Accessed September 30, 2020. http://image-net.org/papers/imagenet_cvpr09.pdf.

31. Vardazaryan A, Mutter D, Marescaux J, Padoy N. Weakly-supervised learning for tool localization in laparoscopic videos. Accessed September 30, 2020. https://link.springer.com/chapter/10.1007/978-3-030-01364-6_19.

32. Fuentes-Hurtado F, Kadkhodamohammadi A, Flouty E, Barbarisi S, Luengo I, Stoyanov D. EasyLabels: weak labels for scene segmentation in laparoscopic videos. *J Comput Assist Radiol Surg*. 2019;14(7):1247-1257.

33. Yu T, Mutter D, Marescaux J, Padoy N. Learning from a tiny dataset of manual annotations: a teacher/student approach for surgical phase recognition. Accessed September 30, 2020. https://arxiv.org/abs/1812.00033.

34. Simonyan K, Vedaldi A, Zisserman A. Deep inside convolutional networks: visualising image classification models and saliency maps. Accessed September 30, 2020. https://arxiv.org/abs/1312.6034.

35. Zhou B, Khosla A, Lapedriza A, Oliva A, Torralba A. Learning deep features for discriminative localization. Accessed September 30, 2020. https://arxiv.org/abs/1512.04150.

36. Al Hajj H, Lamard M, Conze PH, Cochener B, Quellec G. Monitoring tool usage in surgery videos using boosted convolutional and recurrent neural networks. *Med Image Anal*. 2018;47:203-218.

37. Howard AG, Zhu M, Chen B, et al. Mobilenets: efficient convolutional neural networks for mobile vision applications. Accessed September 30, 2020. https://arxiv.org/abs/1704.04861.

38. Tan M, Le Q. EfficientNet: rethinking model scaling for convolutional neural networks. Accessed September 30, 2020. https://arxiv.org/pdf/1905.11946v3.pdf.

39. Hou L, Zhang R, Kwok JT. Analysis of quantized models. Accessed September 30, 2020. https://openreview.net/pdf?id=ryM_IoAqYX.

NATURAL LANGUAGE PROCESSING 5

5

Leo Anthony Celi, Daniel Gruhl, Euma Ishii,
Chaitanya Shivade, Joseph Terdiman, and Joy Tzung-yu Wu

HIGHLIGHTS

- Natural language processing (NLP) is a collection of tools and computer algorithmic techniques that aim to help humans "structure" and gain an in-depth understanding of free text information.

- Overview of different types of NLP tools:

  - **Vocabulary- and rule-based NLP** is the oldest but most easily interpretable type of NLP. Complex clinical NLP pipelines take a lot of resources and years to build and are often difficult to adapt to different clinical domains. However, simple look-up–type techniques can be useful in many clinical auditing cases where precision is more important than recall.

  - **Supervised NLP** is powerful as long as there is a large enough human labeled data set to train the machine learning model. However, task-specific and large well-labeled data sets take substantial clinical resources to curate.

  - With **unsupervised NLP**, there is no need for labeling because these machine learning models can automatically discover patterns in the data and propose groups or classes. However, a human needs to interpret the resulting groups to figure out the "why" and "what."

  - **Expert-in-the-loop NLP:** What if we make the experts more efficient at helping the machine learn a task? The challenge is to present questions or uncertainties from the machine models to the human in a user-friendly and interactive manner.

- In health care, there is no one-size-fits-all NLP solution. There are many tasks in the clinical domain amenable to different types or combinations of NLP methods. Understanding the performance requirements of the clinical task and the limitations of different NLP tools can help with implementing the most appropriate NLP solution.

▌INTRODUCTION

In health care, natural language is still the most common communication tool for conducting and recording patient-provider and provider-provider interactions in the electronic health records (EHRs). Computers, however, prefer structured data. Lists of diagnosis codes, medication codes, and procedure codes are easy to search, tabulate, and aggregate, and thus are the go-to sources for data science and analytics performed on clinical records. However, such clinical coding is historically based on administrative and billing requirements, where typically only the top 1 or 2 issues per patient visit are structured or "coded" in the form of International Classification of Diseases (ICD), Current Procedural Terminology (CPT), diagnosis-related group (DRG), and other billing codes.[1] However, many clinically important observations are not absolutes or discretes that lend themselves to be structured (coded) in check boxes on a form. As such, the bulk of recorded health care information about patients is currently stored as unstructured data in the EHR.[2,3] Any free text documentation, such as clinical notes or investigation reports, is unstructured data, which cannot be easily automatically analyzed to provide valuable insights into improving clinical care.

Because computers were previously quite expensive, the focus of their use was to maximize financial reimbursement of the patient-provider encounter.[4] As a result, the structured portion of the EHR still disproportionately captures diagnoses and health care interventions for billing purposes. However, the billing codes were not designed to capture patient characteristics and disease contexts that are relevant to explain the reasons behind clinical decisions.[5] In general, only a single DRG code is assigned to what may be a hospitalization from a complex medical situation. Consider a major motor vehicular crash victim with multiple injuries, who had preexisting conditions that were triggered by the trauma and who has psychological issues that arise from survivor guilt. By organizing a complex medical case into 1 or 2 codes, a tremendous amount of clinical information is lost.[6]

Such structuring not only condenses the available clinical information but at times also alters it. Limited discrete coding options can force the provider to select the closest code instead of the correct code. For example, a physician may order a head computed tomography (CT) scan for a young patient with recent long-term memory loss. In many EHR systems that track provider orders, the order may need to be matched with a suitable reason-for-exam code in the EHR. Yet, there may not be a matching code for ordering a head CT in the EHR for this common situation presenting in a rare population. As a result, the physician may be forced to pick the closest code (eg, dementia), which may or may not be on the physician's differential diagnosis for the case. Consider another example of a health plan that requires a cardiac diagnosis before a patient can be referred to a cardiologist. The attending primary care provider may pick a code that sounds reasonable for the referral, even if it is not completely correct. These examples highlight problems of treating structured data in the EHR as "ground truth" for retrospective analysis. In contrast, if health care professionals are able to retrospectively read all the unstructured documentation in the clinical notes for all their patients, then the likelihood of correctly understanding and interpreting the recorded information in the EHR would be higher.

One of the more promising approaches for effective medical information retrieval is the use of **natural language processing (NLP)**. NLP is a collection of tools and computer algorithmic techniques that aim to help humans automatically structure and model relationships between words to gain an in-depth, contextual understanding of free text information.[7] Such automatic structuring of concepts and relationships in free text is critical for efficiently extracting and understanding clinically meaningful information and statistics in the EHR.

Although promising, NLP technology is not perfect. NLP models or systems are task specific and can have problems with generalization to other data sets. An NLP model may only extract the concepts or relationships accurately and reliably when applied to the originally intended task. Therefore, the model is likely to incur a performance loss if applied to a new data set that is very different from the source data set on which the model was developed. For example, in the evaluation of a patient's smoking status, the phrase "is smoker" can have dozens of real-life implications depending on the context of the clinical encounter and the source patient population.[8] Is someone who stopped smoking a few days ago still a smoker during that hospitalization? What about in the context of an outpatient visit? Such criteria would need to be very clear when developing an NLP algorithm to extract smoking status, which exemplifies the nature of the task specificity required for many current NLP models. Such an algorithm would perform best for this particularly defined task when deployed in similar contexts (ie, a model for smoking status could be deployed selectively for a pulmonology outpatient visit vs an inpatient trauma hospitalization). Given the limitations of NLP systems, it is important for clinicians to understand how these NLP models were developed to better anticipate the appropriate use and interpretation of these systems, including identifying how such systems might fail.

There are many potential use cases for NLP in clinical medicine, and this chapter surveys the historical foundations, current trends, and future potential of this technology. The remainder of this chapter is split into the following 4 sections to cover the history, development, and application of different types of NLP systems:

- Vocabulary- and rule-based NLP
- Supervised NLP
- Unsupervised NLP
- Expert-in-the-loop NLP

▍VOCABULARY- AND RULE-BASED NLP

History

The idea of using computers to analyze the textual documentation of clinical reports dates back to the 1960s.[9,10] Most early NLP systems were manually programmed, rule-based expert systems. They focused on extracting predefined phrases and keywords (vocabulary) from specific documents, such as pathology reports,[11] and encoding diagnoses from natural language text. As technology evolved and NLP systems became more facile at processing text in general (ie, outside the field of medicine), the field of medical text processing (also known as clinical NLP) also matured. There are now well-developed computer programs that can process free text by following a methodical pattern of segmenting text documents into sentences—identifying words within the sentence and understanding the grammar of the sentence—and then performing a task of interest, such as encoding medical concepts.[12]

These early clinical NLP systems focused on the task of extracting (ie, search and find) specific terms of interest from documented clinical narratives, which may be followed by context interpretation. The task of named-entity recognition (NER) is a key technique in identifying clinical concepts. However, it is also often necessary to identify whether a term is negated (eg, "no hypertension"). Negex is an example of a simple rule-based algorithm that looks for predefined negation cues in words surrounding the clinical term of interest and has been very effective for negation context detection.[13] Other NLP tasks that build on top of NER include determining relationships[14] between 2 or more concepts (eg, parent-child or IS-A relationship between pneumonia and lung infection) and determining the temporal order of occurrence among 2 or more concepts[15] (eg, palpitations after admission), among many others.

Vocabulary- and rule-based NLP technology has made steady advances in the biomedical domain with the curation of expert controlled vocabulary. To this end, since 1986, the National Library of Medicine has been spearheading the curation effort through a long-term project to develop the Unified Medical Language System (UMLS).[16] In essence, these knowledge sources are machine-readable (although manually curated) dictionaries that encode human clinical understanding and are invaluable in aiding the ability of computer systems to better process and understand clinical texts. The expert-validated vocabulary documents lexical variations of specific medical concepts (eg, "high blood pressure," "hypertension," and "HTN" as different ways to refer to the same concept). One can also define properties of medical concepts (eg, "cough" is a symptom and "pneumonia" is a disease) and encode relationships between different medical concepts (eg, "fever" can be a "sign" or "symptom" of "pneumonia") to create computationally useful taxonomies or ontologies, which NLP systems can use. Such knowledge resources enabled NLP systems such as cTakes[17] and MetaMap[18] to extract useful concepts from clinical text documents.

Due to the interdisciplinary nature of the field, researchers contributing to this field have varying backgrounds in areas such as computer science, data science, and medicine. This has given rise to the interdisciplinary field of biomedical informatics,[19] which focuses on the larger goal of leveraging computer science in the biomedical sciences.

Technology

A vocabulary- and rules-driven system is perhaps the most humanly interpretable type of NLP. Such NLP systems typically use a knowledge base of domain-specific vocabularies (eg, UMLS or Systematized Nomenclature of Medicine–Clinical Terms [SNOMED-CT] for the biomedical domain) to extract (ie, spot) named entities (ie, clinical concepts) from unstructured free text. A series of programmatic rules that interpret written language structures can then be applied to do standard context interpretation in free text, such as negation detection.

For example, to detect whether a simple concept such as pneumothorax is mentioned in radiology reports, one would need a "dictionary" (ie, a list of words or phrases) for the concept, indicating to the NLP system all the different ways that the concept can be written in free text reports. The NLP system can automatically search terms in the dictionary in all the documents of interest in the EHR. To have high recall (ie, sensitivity), the dictionary will need to include any plurals (eg, "pneumothoraces"), abbreviations (eg, "ptx"), misspellings (eg, "pneumothorox"), and semantically equivalent descriptions or patterns (eg, "pleural line with absence of vascular markings outside the line"). However, to also have high precision (ie, specificity), the NLP system needs to have rules to interpret the context in which the named entity was identified in free text (eg, "pneumothorax has resolved" is a negated mention of pneumothorax). For example, one possible negation rule could be as follows: IF a sentence mentions any terms in the "pneumothorax" dictionary and none of the terms in the "negation" context dictionary, THEN the concept is present positively in the notes.

Vocabulary- and rule-based NLP systems can sound simple. However, clinical contexts can quickly become more complicated; for example, the phrases "patient has a past medical history of pneumothorax" or "the patient's mother had a pneumothorax" clearly do not suggest that the patient currently has a pneumothorax but also do not contain clear negating terms. Even the negation context alone can have many variants (eg, "pneumothorax is no longer seen," "no pneumothorax") and room for potential false-negative detection (eg, "no change in pneumothorax"). To achieve higher precision in these cases, the NLP system would need to recognize multiple different types of contexts, such as "negation," "past medical," and "family history." To make the NLP task easier, one can develop dictionaries (as with NER) to recognize the different contexts and then use NLP sentence parsers to produce a graph of the sentence that assigns the target named entity to the correct context, as shown in Figure 5-1. Instead of working with just the raw text, parsing the sentence first means you can write programmatic rules against the "sentence diagram" of the text with the added structural information. In the "no pneumothorax" case, one can use the added information in the parsed sentence to check whether pneumothorax appears in a negated clause.

It is also important to appreciate that clinical language is very specialty specific when developing NLP systems. The same term can have

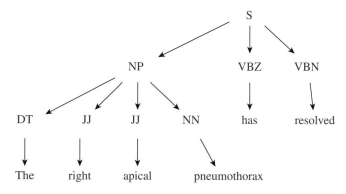

Figure 5-1 • A sentence graph generated by using treebank tagging. Many open source Python libraries (eg, SpaCy and Natural Language Toolkit) can do this. DT, determiner; JJ, adjective; NN, noun; NP, noun phrase; S, sentence; VBN, verb; VBZ, verb.

different clinical meanings and implications for clinicians in different sub-specialties. For example, should "adhesive tape" be considered a medication? For a dermatologist or a plastic surgeon, it may be, but it may not be considered so by other clinical specialties. But just like regular medications, Band-Aids, a type of adhesive tape for wound dressing, can be prescribed with dosing intervals by doctors, can be dispensed by pharmacists, may have medically active ingredients in them, and can also cause side effects (eg, rash)! Therefore, the inclusion and exclusion of terms in a controlled vocabulary tend to be task specific and can affect the performance of the NLP system. This is one reason why relying only on even medicine-specific vocabularies such as UMLS for vocabulary control may not achieve the best result for some clinical applications—such vocabularies may be curated by different groups for their own tasks.

This whole process becomes more complex as the note quality degrades. One might expect a note from a specialist to a referring provider or an operative report to be fairly well written, with proper grammar and spelling, but that is not always the case. A note jotted on a chart during rounds, a report dictated into a speech-to-text recognition system (which can have transcription errors), or a quick message texted into an EHR by a physical therapist may show a more relaxed approach to formal clinical writing. NLP systems that depend on the structure of language for information extraction often fail in such domains.

Finally, authoring such systems requires expertise in computer science, linguistics, and a medical specialty. Understandably, the population of such polymaths is limited.

Clinical Application With Examples

Vocabulary- and rule-based NLP has been used in medicine for many years. One of the earliest systems was the Medical Language Processor (MLP), which was introduced in 1981. The MLP system used even earlier NLP work on grammar-based parsing of the English language (Linguistic String Analysis, circa 1965) to turn free text clinical notes into structured data.

Perhaps the most famous example of an early NLP system for clinical texts is the Medical Language Extraction and Encoding (MedLEE) System,[20,21] which has been integrated with the EHR of some hospital systems, including the Columbia University Medical Center since 1995. The MedLEE system reviews the medical records of patients and can perform complex NLP tasks such as indicating when there are potentially reportable diseases, suggesting appropriate clinical testing, checking the need for vaccination, and indicating when there may be a local outbreak of diseases.

Complex NLP systems such as MLP and MedLEE require a lot of resources and take years to develop. However, there are actually many day-to-day clinical use cases that can be addressed with simple NLP techniques that do not require building a complex NLP pipeline. For example, if a surgeon is interested in auditing the documentation of "sponge checks" in operating room notes, running a simple look-up–type NLP with a relevant but limited vocabulary list on all the notes will be able to output that statistic. Another example may be extracting measurement values from reports, such as HR 120 or BP 117/92, using regular expression rules, which gives added flexibility for matching named entities in free text. Regular expression allows one to write rules to match and extract specific patterns, such as "look for HR then extract numerical values that occur after it" (eg, Python code below). Finally, using sentence parsing allows one to write simple rules against the sentence structure for context detection, such as negation.

```
report_text = "Reason for Exam: Endocarditis.
               BP (mm Hg): 155/70
               HR (bpm): 89
               Status: Inpatient
               Test: TEE (Complete)
               Doppler: Full Doppler and color Doppler
               Contrast: None
               Technical Quality: Adequate"

regular_expression_query = r'(HR).*(\d\d)'
hit = re.search(regular_expression_query, report_text)

if hit:
        print(hit.group(0))
        print(hit.group(1))
        print(hit.group(2))
else:
        print('No hit for the regular expression')
```

Simple NLP systems like these have a lot of potential for structuring free text information in the EHR as required by specific clinical study requirements. They are also the go-to NLP techniques when there are many different concepts or named entities that need to be extracted from text, such as when extracting different observations, or findings, from imaging reports as image-level labels for training deep-learning imaging diagnostic algorithms.[22]

Although manually intensive, these rule-based systems often have very high precision, at the expense of requiring a large amount of human effort to develop. This may be acceptable for tasks in which high precision is important. High precision is especially suitable for quality improvement projects, such as vaccination checks, in which the goal is to notify a provider to verify that the patient's vaccines are up to date based on automatically extracted information. Moreover, there is a low incremental cost associated with the task, especially if a provider was going to have to check anyway, and a high potential for saving time over a manual vaccine check that could involve reading through multiple years' worth of clinical notes.

Limitations and Challenges

Although highly specific and interpretable, these vocabulary- and rule-based NLP systems do require substantial work to move to a new domain. The bottleneck for developing a reliable vocabulary- and rule-based NLP system is 2-fold. First, the clinical expert will have to curate and validate an exhaustive list of terms that can be specifically mapped to the target concept or relation. This is a challenge because health care notes are notoriously written with many shorthand terms and abbreviations that are often specialty and institution specific. It is also difficult for clinicians to anticipate all the different ways that a concept can be spelled in clinical notes. Second, multiple programmatic rules are often required to correctly use the vocabulary on unstructured text, which can require significant programming resources. For vocabulary- and rule-based NLP systems to perform well, both the vocabulary and rules need to be domain specific for the task. As such, in the medical domain, clinical experts are highly valuable in this development process because they possess the requisite knowledge to create functional systems.

▌ SUPERVISED NLP

Supervised NLP is a type of machine learning where a system is given a (large) number of human annotated examples for the purpose of training the system. Compared to the previously described rule-based method, this technology does not require task-specific rules to be written by a computer scientist or linguist. Instead, there are off-the-shelf machine learning libraries that implement the NLP solution. However, with supervised learning, a subject matter expert is needed who can design the experiment and perform the manual annotation to teach the machine (see Chapter 3).

History

There are several factors that increased the popularity of using machine learning methods to solve increasingly more complex NLP task formulations. First, the widespread adoption of EHR systems enabled the dawn of big data–driven NLP in the clinical domain. Nowadays, large amounts of digitalized clinical data combined with faster and cheaper computer processors has made it possible to solve NLP problems with machine learning methods in the clinical domain as well.

Second, as NLP technologies have matured, task requirements have increased in complexity, from dealing with word- and phrase-level analyses (eg, NER and negation detection tasks) to sentence- and paragraph-level analyses (eg, question answering and natural language inference tasks). Document-level NLP formulations (ie, inferring information from understanding a whole document) are an even more complex task. Many of these complex NLP problems demand more advanced methodologies and solutions than those that can be offered by vocabulary look-up and rule-based NLP systems.

Finally, in recent years, a focus of NLP research has been to solve text extraction problems in an end-to-end manner, inferring additional information from prior domain knowledge, and to be more interactive with human users. The interactive objectives are driven by the need to integrate artificial intelligence (AI) systems more naturally into the workflow of clinical experts with the eventual goal of providing real-time clinical information to physicians. Machine learning–based NLP methods enable models to automatically "learn" crucial prior knowledge from existing large records of human language in the open domain (eg, the World Wide Web) or medical language in the clinical domain (eg, all the clinical notes in the EHR).

NLP techniques such as question answering evolved to build end-to-end models that can interact with human users.[23] This type of NLP research involves the automatic extraction of the correct answer from a document to questions asked by a user. This is the kind of information-retrieval technology that produces "Barack Obama" as an explicit answer when a user searches for "Who was the 44th president of the United States?" Prior to the development of this technology, ranking-type search algorithms would have only produced a list of relevant pages for users to browse in order to determine the correct answer themselves. In the biomedical domain, question answering has been developed using different sources of documents, such as scientific articles[24,25] and clinical notes in the EHR.[26] Although question answering engines may not be suitable for all clinical use cases, they are suitable for scenarios where the user might want to develop a humanly accessible engine, where experts can directly question the EHR and get answers to a question such as, "When did this patient quit smoking?"

Another deceptively simple but challenging problem is that of natural language inference (NLI) or recognizing textual entailment.[27] Given 2 sentences—a premise and a hypothesis—the task is to classify the hypothesis as an entailment (definitely true given the premise), a contradiction, or neither. For example, using the premise, "The patient has type 2 diabetes," the task involves classifying hypotheses—"The patient has a chronic disease," "The patient's insulin levels are always normal without taking medications," and "The patient has hypertension"—to be true, a contradiction, or neither. A related task to NLI is that of determining whether 2 phrases or questions are equivalent.[28] This is especially useful in a setting where questions are sourced from patients. For example, the question, "I have had retinitis pigmentosa for 3 years. I'm suffering from this disease. Please let me know if there is any way to treat my eyes such as stem cell injections" is equivalent to "Are there treatments for RP?"

As with vocabulary- and rule-based NLP, supervised machine learning is simply another computational methodology that can be used to solve different types of NLP task formulations, such as concept extraction, context interpretation, question answering, and NLI. These high-level NLP task formalizations help define the technologic research challenges across domains. Understanding how to formulate NLP tasks is useful for determining the best methodology one can use to build immediate practical applications. For example, automatic deidentification of clinical text is usually formulated as an NER-type NLP task because protected health information is typically mentioned only at the word and phrase level.[29] However, identifying adverse drug reactions will need context detection on top of NER because it could be negated or may not even refer to the patient.[30] Both tasks can be solved by using vocabulary- and rule-based NLP or supervised machine learning NLP methods. More complex tasks, such as examining patient records in the EHR to see whether a patient fulfills diagnostic criteria for a study, may be better formulated as an end-to-end question answering and NLI task. Predicting patient outcomes using clinical narratives from an entire longitudinal record will need to be formulated as a document-level NLP task. These more complex NLP task formulations tend to be better addressed using supervised machine learning methods.

Technology

Machine learning techniques have transformed the field of NLP. The biggest advantage of a supervised NLP algorithm is that NLP scientists can now "train" machines to "learn" the vocabularies and rules required to extract, or classify, the concepts, relations, answers to questions or entailments, and so on, of interest directly from free text. NLP scientists no longer need to program and handcraft every single rule. However, the domain experts still need to curate examples that they wish the machine learning model to learn.

What does it mean to train a machine learning model? Machine learning is fundamentally a collection of different curve fitting optimization techniques. The simplest example is a linear regression model, which is frequently used in quantitative clinical research for knowledge discovery or outcome prediction. Figure 5-2 (generated from the SOCR Data Major League Baseball HeightsWeights data set)[31,32] shows a 2-dimensional scatter plot that is fitted by a simple linear algebra equation.

However, a linear model, although effective for many applications, is not the only way to model data. To generalize the methodology, machine learning scientists tend to depict a model as the infamous black box (Figure 5-3), which takes some input and produces some output. This

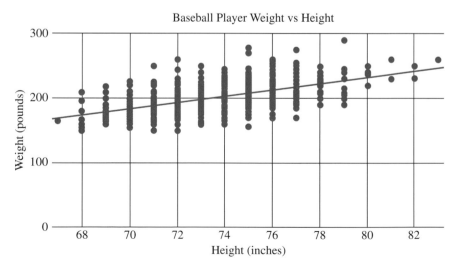

Figure 5-2 • A sample fitted scatter plot for a simple linear regression model: $y = B * x + C$.

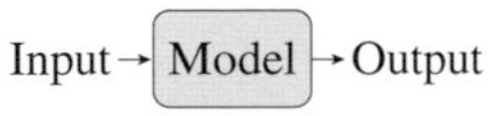

Input → Model → Output

Figure 5-3 • A typical input-output depiction of a machine learning model.

model can use a linear equation, a random forest, a neural network, or many other analytic methods. Finally, a deep neural network is simply made of varying layers of connected linear models that in theory have the potential to fit any given data pattern if given a large enough training data set (see Chapter 4).

We can gain some high-level understanding of how machine learning models work with some research language domain adaptation. In the equation provided in the caption for Figure 5-2, the class, target label, or output in a machine learning problem would usually be the outcome or dependent variable (ie, y) that clinicians are interested in predicting. The features or input is closest to the independent variables or predictors in traditional clinical research (ie, x). And learning or fitting the model can best be explained as the process of finding the best weights, coefficients, or B for each feature (x_i). If this output is explicitly labeled in the data set by a human, then we call this supervised machine learning; if not, then the learning is unsupervised.

At a very high level, modeling an NLP task with machine learning is not so different from, for example, using a linear regression model to predict how long a patient is likely to live with or without a new treatment. This also means that one needs to be careful about the usual caveats of bias and generalizability as in any other scientific research.

There are some philosophical or methodologic differences between machine learning and traditional clinical research approaches to data modeling. Clinical research methodologies draw heavily from the discipline of frequentist statistics. When modeling data, one often assumes there is one underlying truth, which lends itself to hypothesis testing. Various initial assumptions are made based on experts' knowledge of the world prior to any modeling of the data in order to control for confounding and avoid P value hunting and overfitting. In comparison, in the age of very large data sets, the computer science discipline tends to think that it is better to empirically measure their model's internal and external validities with proper data modeling methodologies. This is one reason why machine learning scientists would simply divide the whole data set into different training, validation, and testing subsets and report the performance on each subset separately. There are also theories and ongoing research to determine how to recognize when a model may not generalize well because it was overfitted to the training and validation data sets.

The basic idea behind training any supervised machine learning model is that the human supervisor would give the model many teaching examples of what is and is not in a class of interest. In the previous pneumothorax concept extraction example, the target class or label (ie, the model's output) would be "pneumothorax present" or not. The model would need to be trained on a data set with a large number of positive and negative examples of clinical notes, with and without "pneumothorax" present. For supervised NLP machine learning models, the predictors or features are usually derived automatically from the raw text, in the form of words, phrases (ie, n-grams), or embedded word vectors. These features are input to the machine learning model for predicting the target output, which is the presence or absence of pneumothorax in notes. Training the model means finding the best weights (ie, coefficients) for the best features (ie, independent variables) that would minimize the model's mistakes. The best input features could potentially be handpicked by experts but can also be automatically derived from the feature selection process during training. Therefore, to have a robust (ie, more generalizable) supervised NLP algorithm, the machine requires many sample clinical notes with different feature variations to demonstrate how each of the output classes could be described in clinical notes.

By definition, supervised machine learning methods require human-generated labeled (ie, structured) data sets. However, there exist a few opportunities where the training and testing data set is already being collected in large quantities from some routine human activities. For example, medical administrative coders routinely enter discreet billing codes in association with the clinical notes in the EHR. This routine administrative coding process produces a labeled data set that can be used to train supervised machine learning models that output billing codes given clinical notes as the input. However, these coding entries are not always correct, and the ultimate NLP model can only be as good as the ground truth data set on which it was trained. In addition, many clinical concepts of interest to researchers and auditors are not always coded in the structured billing codes. Therefore, de novo gold standard data set creation is still often required to develop NLP models specific to different clinical applications.

Clinical Application With Examples

There are many tasks in the clinical domain that can be addressed with supervised NLP. Numerous open-source Python libraries are available to implement supervised machine learning algorithms. Commonly used NLP-specific Python libraries include Natural Language Toolkit,[33]

StanfordNLP,[34] and SpaCy.*[35] These libraries offer toolkits to implement standard NLP preprocessing tasks (eg, tokenizing and parsing sentences), using supervised machine learning methods.[36] Deep-learning Python frameworks, such as Pytorch, Tensorflow, and Keras, can be used for building customized deep-learning–based NLP models. In many cases, as long as there is a large enough labeled data set, training a standard supervised NLP model is a matter of preprocessing the data set into a suitable format and then calling the appropriate programming libraries.

Concept extraction is a common application of supervised NLP on clinical notes. For example, Li et al[37] annotated 878 EHR notes with 76,577 sentences to identify bleeding events in patients on anticoagulant therapy for cardiovascular disease. This is an example where a sentence-level annotated data set was used to train and validate several NLP models, including both supervised and unsupervised models. The supervised model used a convolutional neural network, which was trained on 1451 sentences annotated as positive for bleeding events and 285 annotated as negations.

Patient phenotyping is another application of supervised NLP that can be very useful for identifying eligible patients for clinical research studies from the EHR.[38] Compared with a vocabulary- and rule-based NLP system that typically works at the phrase or sentence level, a supervised model has more flexibility with analyzing the patient phenotype at the document level[39] or potentially the whole patient record level. Using supervised NLP methods avoids having to write multiple rules when the clinical task is to find patients who fulfill a set of complex clinical criteria. However, even with the most advanced supervised NLP algorithms, analyzing patient phenotypes at the document and longitudinal record level is still difficult to do accurately (eg, identifying whether a patient diagnosis is historical or family history related). Properly interpreting a longitudinal patient record requires common sense medical knowledge. For example, a patient diagnosed with diabetes mellitus last year is still diabetic, whereas a broken leg diagnosed 1 year ago would likely no longer be an active diagnosis *if* the patient is otherwise healthy. Ultimately, current NLP systems can help the clinical expert accelerate the cohort selection process but still cannot reliably make the final decision without human oversight.

Beyond concept extraction and patient phenotyping, supervised learning with textual data has also been used to perform clinical prediction-type tasks, such as assessing risks of developing future diseases[40] and predicting drug interactions.[41] However, implementing these predictive machine learning models in the clinical workflow is still an ongoing challenge.[42-44]

---

*https://github.com/allenai/scispacy is a version of SpaCy trained for biomedical documents.

Limitations and Challenges

There are several challenges for building supervised NLP algorithms, most of which center around curating the appropriate data set to train a model for the given clinical application. Collecting such annotations is a challenging cross-disciplinary task and has to be done carefully with medical experts following specific guidelines.[45] The research community in the clinical NLP field has made significant advances on curating annotated data sets for various fundamental tasks[46] and making a comprehensive anonymized EHR available for research.[47]

De novo curation of the training and testing data set often requires a high clinical time investment. Unfortunately, there is often a chicken-and-egg problem when sampling data points for the human expert to annotate the training and testing data set. This is because the prevalence of positive examples to teach the network is often very low if the examples were randomly drawn from the population of interest. Besides the suboptimal clinician time spent on curating too many negative examples, the resulting "unbalanced" data set (ie, more negative than positive examples) also poses a problem for good machine learning science. To illustrate this simply, suppose only 5% of the training and testing data are positive; then, the NLP model can almost always output a correct prediction simply by "guessing" the output as the negative class all the time. The model's performance would be excellent without having learned any useful features associated with either classes. Furthermore, even if sampling or data augmentation techniques are used to balance the positive and negative classes, we still cannot always expect the NLP model to generalize well outside the curated data set, particularly if the model had only seen a very small number of examples of what the positive class may look like.

Arriving at an agreement on what is and is not a target example between domain experts is another challenge for data set curation. In general, creating a well-annotated data set for supervised learning is a challenging cross-disciplinary task that has to be performed carefully with medical experts following specific guidelines.[45] Agreement between clinicians can be very difficult due to the uncertain nature of many clinical cognitive tasks. For example, is the note a positive example of "nonadherence" if it describes an intoxicated patient who was "noncompliant with neuro examination"? What if the patient was suspected to have had a stroke instead? Therefore, one way to improve interannotator agreement when creating the data set is to clearly define the clinical criteria for each class at the start and to then have the annotators go through a few clinical notes together. However, as with many situations in medicine, unexpected edge cases are often unavoidable, and multiple experts' opinions may be required to obtain the final consensus.

Another major challenge for supervised NLP algorithms is explainability, the lack of which is a barrier for some clinical implementations. A disadvantage of more complex mathematical models is that they make many supervised NLP models less humanly interpretable compared to the vocabulary- and rule-based NLP techniques. In contrast, no specific rules need to be programmatically coded to use textual features in supervised machine learning. Supervised models can often use features that were not selected a priori by the human experts to predict the output. In linear models, explainability is fairly straightforward by observing coefficients of the variables that enable prediction. However, in the case of deep learning, these features could be combined in humanly uninterpretable ways between layers in the network, and sometimes, all we can see is the final prediction performance without understanding how that prediction was achieved. It is an ongoing area of research to figure out the textual features that had the most impact or weight on the final prediction. By developing methods to review these features (ie, words or phrases) manually,[39] the experts can gain some insight into what went on in the black box and decide whether the NLP algorithm's prediction can be trusted.

The research community in the clinical NLP field has made significant advances on curating annotated data sets for various fundamental tasks[46] and making a comprehensive anonymized EHR available for research.[47] However, another significant ongoing barrier to the advancement of the field has been the inability to make these resources publicly available due to concerns of patient privacy. The community has endeavored to overcome these barriers[48] through data deidentification and organizing shared annotation tasks. These efforts helped make annotated data sets increasingly available for development and benchmarking of clinical NLP systems. The open-sourced data sets also encouraged the development of open-sourced clinical NLP systems,[17] fostering further research.

UNSUPERVISED NLP

When confronting the challenges of obtaining the vast number of accurate labels required for supervised NLP, the obvious question arises: Would it be possible to learn without such labels? The answer is, surprisingly, yes. Any written human language has certain structures and expressed knowledge about the world. If given a large collection of reasonably coherent sample texts (ie, a corpus), a computer can begin to identify patterns in the data without any additional human labeling. This is NLP with unsupervised machine learning.

History

One of the most exciting applications of unsupervised learning to NLP emerged in 2013 with the advent of word2vec-style word embeddings. The idea is to use a shallow neural net to learn the context of words in a corpus. With surprisingly small networks (eg, ~300 dimensions) such systems can do remarkably well at finding similar words. This can be very helpful to, for example, find a large list of symptoms, drugs, or diagnoses, given a few starting examples. As long as a concept is linguistically coherent, this method can work.

However, word2vec is limited in the length of the phrases it can find. This can be a problem in medicine, where a long phrase such as "early-stage ER+/HER2– breast cancer" is a single concept. In these cases, pattern-based systems such as the Domain Learning Assistant can be used.[49,50]

Clustering algorithms is another promising group of unsupervised methods that has recently emerged in the clinical domain for grouping similar documents, concepts, or patients. The hope is that, after the computer suggests the clusters of documents automatically, a human expert can then look at the documents and identify whether there is an interesting reason that they were classified together (eg, they are all discharge summaries or phlebotomy reports).

However, not all of the features or groups that clustering algorithms suggest would make clinical sense. Take a plausible clustering task of dividing all the patients in the EHR into 2 groups. A human would likely try to do this by picking some meaningful features, such as sex or acuteness of presentation. A clustering algorithm would just suggest 2 groups based on patterns in the data it is optimizing without any explanation. It would be up to the human to figure out why. Sometimes, the reason (ie, data pattern) could be interesting, but the reason can also be either not useful or not interpretable.

Technology

At a high level, all of these unsupervised learning methods deal with finding similarity or maximum differences in the underlying data. To implement any unsupervised learning algorithm with textual data, the data need to be re-represented mathematically as vectors for a computer. After this step, other types of learning algorithms, such as clustering, can then be implemented to capture the underlying data patterns.

Creating a word embedding is the process of representing words in a corpus as vectors (ie, a set of numbers). Word2vec is a particular group of methods to efficiently create word embeddings (or representations) for a

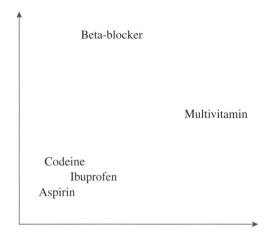

Figure 5-4 • Illustration of drug terms in vector space of a semantic word embedding.

corpus of text, such as Wikipedia or all the radiology reports in an EHR. The vectors are based on one or more surrounding words preceding and following each word. Thus, each word is represented by a vector in vector space, where semantically similar words are clustered together by their similar contexts. A medically related illustration for this semantic vector space of words can be demonstrated by Figure 5-4.

There are 2 methods used by word2vec to train word embeddings: continuous bag of words (CBOW) and skip-gram. The CBOW method takes a surrounding window of context words as input and learns to predict the target word as output using a neural network as the processing layer. The skip-gram method inputs a target word and outputs probabilities of the surrounding window of context words. Word2vec is the original programming implementation of CBOW and skip-gram. GenSim and Glove are Python libraries that have subsequently reimplemented the core ideas from word2vec with added features, such as using additional sentence parsing information to improve the word embedding representation. For further details on this topic in the biomedical domain, we recommend a paper by Chiu et al[51] as a helpful resource in establishing the optimal parameters for training word embeddings. Once the word embedding is trained, other unsupervised learning methods, such as clustering or topic modeling, can be implemented to automatically group documents or patients, depending on the task. But again, thereafter, it is still up to a human to interpret and make sense of these groups or classes.

A trained word embedding can be directly useful in some applications. Open domain examples that use word2vec-type embeddings are the messaging applications on cell phones that employ next-word prediction when a user is typing a message. The messaging application predicts and displays the most probable choices of what the next word will be in the typed message, based on the meaning of one or more of the preceding words that have already been typed. However, clinical language is typically quite different from everyday language. Training a word embedding specifically on a clinical notes corpus can prime a system with word representations that have clinical domain–specific correlations. For example, if an NLP system using word2vec has been trained on mammography reports containing text such as "core needle biopsy," the system would predict in a new report that the word following "core needle" would be "biopsy."

Word sense disambiguation is another application of word embeddings.[52] In natural language, the same words or phrases can mean different things in different contexts. For example, "apple" as a fruit and "Apple" as a company. This is a well-recognized issue in the clinical domain, where terminologies used by one specialty can refer to totally different concepts in a different specialty[53] (eg, CVA could mean cerebrovascular accident as in a stroke or costovertebral angle as in CVA tenderness).

Clinical Application With Examples

Unfortunately, the field of unsupervised learning in NLP is still fairly young, and it is currently hard to find an immediately practical clinical use case that can be built with only unsupervised techniques. However, people are still excited that computers are beginning to be able to draw conclusions directly from the data without the prior bias or ambiguity that can be introduced by domain experts through the labeling process. Although the results are hard to interpret, the technology is still promising because of its potential to discover prior unknown patterns in the data, which could add to clinical understanding in a data-driven health system.

The greatest near-term promise of unsupervised methods is as an adjunct to other models. For example, unsupervised methods can be very helpful for generating more useful features for training a supervised machine learning model. Word2vec can be specifically trained on clinical documents to learn specialized word representations (ie, features) in the clinical domain, which can be quite different compared to the open domain. These features can then be used to learn another supervised task in the clinical domain, such as patient phenotype prediction from clinical notes (eg, whether the patient has advanced heart failure or not).[39]

In fact, unsupervised methods can be used to create embeddings for more than just words. The unit of representation can be a sentence, a document, or a patient's entire EHR record. By creating a higher dimensional representation of patient data with unsupervised methods, you could effectively group together similar patients as they would appear to a computer. It is important to note that this similarity metric is derived automatically without a human specifying which features should or should not be considered. Despite the lack of human feedback, it has been demonstrated that the computer can sometimes learn to make better clinical predictions in a supervised learning task (eg, predicting a patient's future diagnosis) when it uses features generated in an unsupervised manner from the underlying data pattern.[40]

Limitations and Challenges

Today, open source packages, such as GenSim[54] and Glove,*[55] can help with easily implementing different kinds of word embedding and clustering techniques for unsupervised NLP. In all these cases, the unsupervised NLP algorithms are finding a natural pattern in the text. Because the computer does not need a human in unsupervised machine learning, the obvious advantage is that clinicians would not have to spend months or years creating the data sets necessary to develop these algorithms. However, the aphorism that "there is no free lunch" is true for any NLP tools—interpreting the "what" and "why" of these unsupervised NLP systems' output is still very difficult. In particular, one should be aware that the clusters or classes automatically learned from the underlying data patterns are often not clinically interpretable and may not be task specific enough for most clinical applications compared to the other NLP techniques.

At the end of the day, these systems are looking for naturally occurring patterns, but they have no sense of why these patterns are occurring. The classic example of a worthless pattern might occur from feeding the machine a pile of reports from yesterday only to have the system find the pattern that "all reports are filed on Thursday." Understanding which patterns are important and which are spurious requires a human with common sense.

▌EXPERT-IN-THE-LOOP NLP

To counter the disadvantages of a purely unsupervised system, we find that it is useful to have an expert work with the AI system. This is the emerging field of human-in-the-loop systems. In medicine, we often speak

---

*GenSim is word2vec (bag of words) reimplemented without sentence parsing. Stanford Glove implements word embedding too but uses additional sentence structure information from the sentence parse tree, giving it better performance on well-written (grammatically) texts.

of the subfield of expert-in-the-loop, where we need the human to have specialized knowledge and well-developed common sense in their clinical field of expertise. In a very broad sense, human-in-the-loop systems seek to use unsupervised methods to identify the areas where human supervision will have the greatest impact for the time spent.

History

The concept of a pattern of interaction between an expert and nonexpert is not new. Anyone who has supervised an internship or residency is used to the pattern of the nonexpert trainee asking questions and learning from the expert. They are also familiar with learning interactions that work well (eg, students asking questions when they are confused) and those that do not (eg, lecturing at students when they do not have the context to make sense of the lecture). Expert-in-the-loop seeks to emulate the best of those interactions to more rapidly train systems (hopefully much more rapidly than traditional supervised machine learning), while keeping the results understandably aligned to real-world concern (unlike unsupervised machine learning).

Technology

Even the best NLP algorithms can fail on ambiguous, confusing, or just poorly written text. A little experience with these systems can give you a good idea of when this is likely to happen. In such cases, it makes sense to have a human reviewing the observations and conclusions of the AI, especially in those cases where the system knows it is confused (Figure 5-5).

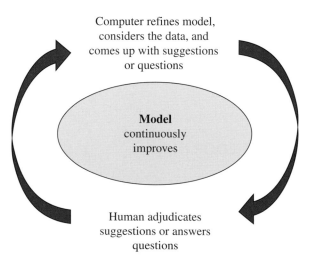

Figure 5-5 • System diagram illustrating human-in-the-loop.

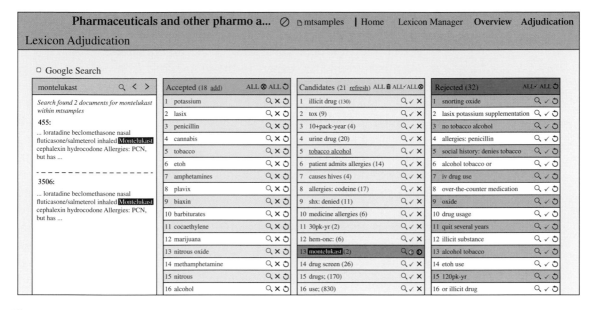

Figure 5-6 • The Domain Learning Assistant is an example of a natural language processing (NLP) system that applies human-in-the-loop methodologies for concept (vocabulary) expansion. With an expert in the loop, this NLP tool can be used in any domain and in any language. This pharmaceutical lexicon example demonstrates words that have been accepted by a human reviewer in the "Accepted" column, words that have been rejected in the "Rejected" column, and candidate words that have been identified by the system but require human review in the "Candidates" column.

A good example of this is lexicon expansion—the task of starting with a small list of items (eg, drugs [we could start with aspirin, acetaminophen, and codeine]) and expanding to a more comprehensive list of terms, as shown in Figure 5-6. An unsupervised machine learning system can examine a large corpus of medical text and find words and phrases that are similar to these seed terms. The terms the system suggests to add to our example of drugs will include obvious additions (eg, penicillin), ones subject to debate (eg, vitamin C), others that are more distant (eg, adhesive tape), and ones that are simply wrong (eg, Monday). A human can quickly accept or reject these suggestions. The accepted and rejected suggestions become labeled examples that the system then can use to reconsider the corpus and come up with new and better suggestions.

The technologies here include traditional unsupervised and supervised methodologies, as well as a surprising amount of work on user experience. A well-designed user interface (UI) for such a task (eg, swipe left to accept, right to reject [or vice versa]) can take the human only a second to adjudicate per term. A less well-designed UI can easily take

2 or 3 seconds per term. Although this may seem minimal, once you begin to consider that the human's time is the dominant cost, a 300% cost difference to develop a lexicon starts to become consequential.

Another area where expert-in-the-loop excels is in cases of "assignment" to categories. Consider the case of adverse event drug coding. A MedDRA (Medical Dictionary for Regulatory Activities) code needs to be assigned to each adverse event report. There are over 100,000 codes that may need to be assigned.[56] It takes quite a while for a human to make such assignments. AI typically will only do a correct assignment approximately two-thirds of the time (making an incorrect assignment one-third of the time). This is clearly too low an accuracy level for an automated system. However, if the AI looks at the text reports and suggests the top 5 categories, the correct answer would be included over 90% of the time (and the human user can easily select the correct one in less than a second). This effectively reduces the manual time for review by a factor of 10.

Active learning is another machine learning research area that complements the human-in-the-loop approach. An active learning approach seeks to identify the one piece of information (eg, usually the fact the system is most confused about at the moment) that will result in the largest improvement of a particular model. Using this in a human-in-the-loop setting optimizes identification of questions on which clinicians should spend their time. The goal is to have a human supervise as small an amount of labeling (eg, a few hours at most) to generate the training data that will result in the best system for a complex task. Typically, with active learning–enhanced human-in-the-loop, the model can be trained in a matter of a few hours to levels that would more commonly take days, weeks, or in some cases months of human training.

Limitations and Challenges

Although these expert-in-the-loop systems do learn more quickly than typical AI systems (as they work to resolve the areas of the clinical tasks the systems are most confused about first), they still require an expert to train them and thus are limited by human agreement about what the "right" answer is; for example, opinions differ on the efficacy of aspirin for reducing cardiac events in the general population.

They also require developers of the systems to identify how to best surface the machine's ideas and confusions to the human (which makes user experience research essential as well) and how to make the most of the feedback the human chooses to provide. For example, is it best for the human to answer a series of yes or no questions, to make free text pronouncements, or to underline the most important part of a chapter?

As the youngest of these fields, there are fewer "canned" solutions in this space. But the technology has the potential to develop impactful AI solutions more rapidly.

SUMMARY

One of the biggest challenges to AI-based NLP in the clinical domain is the availability of large corpora of clinician-annotated examples that capture all the nuances of the domain of interest. This limitation means that, in many cases, fully automated AI NLP systems are impossible; there are simply not enough examples to train such a system to run on its own against all possible patients and situations. In these cases, human-in-the-loop systems, where the AI assists the human in tagging or scoring information, can be useful because they can accelerate the already existing human processes. In these cases, the AI system acts as an assist to the human. This allows a human to review, for example, a few thousand surgical cases an hour for a feature of interest instead of the more time-consuming task of reviewing entire cases (which could take an hour or more per case). For studies of an exploratory or one-shot nature, this approach especially makes sense as it would take substantially more than an hour to code a system that would even have a chance at coming close to the accuracy of a human.

Finally, it is worth noting that irony, implication, and subtle shadings are very difficult for a computer to grasp. A note that says, "Patient was admitted to the ICU 3 days ago for acute pneumonia. Patient has been a nonsmoker for 3 days" is not actually a clinical assertion that the patient is a nonsmoker. Using NLP in health care requires a good sense of pragmatism. Recognizing that such systems, although powerful, have limits and identifying where they can be used to have the greatest impact are currently more of an art than a science.

REFERENCES

1. Wei WQ, Teixeira PL, Mo H, et al. Combining billing codes, clinical notes, and medications from electronic health records provides superior phenotyping performance. *J Am Med Inform Assoc.* 2015;23(e1):e20-e27.
2. Capurro D, van Eaton E, Black R, et al. Availability of structured and unstructured clinical data for comparative effectiveness research and quality improvement: a multisite assessment. *EGEMS.* 2014;2(1):1079.
3. Rosenbloom ST, Denny JC, Xu H, et al. Data from clinical notes: a perspective on the tension between structure and flexible documentation. *J Am Med Inform Assoc.* 2011;18(2):181-186.

4. Topaz M, Shafran-Topaz L, Bowles KH. ICD-9 to ICD-10: evolution, revolution, and current debates in the United States. Perspectives in Health Information Management/AHIMA, American Health Information Management Association. Accessed October 6, 2020. http://library.ahima.org/doc?oid=301221#.X30wcWhKjIU.

5. Rea S, Pathak J, Savova G, et al. Building a robust, scalable and standards-driven infrastructure for secondary use of EHR data: the SHARPn project. *J Biomed Inform*. 2012;45(4):763-771.

6. Benesch C, Witter DM, Wilder AL, et al. Inaccuracy of the International Classification of Diseases (ICD-9-CM) in identifying the diagnosis of ischemic cerebrovascular disease. *Neurology*. 1997;49(3):660-664.

7. Demner-Fushman D, Chapman WW, McDonald CJ. What can natural language processing do for clinical decision support? *J Biomed Inform*. 2009;42(5):760-772.

8. Uzuner Ö, Goldstein I, Luo Y, et al. Identifying patient smoking status from medical discharge records. *J Am Med Inform Assoc*. 2008;15(1):14-24.

9. Hirschman L, Grishman R, Sager N. From text to structured information: automatic processing of medical reports. In Proceedings of the June 7-10, 1976, National Computer Conference and Exposition, pp 267-275. Accessed October 6, 2020. https://dl.acm.org/doi/10.1145/1499799.1499842.

10. Gell G. Free text processing in clinical documentation. *J Clin Comput*. 1982;10(5-6):170.

11. Rothwell DJ, Hause LL. SNOMED and microcomputers in anatomic pathology. *Med Inform*. 1983;8(1):23-31.

12. Friedman C, Alderson PO, Austin JH, et al. A general natural-language text processor for clinical radiology. *J Am Med Inform Assoc*. 1994;1(2):161-174.

13. Chapman WW, Bridewell W, Hanbury P, et al. A simple algorithm for identifying negated findings and diseases in discharge summaries. *J Biomed Inform*. 2001;34(5):301-310.

14. Uzuner Ö, South BR, Shen S, et al. 2010 i2b2/VA challenge on concepts, assertions, and relations in clinical text. *J Am Med Inform Assoc*. 2011;18(5):552-556.

15. Sun W, Rumshisky A, Uzuner O. Evaluating temporal relations in clinical text: 2012 i2b2 challenge. *J Am Med Inform Assoc*. 2013;20(5):806-813.

16. Bodenreider O. The unified medical language system (UMLS): integrating biomedical terminology. *Nucleic Acids Res*. 2004;32(suppl 1):D267-D270.

17. Savova GK, Masanz JJ, Ogren PV, et al. Mayo clinical Text Analysis and Knowledge Extraction System (cTAKES): architecture, component evaluation and applications. *J Am Med Inform Assoc*. 2010;17(5):507-513.

18. Aronson AR. Effective mapping of biomedical text to the UMLS Metathesaurus: the MetaMap program. Accessed October 6, 2020. https://ii.nlm.nih.gov/Publications/Papers/metamap_01AMIA.pdf.

19. Bernstam EV, Smith JW, Johnson TR. What is biomedical informatics? *J Biomed Inform*. 2010;43(1):104-110.

20. Friedman C, Hripcsak G, DuMouchel W, Johnson SB, Clayton PD. Natural language processing in an operational clinical information system. *Nat Lang Eng*. 1995;1(1):83-108.

21. Friedman C, Shagina L, Lussier Y, Hripcsak G. Automated encoding of clinical documents based on natural language processing. *J Am Med Inform Assoc.* 2004;11(5):392-402.

22. Irvin J, Rajpurkar P, Ko M, et al. Chexpert: a large chest radiograph dataset with uncertainty labels and expert comparison. arXiv:1901.07031. Accessed October 6, 2020. https://arxiv.org/abs/1901.07031.

23. Demner-Fushman D, Lin J. Answering clinical questions with knowledge-based and statistical techniques. *Comput Linguist.* 2007;33(1):63-103.

24. Lee M, Cimino J, Zhu HR, et al. Beyond information retrieval—medical question answering. *AMIA Annu Symp Proc.* 2006;2006:469-473.

25. Šuster S, Daelemans W. Clicr: a dataset of clinical case reports for machine reading comprehension. arXiv:1803.09720. Accessed October 6, 2020. https://arxiv.org/abs/1803.09720.

26. Pampari A, Raghavan P, Liang J, et al. emrQA: a large corpus for question answering on electronic medical records. arXiv:1809.00732. Accessed October 6, 2020. https://arxiv.org/abs/1809.00732.

27. Romanov A, Shivade C. Lessons from natural language inference in the clinical domain. arXiv:1808.06752. Accessed October 6, 2020. https://arxiv.org/abs/1808.06752.

28. Abacha AB, Demner-Fushman D. Recognizing question entailment for medical question answering. *AMIA Annu Symp Proc.* 2017;2016:310-318.

29. Stubbs A, Kotfila C, Uzuner Ö. Automated systems for the de-identification of longitudinal clinical narratives: overview of 2014 i2b2/UTHealth shared task Track 1. *J Biomed Inform.* 2015;58:S11-S19.

30. Segura Bedmar I, Martínez P, Herrero Zazo M. Semeval-2013 task 9: extraction of drug-drug interactions from biomedical texts (ddiextraction 2013). Accessed October 6, 2020. https://www.semanticscholar.org/paper/SemEval-2013-Task-9-%3A-Extraction-of-Drug-Drug-from-Segura-Bedmar-Mart%C3%ADnez/a9a5b40e179ed22e3d59b7823bffc9d3aaa65474?p2df.

31. Saint Onge JM, Krueger PM, Rogers RG. Historical trends in height, weight, and body mass: data from US Major League Baseball players, 1869–1983. *Econ Hum Biol.* 2008;6(3):482-488.

32. Saint Onge JM, Rogers RG, Krueger PM. Major league baseball players' life expectancies. *Soc Sci Quart.* 2008;89(3):817-830.

33. Loper E, Bird S. NLTK: the natural language toolkit. Accessed October 6, 2020. http://ed.loper.org/publications/nltk_acl04.pdf.

34. Manning C, Surdeanu M, Bauer J, et al. The Stanford CoreNLP natural language processing toolkit. In Proceedings of 52nd Annual Meeting of the Association for Computational Linguistics: System Demonstrations. Accessed October 6, 2020. https://www.aclweb.org/anthology/P14-5010/.

35. Choi JD, Tetreault J, Stent A. It depends: dependency parser comparison using a web-based evaluation tool. In Proceedings of the 53rd Annual Meeting of the Association for Computational Linguistics and the 7th International Joint Conference on Natural Language Processing (Volume 1: Long Papers), 2015, pp 387-396. Accessed October 6, 2020. https://www.aclweb.org/anthology/P15-1038.pdf.

36. Srinivasa-Desikan B. *Natural Language Processing and Computational Linguistics: A Practical Guide to Text Analysis With Python, Gensim, spaCy, and Keras.* Packt Publishing Ltd; 2018.

37. Li R, Hu B, Liu F, et al. Detection of bleeding events in electronic health record notes using convolutional neural network models enhanced with recurrent neural network autoencoders: deep learning approach. *JMIR Med Inform.* 2019;7(1):e10788.

38. Miotto R, Weng C. Case-based reasoning using electronic health records efficiently identifies eligible patients for clinical trials. *J Am Med Inform Assoc.* 2015;22(e1):e141-e150.

39. Gehrmann S, Dernoncourt F, Li Y, et al. Comparing deep learning and concept extraction based methods for patient phenotyping from clinical narratives. *PloS One.* 2018;13(2):e0192360.

40. Miotto R, Li L, Kidd BA, Dudley JT. Deep patient: an unsupervised representation to predict the future of patients from the electronic health records. *Sci Rep.* 2016;6:26094.

41. Tatonetti NP, Patrick PY, Daneshjou R, et al. Data-driven prediction of drug effects and interactions. *Sci Trans Med.* 2012;4(125):125ra31.

42. Dahlem D, Maniloff D, Ratti C. Predictability bounds of electronic health records. *Sci Rep.* 2015;5:11865.

43. Bellazzi R, Zupan B. Predictive data mining in clinical medicine: current issues and guidelines. *J Am Med Inform Assoc.* 2008;77(2):81-97.

44. Wu J, Roy J, Stewart WF. Prediction modeling using EHR data: challenges, strategies, and a comparison of machine learning approaches. *Med Care.* 2010;48:S106-S113.

45. Wu JT, Dernoncourt F, Gehrmann S, et al. Behind the scenes: a medical natural language processing project. *Int J Med Inform.* 2018;112:68-73.

46. Albright D, Lanfranchi A, Fredriksen A, et al. Towards comprehensive syntactic and semantic annotations of the clinical narrative. *J Am Med Inform Assoc.* 2013;20(5):922-930.

47. Johnson AE, Pollard TJ, Shen L, et al. MIMIC-III, a freely accessible critical care database. *Sci Data.* 2016;3:160035.

48. Chapman WW, Nadkarni PM, Hirschman L, et al. Overcoming barriers to NLP for clinical text: the role of shared tasks and the need for additional creative solutions.

49. Coden A, Gruhl D, Lewis N, et al. SPOT the drug! An unsupervised pattern matching method to extract drug names from very large clinical corpora. In 2012 IEEE Second International Conference on Healthcare Informatics, Imaging and Systems Biology, September 27, 2012, pp 33-39. Accessed October 6, 2020. https://ieeexplore.ieee.org/document/6366185.

50. Gentile AL, Gruhl D, Ristoski P, et al. Explore and exploit. Dictionary expansion with human-in-the-loop. In European Semantic Web Conference, June 2, 2019, pp 131-145. Accessed October 6, 2020. https://link.springer.com/chapter/10.1007/978-3-030-21348-0_9.

51. Chiu B, Crichton G, Korhonen A, et al. How to train good word embeddings for biomedical NLP. In Proceedings of the 15th Workshop on Biomedical Natural Language Processing, August 2016, pp 166-174. Accessed October 6, 2020. https://www.aclweb.org/anthology/W16-2922.pdf.

52. Liu H, Lussier YA, Friedman C. Disambiguating ambiguous biomedical terms in biomedical narrative text: an unsupervised method. *J Biomed Inform.* 2001;34(4):249-261.

53. Sheppard JE, Weidner LC, Zakai S, et al. Ambiguous abbreviations: an audit of abbreviations in paediatric note keeping. *Arch Dis Child.* 2008;93(3):204-206.

54. Rehurek R, Sojka P. Software framework for topic modelling with large corpora. In Proceedings of the LREC 2010 Workshop on New Challenges for NLP Frameworks 2010. Accessed October 6, 2020. https://is.muni.cz/publication/884893/en/Software-Framework-for-Topic-Modelling-with-Large-Corpora/Rehurek-Sojka.

55. Pennington J, Socher R, Manning C. Glove: global vectors for word representation. In Proceedings of the 2014 Conference on Empirical Methods in Natural Language Processing (EMNLP), October 2014, pp 1532-1543. Accessed October 6, 2020. https://www.aclweb.org/anthology/D14-1162/.

56. Brown EG, Wood L, Wood S. The medical dictionary for regulatory activities (MedDRA). *Drug Saf.* 1999;20(2):109-117.

COMPUTER VISION IN SURGERY: FUNDAMENTAL PRINCIPLES AND APPLICATIONS

6

Daniel A. Hashimoto, Amin Madani,
Allison Navarrete-Welton, and Guy Rosman

HIGHLIGHTS

- Although computer vision functions in a manner unique from biologic vision, many principles were influenced by biologic systems.
- Digital images are composed of fundamental units and shapes represented on a coordinate system. Digital images are represented by a matrix of values that contain information (eg, color, transparency) that affects the way we perceive the images.
- Videos are composed of a series of still images, of which a single image is referred to as a video frame. Many principles of computer vision relating to still images thus apply to video but with the added component of time.
- Computer vision problems often rely on detection of features, which are attributes in the data that can be used to assist in modeling.

▌ WHAT IS COMPUTER VISION?

Computer vision refers to machine understanding of visual data (ie, images and videos). Although computer vision is a field in and of itself, it also heavily intersects with machine learning and related fields such as image processing, signal processing, optics, and the cognitive sciences such as psychology and neuroscience.[1] While object detection/recognition (eg, identifying items, animals, or people in an image) has become more popular in our daily lives through social media and other platforms, computer vision encompasses a field of work that is quite broad and includes research on describing and analyzing the visual world in numerical or symbolic form to allow for interpretation of images for subsequent action (eg, analyzing visual information for computer-assisted driving). Research and applications in computer vision have embodied the intersectional spirit of the field as techniques have drawn methodology from various schools of machine learning, including deep learning.

In this chapter, we will cover fundamental principles necessary for a foundational understanding of computer vision, particularly as it applies to surgery. As with other chapters in this section, the information in this chapter is not intended to imbue expertise, as entire series of textbooks are needed to cover aspects of computer vision; rather, it is intended to provide knowledge on the principles of computer vision so that the reader may be better informed when reading and assessing surgical literature that may use computer vision in its methodology. Additional resources are available in the appendix for further study and a deeper dive into topics in computer vision.

█ HUMAN VISION IN BRIEF

Although an in-depth review of the human visual system is outside of the scope of this chapter, a brief review of the human visual system can help provide context to understanding the similarities and differences between our own visual systems and that of computers.[2]

Optical reception within the human visual system occurs in the eye as light passes through the cornea and lens and onto the retina (Figure 6-1). The retina is composed of a number of cell types (eg, rods, cones, bipolar and ganglion cells) that serve as a neural network (Figure 6-2) to process optical information entering the eye and transmit it via neural pathways to the visual cortex. Within the retina, distinct cell types contribute to the perception of vision. Rods are attuned to detect low-intensity light, whereas cones detect high-intensity light that contributes most to sharp vision and color detection. Cones are attuned to respond to light waves at frequencies corresponding to red, green, and blue—the 3 primary colors. The perception of color is therefore thought to be a product of the relative frequency of signals from each of the different cones. Thus, to oversimplify for the sake of example, in the visual system in humans, a differential signal from different neurons, along with subsequent modulation of that signal by other neurons, leads to the eventual perception of vision by the brain.

As first introduced in Chapter 3 and further described in Chapter 4, inspiration for some machine learning methodologies comes from the

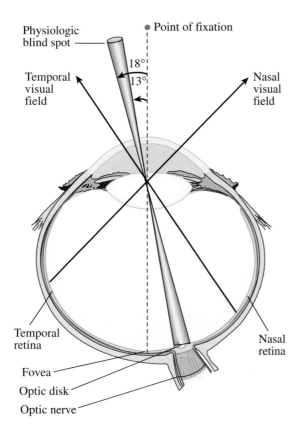

Figure 6-1 • Illustration of the eye demonstrating passage of light through the cornea and lens and onto the retina. (Reproduced, with permission, from Waxman SG. *Clinical Neuroanatomy.* 28th ed. McGraw-Hill; 2017.)

biologic nervous system, and such methods are some of the most popular techniques in computer vision at this time due to their ability to process large amounts of information. Similar to the human visual system, "neurons" within a neural network fire depending on the type and weight of a feature from an image with the resultant output of the network being somewhat analogous to perception by a person's brain, such as in our earlier example.

In the next section, a description of the anatomy of an image, particularly a digital one, helps to provide a better understanding of the features of an image that can be detected by a computer vision system.

▌ANATOMY OF AN IMAGE

Images, whether 2-dimensional (2D) or 3-dimensional (3D), are represented by a number of features ranging from low-level characteristics such as color and texture to high-level information, loosely termed semantics,

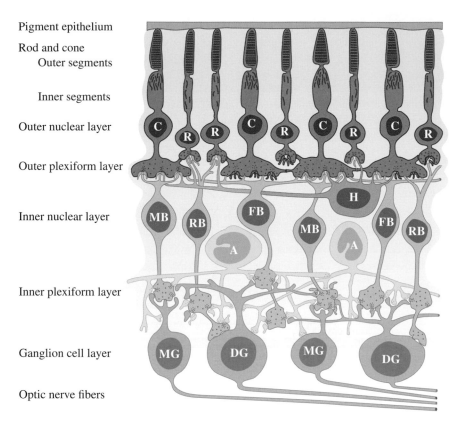

Pigment epithelium

Rod and cone
   Outer segments

   Inner segments

Outer nuclear layer

Outer plexiform layer

Inner nuclear layer

Inner plexiform layer

Ganglion cell layer

Optic nerve fibers

Figure 6-2 • Illustration of the network of cells that comprise the retina. (Reproduced, with permission, from Waxman SG. *Clinical Neuroanatomy*. 28th ed. McGraw-Hill; 2017.)

that provides cues on the context of the image or the intentionality of an object within an image. Behind each element of an image is a world of mathematics that is used to describe and analyze the element. We will focus here on the basic concepts that are necessary to obtain an understanding of the field and provide additional references for readers who are interested in pursuing more in-depth reading on mathematical topics related to image construction.

Image and Video Capture

A camera captures light that streams through a lens and onto film. For digital images, film is replaced by an image sensor, such as a charge-coupled device or active pixel sensor (eg, complementary metal-oxide semiconductor [MOS]), in which MOS capacitors convert photons into electrical charges. The image sensor then outputs the electric signal to a frame grabber, which digitizes the signal and stores it in a frame buffer. The frame buffer is a portion of the random-access memory (RAM), which stores the bitmapped image created by the frame grabber. The frame buffer can then send the image to a processor for graphic display, further manipulation, or analysis.

Image Geometry

Perhaps one of the most readily conceptualized frameworks of space and position is the Euclidean coordinate system comprising 2 axes—x and y—on a 2D plane with the addition of a third axis (z) for 3D structures (Figure 6-3).

Digital images are composed of fundamental units and shapes represented on a coordinate system. The pixel is often considered the smallest component of a digital image, and a single pixel denotes a single point on an image. A line can then be constructed by aligning 2 or more pixels, whereas a plane is a flat surface. These 3 elements can be modified to create all of the elements in 2D and 3D images, such as curves, surfaces, conics, and volumes.[3]

Image processing can involve various types of geometric transformations to create slightly different perspectives on the same image. Although transformations serve a variety of purposes, the primary use that surgeons may encounter is for augmenting a data set of surgical images. While most of the transformations are best described mathematically through matrix manipulation, Table 6-1 provides definitions and examples of common geometric transformations.

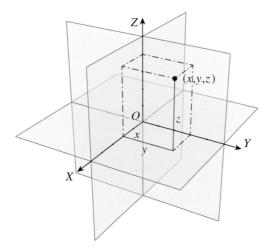

Figure 6-3 • Euclidean coordinate system with x, y, and z axes denoting 3-dimensional space.

Table 6-1	EXAMPLES OF COMMON GEOMETRIC TRANSFORMATIONS		
Transformation	Definition	Maintains	Example
Translation	Every point moves by the same distance in a given direction.	Orientation	▲ → ▲
Rigid (Euclidean)	Preserves Euclidian distance between all points. Includes rotation, reflection, or a combination of both.	Length	↗ → ↖ → ↘
Affine	Maintains collinearity of points and the ratio of distances between points. Includes expansion, dilation, and shear.	Parallelism	▢ → ▱
Projective transformation	Maps lines to lines without preserving parallelism.	Straight lines	▱ → ⏢

Note: A transformation maintains the characteristics of the transformations that are listed below it as well (eg, translation maintains orientation *and* length, parallelism, and straight lines).

Adapted from Szeliski R. *Computer Vision: Algorithms and Applications (Texts in Computer Science series)*. Springer; 2011, Table 2.1.

Image Resolution

Locations in the image plane are often described in terms of pixel (picture element) coordinates, placing the image on a grid with a fixed scale, or resolution. The resolution of 2D digital images can be described by the number of pixels in width by the height. Thus, commonly used descriptions of the resolution of digital images (particularly video) include 720p or 1080p, which refers to images that are 1280 × 720 pixels and 1920 × 1080 pixels, respectively. Originally, resolutions would match the size of the image sensor. Since an image is captured by a camera, the 3D image is mapped into 2 dimensions by the image sensor. However, images are often resized for a variety of reasons, such as ease of view or processing. The greater the number of pixels, the "higher definition" or more closely a digital image can represent its intended scene, object, or person. Of course, greater pixel density also means there is more information to store, so the file size of images with more pixels is larger.

The position of a given pixel is most commonly reported in the form of pixel coordinates (x, y), with $(0, 0)$ representing the top left corner.

Therefore, when images undergo semantic or pixel-wise segmentation (see later section "Semantic Segmentation"), the location of an annotation is communicated through pixel coordinates.

Video Frames

Each video is composed of a series of still images, of which a single image is referred to as a video frame. A video will also have a frame rate that is reported in frames per second (fps). The most common frame rates are 24, 25, and 30 fps, with most surgical video systems recording at 25 or 30 fps. Due to conventions in broadcast television and playback used internationally, North American video systems typically record at 30 fps (National Television System Committee standard), whereas European systems typically record at 25 fps.

For video, the aspect ratio (AR) is often reported. The AR simply refers to the ratio of a video's width to height. The "standard," or traditional, AR is 4:3, whereas the more modern or widescreen AR is 16:9. The AR is derived from the resolution. Thus, 480p video (720 × 480 pixels) is considered standard definition, whereas 720p and higher resolution video is considered high definition. As with any still image, a video frame's pixel positions are characterized by pixel coordinates.

Color

The simplest image form is that of a binary image composed of pixels that are either black (1) or white (0). These images are often sufficient to represent the outline or general shape of an image. Grayscale images further increase the amount of information available by providing a scale of 256 shades of gray ranging from 0 (black) to 255 (white). Both binary and grayscale images are considered monochromatic (ie, they are composed of shades of one color). However, not all monochromatic images are grayscale because images can be composed of monochromes in different colors. In fact, most color images are created through a combination of 3 bands of monochromatic images—red, green, and blue (RGB). Color images thus contain greater information with 256 shades (or greater) per each of the 3 colors.

Color can be reported in bits, where 1 bit is the amount of information held for a binary digit. Thus, 1 bit (2^1) can store 2 colors (black and white), 8 bits (2^8) 256 colors, and 24 bits (2^{24}) 16,777,216 colors. Although higher bit color images exist, 24-bit color is considered "true color" because the human retina is estimated to be able to discern 10 million colors. Finally, some images will have an extra 8 bits for the alpha channel, which stores information on the opacity of a color. Thus a 32-bit image is 24 bits for color and 8 bits for the alpha channel.

IMAGE PROCESSING

While geometric transformations were introduced earlier as a type of image processing, additional types of processing can be applied to further manipulate an image. Many of these processes, such as adjustment of brightness and contrast and application of filters, are common even outside of computer vision because they are commonly used to adjust photographs and videos (eg, Instagram, Adobe Photoshop Lightroom, Apple iMovie). Aside from beautifying an image, these processes are also helpful in optimizing results that can be obtained from computer vision studies.

Point Operations

Point operations are image transformations in which the output of a pixel's value is dependent only on that pixel's input value. Thus, point operations include adjustments in brightness/contrast (ie, bias and gain) and color correction (ie, adjustments to intensity, hue, and saturation). These point operations can be conducted globally to make adjustments across an entire image, such as when one manually adjusts the brightness slider on an image, or they can be performed in an optimized manner specific to the particular image (eg, the auto adjust setting on photograph applications such as Google Photos). Optimization techniques vary, but a commonly used set of methods is histogram equalization, where pixel values are plotted across the whole image in a histogram and values are subsequently adjusted based on the overall distribution of values (Figure 6-4). Such adjustments can be made globally across an entire image or in a locally adaptive manner with the whole image divided into sections for subsequent equalization. Locally adaptive histogram equalization is no longer considered a point operation but rather a local or neighborhood operation where the value of surrounding pixels plays a role in determining the pixel's final output after transformation.[3]

Filters

Histogram equalization techniques are helpful in normalizing images for subsequent use in machine learning. For example, a data set of an operative video of laparoscopic cholecystectomy can have a wide range of pixel

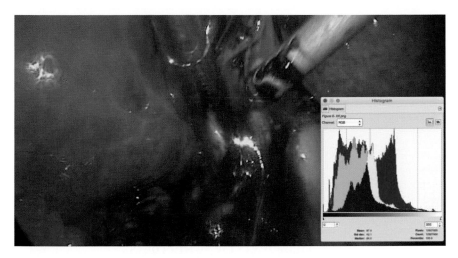

Figure 6-4 • Example of an RGB (red, green, and blue) histogram on a surgical image.

intensity values based on the white balance of the laparoscopic camera, the light intensity, and the resolution, among other factors. Normalization of values across the entire data set can yield more uniform training on the data set that is less susceptible to noise from any issues inherent to video or image capture quality. This leads us to a discussion on the use of filters in image processing.

Filters act to adjust images at the local level, with adjustments made to a pixel based on surrounding pixel information. These local operations can be used to denoise, sharpen, blur, or otherwise modify specific sections or an entire image. As with any image manipulation, it is important to recall that the modifications are not simply visual changes that one sees in an image; rather, underlying changes to the numerical values describing each pixel are occurring. For example, in the case of linear filters, a small matrix ω, known as a kernel or mask, is convolved with the matrix that represents an image of interest. Although a deep dive into matrix mathematics is outside the scope of this book, recall that a convolution is a mathematical operation that expresses how 2 functions modify each other's shape. Thus, in the case of an image, a convolution determines the value of a pixel by considering the weighted values of all of its neighboring pixels (Figure 6-5). For example, a "blur" filter can be applied by taking an average pixel color of neighboring pixels (within that matrix of pixels) and applying it to a target pixel to smoothen aspects of an image. Although filters are used at a consumer level to modify photographs and videos, they can also be applied by neural networks to assist in image analysis, as described later in this chapter.

29	40	14
51	32	17
49	22	13

A

*

0	1	0
0	0	0
0	0	0

B

=

29*0	40*1	14*0
51*0	32*0	17*0
49*0	22*0	13*0

C

=

	40	

D

Figure 6-5 • Simplified illustration of image convolution of an image matrix (**A**) by kernel ω (**B**). The green box represents the central pixel under manipulation in the convolution, whereas matrix **C** represents the intermediate calculation of each pixel and matrix **D** is the resulting value of the central pixel. ω is then moved along to the next pixel, and the process is repeated for all pixels.

▮ FEATURE DETECTION AND DESCRIPTORS

With a basic understanding of filters, one can understand how feature detection can be accomplished on digital images. As introduced in Chapters 3 and 4, features are attributes in the data that can be used to assist in modeling. In images, features can be components of an object or scene (eg, the vertical edges of a water bottle) or a composite of components that describe a point of interest in an image (eg, the ears of a dog, the peak of a mountain). Think of a jigsaw puzzle. How does one go about determining which pieces go together where? Most commonly, people will look for key features like corners, edges, and colors to help determine how the pieces come together into a recognizable image. The specific feature's points of interest will change depending on the task at hand (Figure 6-6). Similarly, information about the feature points is often described as a high-dimensional vector that captures the "essence" of what this feature point looks like.

There are numerous available algorithms to achieve feature detection and description, and the use of each depends on the particular interests and experience of the investigator(s). For example, the Harris corner and Shi-Tomasi corner detectors are designed to, as their names suggest, detect corners in images. Scale-invariant feature transform (SIFT) and speeded up robust features (SURF) are 2 local feature detectors. Their design comes from careful analysis of what are considered nuisance factors in the task of object and scene recognition and a choice of features that is invariant to transformations; for example, the keypoint measures and the feature descriptors are selected to be invariant to scale changes, rotation, translation, and other transforms. Finally, it is worth noting that, as in many other computer vision tasks, novel descriptors take a learned approach.[4]

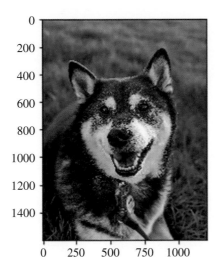

Figure 6-6 • Example of feature detection in a photograph of a dog.

Edge and Texture Detection

Edges in an image divide 2 adjacent sections of an image, such as separating one object from another. That is, there is a transition in the value of adjacent pixels to denote a transition from one object to another (or from an object to the background). Thus, it is possible to use convolutions to measure the weights of surrounding pixels to determine whether an edge exists in a given portion of an image. As an example of how this works, consider the Sobel filter, which is a 3×3 kernel designed to detect either horizontal or vertical edges (Figure 6-7). This filter can be convolved with a target image to detect edges that can assist with further computer vision tasks such as image classification, localization, and semantic segmentation (Figure 6-8).

1	2	1
0	0	0
−1	−2	−1

A

1	0	−1
2	0	−2
1	0	−1

B

Figure 6-7 • (**A**) demonstrates a horizontal Sobel filter, whereas (**B**) demonstrates a vertical Sobel filter to detect edges. These filters are convolved over a target image.

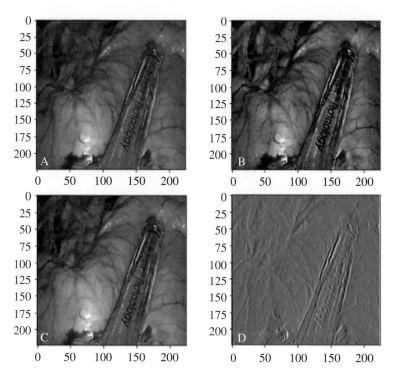

Figure 6-8 • Demonstration of the application of Sobel filters to detect edges in an image.

Edge detection has been incorporated in a number of different types of algorithms dating back decades. For example, the Canny edge detection algorithm, developed in the 1980s, works by considering edges detected by changes in intensity of pixels; however, this approach only considers local data from neighboring pixels without the overall "macro" view of the entire image. More recent approaches have used deep learning to accomplish edge detection and subsequently object detection, as detailed in later sections of this chapter.

For images, texture refers to the perceived surface quality of an object. If thinking about texture from a structural perspective, texture is created from a set of texels, or a set unit of elements defining a given structure, that is repeated to create a pattern. The size and character of texels can vary based on the texture being represented. For example, representing sand requires a finer granularity than representing texture like a jar of marbles. The regularity (or lack thereof) of the pattern can also vary (eg, bricks are quite regular). For many images, identifying a texel may be difficult if patterns are not regular (eg, wood grain). Therefore, in most modern computer vision applications, approaches to texture detection are centered around detecting edges from pixels. The density and direction of pixels can provide information about the given texture of a surface, and differences in texture can help distinguish different objects within an image.[5]

Feature Detection in Video

Feature detection in video is not fundamentally different from that of images. Differences arise in the way that these features are detected and tracked over time because video is a series of images that are rapidly displayed over time. Algorithms can be used to track simple features such as color over time to track objects that may move across a video. More effective but complex algorithms can track objects or locations within a video based on techniques such as matching features in different frames of a video or estimating optical flow (ie, the apparent motion of an object that is perceived by changes in position of that object or the camera in 2 consecutive frames).

MULTIPLE VIEW GEOMETRY AND 3-DIMENSIONAL SPACE

In many cases, we need to reason about 3D scenes from 2D camera images. It is important to consider the frame of reference to which objects in a scene are placed because, unlike a 2D image, the "view" may change depending on the perspective of the viewer. A world-coordinate frame of reference considers the coordinate system of the overall scene and where objects are within that coordinate system with x_w, y_w, z_w coordinates. An object-coordinate frame of reference considers a point of interest relative to a reference object in the 3D image (eg, the orientation of the key relative to the keyhole in the door), whereas a camera-coordinate frame represents objects relative to the location of the camera (Figure 6-9). Each of these coordinate frames is actually present in real life as we interact with objects. The world- and object-coordinate frames of reference reflect our environment, and the camera-coordinate frame reflects our perception of our 3D environment. These frames are transformed and translated progressively into a captured image that can be either 2D or 3D, with pixel coordinates representing the final 2D frame of reference.[6]

This joint 3D representation of the image and scene allows us to explain the image formation and extend it to the case of multiple images from either consecutive camera frames or separate cameras. These are useful either for systems with multiple cameras or for analyzing video feeds.[7] The

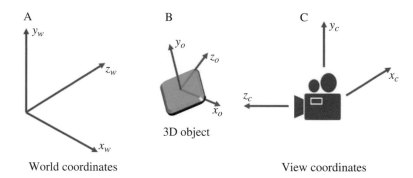

Figure 6-9 • A demonstrates a world-coordinate frame of reference, **B** demonstrates an object-coordinate frame of reference, and **C** demonstrates a camera-coordinate frame of reference. 3D, 3-dimensional.

relationship between the multiple viewpoints, as well as other cues, allows us to reconstruct 3D measurements and reason about 3D object shapes and sizes, as well as understand the position of the camera, a process that has its roots in mapmaking and photogrammetry.[8,9] In addition, the geometrical reasoning allows us to easily match objects and keypoints between different images, lending itself to understanding and tracking parts of the scene. Many of the operations involving multiple view geometry, such as transforming 3D world coordinates into 2D image coordinates, are often formalized via homogeneous coordinates, making many of the mathematical operators easier to express and compute.[10]

▌IMAGE COMPRESSION

In any discussion of digital images, a brief word on image compression is necessary to familiarize readers with the major topics associated with compression (reduction in the size of data) of images and video. Lossless compression methods, in which the original form of the image can be reconstructed perfectly from the compressed file, are preferred for situations, such as medical images, where preservation of fidelity is of utmost importance. Lossy compression methods introduce noise into the original files; however, they result in significantly smaller file sizes (Table 6-2).

Video codecs perform the compression and decompression of video (codec is derived from a combination of *encoder* and *decoder*). Video content can be bundled together with audio within a container of multimedia data. The container (eg, MP4, FLV, WMV, MOV) merely serves to store the data within a file. Therefore, file types do not necessarily provide information on the actual codec used for a video.

Table 6-2	EXAMPLES OF COMMON LOSSLESS AND LOSSY FORMATS	
	Lossless Formats	**Lossy Formats**
Audio	WAV, AIFF	MPEG3, AAC, AC3
Image	PNG, TIFF	JPEG, GIF
Video	H.264 Lossless, H.265 Lossless	H.264 Lossy, MPEG4[a]

[a]MPEG4 is a case where both lossless and lossy compression are possible because the standards for MPEG4 allow for lossless compression.

CLASSIFICATION AND SEGMENTATION OF IMAGES

With a basic understanding of the construction and processing of digital images, we can now begin to approach the various types of tasks typically assigned to computer vision. Some of the most common tasks revolve around the detection of objects (including people and animals) in images. Image classification is perhaps the simplest form of these detection tasks, where a model is asked to simply classify an image as having or not having an object of interest. Object detection extends the classification one step further and localizes where on an image an object is likely to be (most commonly through use of a bounding box). Object detection can be further defined to include segmentation, where the target object boundaries are indicated by highlighting the specific pixels that correspond to that object (as opposed to using more general bounding boxes). Segmentation has been its own large field of research (eg, in medical imaging modalities such as computed tomography and magnetic resonance imaging) based on the clear definition of objects in various imaging modalities and how they translate to clear mathematical definitions.[11,12] Finally, instance segmentation refers to highlighting of the pixels of multiple objects of the same target class such that each instance of the object is identified separately on the same image (Figure 6-10).

There are many potential methodologies to apply computer vision for improving the quality and safety of surgical care, and we will discuss a few examples throughout the rest of the chapter. Although traditional machine learning techniques can and have been applied to surgical research, the vast majority of applications are currently using deep-learning methods. Thus, we will focus on building a basic understanding of how deep neural network architectures have paved the way to give algorithms the means to identify objects and scenes throughout the operating room and make clinically meaningful inferences.

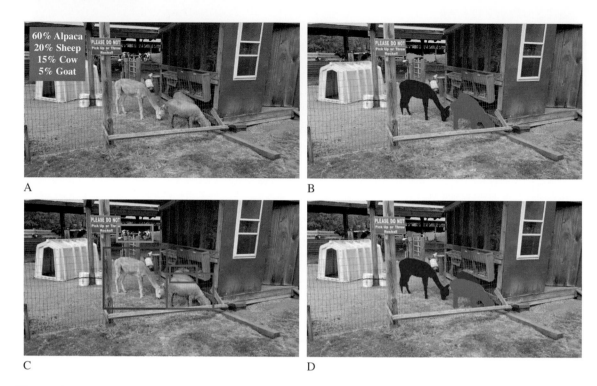

Figure 6-10 • Illustration of the differences in (**A**) image classification, (**B**) semantic segmentation, (**C**) object detection, and (**D**) instance segmentation.

Chapter 4 provided an overview of deep learning and described deep neural networks as the basis for some of the latest advancements in machine learning. Deep neural networks are extremely "data hungry," and their ability to develop a digital footprint that corresponds to a specific output (eg, identification of a specific object) can best be accomplished by providing it with large sets of variations and instances. Through repeated iterations of forward propagation and backpropagation, the network adjusts and fine-tunes its connections in order to minimize the cost function (ie, the discrepancy between the predicted and actual results). The recent widespread on-demand availability of images and videos in the digital era has led to tremendous and accelerated advancements in the field of computer vision and the ability to develop algorithms that are capable of human-level object detection.

Deep neural networks whose objective is to identify spatial data are largely dependent on using convolutions (hence, the term convolutional neural network [CNN]). Conceptually, using CNNs for object recognition is analogous to a flashlight sliding across an image in a dark room, whereby subcomponent features of the image are identified until sense is made of the entire image. As briefly introduced in Chapter 4 and earlier in this chapter,

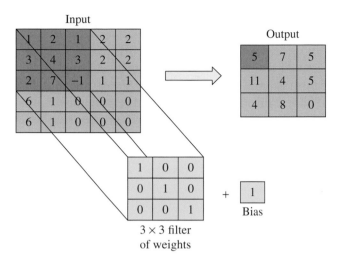

Figure 6-11 • Visualization of a 3 × 3 convolutional filter operating on a 5 × 5-sized input producing an output of size 3 × 3.

a convolution is a mathematical operation describing the combination of 2 functions in order to produce a third function. For image recognition, a convolutional matrix, or "kernel" (small $n \times n$ matrix of pixels that represents a specific localized portion of the image and their associated weights; Figure 6-11), is applied to the entire data set, by sliding pixel by pixel. Kernels run a mathematical function for every matrix of pixels in that particular image, producing a single output for each matrix to create a modified view of the data—a process photo applications and smartphones similarly use to apply filters for images. By using kernels, the neural network can make sense of pixels—not as individuals in their own positions, but as groups of neighboring pixels—thereby allowing it to find patterns in images and videos. In deep learning for image recognition, the original pixels in an image run through multiple filters, and at each stage, the data are condensed, where the deepest layers of the neural network contain increasingly fewer neurons.

Many different types of filters and functions have been developed, allowing for the identification of various image features (eg, edges, contrast, circles, etc.). Each layer of computation in a neural network uses mathematical operations to extract features of increasing complexity with the goal of identifying a digital pattern that represents target objects or scenes. This is critical because in order to recognize a particular target, a robust network must be able to account for many different variations. For instance, if the purpose is to develop facial recognition software, the network needs to account for various alterations in the subject's facial appearance (eg, different hairstyle, facial expression, ambient light, background, angle and position of face).

Image Classification

Perhaps the most common computer vision task is that of image classification, where an algorithm is trained to be able to label a set of images with a particular category. Image classification algorithms have shown very promising early results with significant potential applications in medicine, such as for screening and diagnostic purposes. For example, using a large data set of 128,000 retinal images, Gulshan et al[13] developed and validated a CNN that is capable of detecting diabetic retinopathy. Their algorithm demonstrated very high sensitivity and specificity for detecting signs of diabetic retinopathy as well as macular edema with subsequent suggestions to make an appropriate referral to an ophthalmologist. Similarly, Esteva et al[14] published the results of a CNN capable of making diagnostic predictions comparable to expert dermatologists using single images of skin lesions. In their study, they used a Google Inception v3 architecture that was pretrained on the ImageNet data set and subsequently trained it on a data set of approximately 130,000 skin lesions. More recently, a Google-funded study evaluated the performance of an algorithm to identify cancerous breast lesions on mammograms. In this paper, the investigators demonstrated the potential to use deep learning and computer vision to decrease the false-positive and false-negative rates to decrease the workload on radiologists.[15] In surgery, image classification can be done to identify specific phases, steps, and actions that occur during an operation or to identify time points of particular events of interest (eg, bleeding or other complications). In this context, deep learning can be used to review surgical videos and intraoperative events for quality improvement and improving surgical performance. This will be covered in more detail in Chapters 7 and 11.

Instance Detection

When designing an algorithm whose task is to localize an object within images or videos, we can either broadly include an entire class of that specific object (class detection) or more specifically detect "instances" of a particular object within a scene. An instance is a subcategory of a particular object (eg, detecting and localizing red cars instead of just cars). The localization of objects has traditionally been done using bounding boxes and labels as an output of either neural networks or other techniques such as visual search.

Although the simplest way to do this is by sliding a kernel across the entire image and running a CNN for every single one (sliding window technique), this is highly computationally expensive and impractical. To overcome this, a variety of methodologies have been developed over the past decade to improve the efficiency and accuracy of computer vision for object detection. The concepts behind the newer object detection techniques is to expand on the use of CNNs by designing a network that is capable of identifying regions of interest (ROIs) within an image and then using the same principles of image classification to determine whether or not the ROI represents a target object. Initially, region-based CNNs (R-CNNs) and their derivative Fast R-CNNs were developed to identify ROIs for focused assessment to identify and classify a particular object.[16,17] Although these techniques have better processing speed than the sliding window technique, the generation of proposed ROIs is nevertheless time consuming for modern applications of object detection and tracking. Faster R-CNN is a more modern incarnation of the R-CNN family and uses a region proposal network module.[18,19] This single unified network scans every location of an image to determine where further processing needs to be carried out to predict the probability of the presence of an object. Faster R-CNN significantly reduces processing time to near real time with high accuracy (in one example, Faster R-CNN performed 38% faster than Fast R-CNN).[18]

More efficient techniques have been developed by avoiding multiple subnetworks such as those in the R-CNN family, which tend to work in isolation. These new techniques include models called You Only Look Once (YOLO), Single Shot Multibox Detector (SSD), and Region-Based Fully Convolutional Networks (R-FCN). YOLO and its new versions YOLOv3 and YOLOv4, use a single end-to-end trained network that offers exceptional processing speed with real-time performance but at the expense of lower predictive accuracy.[20,21] The input image is split into a grid, and each cell within that grid provides a prediction probability for a prespecified number of bounding boxes. This produces a class probability map that is merged with the bounding boxes into a final output of bounding boxes with class labels. Because the entire pipeline uses only a single network (unlike the R-CNN family with multiple subnetworks), it is much more computationally efficient. Nevertheless, the model learns very general representations of objects.

▌ SEMANTIC SEGMENTATION

Semantic segmentation is a process whereby clusters of pixels in an image can be grouped and subsequently labeled or classified. In contrast to bounding boxes, classification of the object and detection of its existence are performed in addition to delineating exact boundaries. This can be highly desirable in medical applications, where the identification of objects does not always seem to fit or provide clinically meaningful information

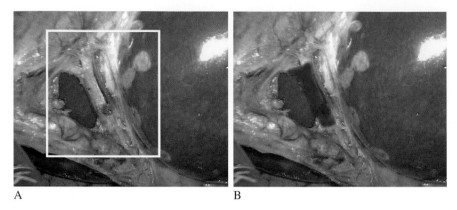

A   B

Figure 6-12 • (**A**) Image of the hepatocystic triangle with a bounding box meant to denote the cystic artery; however, the box overlaps with the cystic duct and other elements of the hepatocystic triangle. (**B**) Image of the hepatocystic triangle with a segment mask over the cystic artery only.

within a bounding box that is cluttered with background noise (Figure 6-12A). The general paradigm to segment images applies a CNN architecture to make dense pixel-wise predictions in order to generate segmentation "maps" that delineate objects at the pixel level. These maps are actually called segment masks. The masks are, similar to kernels described previously, small matrices that are designed to detect the specific objects of interest and highlight those pixels with an overlay (Figure 6-12B).

To improve efficiency, the original image resolution is down-sampled for pixel-wise prediction and up-sampled for learning within the network. When this is done with fully convolutional networks (FCNs), segmentation maps can end up coarse and inaccurate due to the loss of data during the pooling process. Nevertheless, this approach provides the means to generate segmentation maps within images. SegNet uses a similar approach using max pooling and an encoder-decoder architecture, paired with a pixel-wise classification layer.[22] Another very common architecture in the encoder-decoder family is U-Net, initially proposed by Ronneberger et al,[23] which has been used for semantic segmentation in medical imaging.

Instance Segmentation

Instance segmentation attempts to detect all objects within an image while providing pixel-wise segmentation of each instance. It expands on semantic segmentation by partitioning different instances within a class (eg, identifying 4 different pedestrians using different colors to differentiate them). This requires more complex tasks than simply computing the probability of whether an object or particular state is present within an image. Instance segmentation has largely been enabled by the Mask R-CNN architecture, initially published by Facebook AI Research.[24] This method extends Faster R-CNN by adding an FCN branch that runs in parallel and outputs a mask for every ROI for predicting whether or not a pixel is part of an object in a binary fashion (hence, a binary mask). Once these masks are generated, they are output along with the classified bounding boxes from the Faster R-CNN to produce semantic segmentation of various objects and instances, with very little added computational cost to the Faster R-CNN algorithm.

Although semantic segmentation and instance segmentation have not been used as widely as image classification and object detection using bounding boxes in medicine, early results are very promising. Their benefits are especially pronounced for computer vision tasks that require the identification of objects with high precision, where the target object cannot be identified within a bounding box without also including background noise. As a result, the use of semantic segmentation becomes a highly desirable task for fulfilling an unmet need, and this is especially true for the identification of structures in a surgical field. Object detection in a surgical field needs to be precise in order to provide any meaningful information in a background of fatty and fibrous tissues and other organs. This can often only be done through pixel-wise segmentation of objects. One such example is with tool tracking, which will be covered in greater detail in Chapter 7. More challenging yet is the identification of target anatomy and structures that are blended in their environment and often do not have precise boundaries unlike surgical tools that can be easily distinguished from their surrounding environment. Madani et al[25] recently used a pyramid scene parsing network, which consists of a CNN encoder-decoder architecture followed by a pyramid pooling module, to segment important anatomic structures during a laparoscopic cholecystectomy. This model was able to identify critical structures with real-time performance, while providing advice on where to dissect ("GO Zone" = safe to dissect) and where not to dissect ("NO-GO Zone" = dangerous area of dissection that can lead to complications). Future research will apply these models in the operating room to determine their effect on patient outcomes and surgical performance.

SURGICAL PHASE AND STEP RECOGNITION

In addition to classification of specific objects within images, images themselves can be classified into temporal elements. That is, a video can be segmented into component parts. Operations can be represented as high-level phases (eg, access, closure) composed of low-level steps (eg, bowel anastomosis) that are further subdivided into tasks (eg, suturing). Algorithms may be designed to recognize any of these categories with the goal of automatically identifying surgical steps for surgical phase recognition.[26]

Classical machine learning (ie, non–neural network based) approaches to surgical phase or step recognition generally divide the task into 2 steps: first, representing the videos, including possible substeps of normalization and sequencing, and second, classifying the representations into surgical phases.

Video representation can be accomplished in many ways. Generally, surgical videos are first preprocessed to remove irrelevant information such as camera motion or zoom variation. This normalization process may be accomplished in a surgery-specific manner, such as tracking the pupil of the eye to register the coordinate system in cataract surgery videos,[27] or through more generic methods, such as segmenting video sequences into subsequences. This may be done by using the presence or absence of surgical tools to distinguish "action" (ie, clinically relevant) from "idle" (ie, clinically irrelevant) clips.[28] In other cases, a "sliding window" of frame sequences may be used. Once the relevant sequence of preprocessed frames has been identified, many methods are available to represent the visual data, including motion histograms based on optical flow[29]; the bag-of-visual-worlds method, which condenses extracted visual features such as color and texture into a dictionary of learned vector representations[30]; spatiotemporal polynomial basis sets[30,31]; and latent Dirichlet analysis.[32] As Volkov et al[30] note, the choice of data representation is key, especially when the amount of training data is limited. Ideally, the number of features should be kept small to reduce overfitting, while the expressiveness of the features should be maximized in order to include the information necessary to achieve high performance.

To achieve automated identification of surgical steps, the previously discussed approaches of using the training data to associate visual features with operative step labels is a popular option.[31] However, an operation is not defined by one image per step. Rather, an operation is composed of a series of actions that occur over time to create an operative step (ie, driving a needle through tissue, throwing the loops of a knot, and cutting excess suture are actions that compose the step of "suturing"). Thus, approaches such as hidden Markov models (HMMs) and long short-term memory (LSTM) rely on modeling the temporal evolution of the surgery and using some information on preceding surgical steps to inform the prediction of the current step.[27,28] The temporal models have routinely been combined with visual feature-based machine learning classification of steps to improve results.[30] A third common approach is content-based video retrieval, which uses a distance metric to measure the similarity of the current video to annotated examples from an archive of previous surgeries and uses the labels of the most similar annotated clips to determine the classification.[27]

More recent work has demonstrated the potential for neural networks to recognize surgical phases with greater accuracy than classical methods, although with the cost of high computational power demands. Significant performance gains on computer vision tasks have been demonstrated with deep learning. Twinanda et al[33] used a CNN architecture called EndoNet to simultaneously detect tools and recognize phases within laparoscopic cholecystectomy videos. Including a tool detection step in the CNN training process was found to increase performance on phase recognition. The CNN output was fed into a support vector machine classifier to generate confidence values for each phase, which were then fed into a hierarchical HMM to incorporate temporal relations. Hashimoto et al[34] described SleeveNet, a method of automatically identifying phases in laparoscopic sleeve gastrectomy using a combination of a residual neural network to process visual features and LSTM to incorporate temporal cues.

CONCLUSION

Computer vision is a field that has started to be applied to surgical research in applications such as automated identification of tools, anatomic structures, and operative steps. By combining the knowledge you have gained from this chapter with the knowledge gained in Chapters 3 and 4 on machine learning and deep learning, you should have the fundamental building blocks with which to learn more about the breadth of research being conducted at the intersection of surgery and computer vision.

REFERENCES

1. Marr D, Poggio T. A computational theory of human stereo vision. *Proc R Soc Lond B Biol. Sci.* 1979;204:301-328.
2. Grill-Spector K, Malach R. The human visual cortex. *Annu Rev Neurosci.* 2004;27:649-677.
3. Szeliski R. *Computer Vision: Algorithms and Applications (Texts in Computer Science Series).* Springer; 2011.
4. Kumar BGV, Carneiro G, Reid I. Learning local image descriptors with deep Siamese and triplet convolutional networks by minimizing global loss functions. Accessed October 5, 2020. https://ieeexplore.ieee.org/document/7780950.
5. Rao R. Computer vision (UW CSE 455). Accessed October 5, 2020. https://courses.cs.washington.edu/courses/cse455/09wi/.

6. University of Nevada. CS491E/791E: Computer Vision. Accessed October 5, 2020. https://www.cse.unr.edu/~bebis/CS791E/.

7. Ullman S. The interpretation of structure from motion. *Proc R Soc Lond B Biol Sci.* 1979;203:405-426.

8. The ISP Commission. IV programme for Helsinki. *Photogrammetria.* 1976; 32:26-28.

9. Agarwal S, Snavely N, Simon I, Seitz SM, Szeliski R. Building Rome in a day. 2009 IEEE 12th International Conference on Computer Vision. Accessed October 5, 2020. http://grail.cs.washington.edu/rome/rome_paper.pdf.

10. Hartley R, Zisserman A. *Multiple View Geometry in Computer Vision.* Cambridge University Press; 2004.

11. Guyader CL, Le Guyader C, Gout C. Geodesic active contour under geometrical conditions: theory and 3D applications. *Numer Algorith.* 2008;48:105-133.

12. Kimmel R. *Numerical Geometry of Images: Theory, Algorithms, and Applications.* Springer Science & Business Media; 2012.

13. Gulshan V, Peng L, Coram M, et al. Development and validation of a deep learning algorithm for detection of diabetic retinopathy in retinal fundus photographs. *JAMA.* 2016;316:2402-2410.

14. Esteva A, Kuprel B, Novoa RA, et al. Dermatologist-level classification of skin cancer with deep neural networks. *Nature.* 2017;542:115-118.

15. McKinney SM, Sieniek M, Godbole V, et al. International evaluation of an AI system for breast cancer screening. *Nature.* 2020;577:89-94.

16. Uijlings JRR, van de Sande KEA, Gevers T, Smeulders AWM. Selective search for object recognition. *Int J Comput Vis.* 2013;104:154-171.

17. Girshick R, Donahue J, Darrell T, Malik J. Rich feature hierarchies for accurate object detection and semantic segmentation. 2014 IEEE Conference on Computer Vision and Pattern Recognition. Accessed October 5, 2020. https://arxiv.org/abs/1311.2524.

18. Ren S, He K, Girshick R, Sun J. Faster R-CNN: towards real-time object detection with region proposal networks. *IEEE Trans Pattern Anal Mach Intell.* 2017;39:1137-1149.

19. Shih K-H, Chiu C-T, Pu Y-Y. Real-time object detection via pruning and a concatenated multi-feature assisted region proposal network. 2019 IEEE International Conference on Acoustics, Speech and Signal Processing (ICASSP). Accessed October 5, 2020. https://ieeexplore.ieee.org/document/8683842.

20. Redmon J, Divvala S, Girshick R, Farhadi A. You only look once: unified, real-time object detection. 2016 IEEE Conference on Computer Vision and Pattern Recognition (CVPR). Accessed October 5, 2020. https://arxiv.org/abs/1506.02640.

21. Shaifee MJ, Chywl B, Li F, Wong A. Fast YOLO: a fast you only look once system for real-time embedded object detection in video. Accessed October 5, 2020. https://arxiv.org/abs/1709.05943.

22. Badrinarayanan V, Kendall A, Cipolla R. SegNet: a deep convolutional encoder-decoder architecture for image segmentation. *IEEE Trans Pattern Anal Mach Intell.* 2017;39(12):2481-2495.

23. Ronneberger O, Fischer P, Brox T. U-Net: convolutional networks for biomedical image segmentation. Accessed October 5, 2020. https://arxiv.org/abs/1505.04597.

24. He K, Gkioxari G, Dollar P, Girshick R. Mask R-CNN. *IEEE Trans Pattern Anal Mach Intell.* 2020;42:386-397.

25. Madani A, Namazi B, Altieri M, et al. Artificial intelligence for intraoperative guidance: using semantic segmentation to identify surgical anatomy during laparoscopic cholecystectomy. Annals of Surgery. 2020. Accepted for publication.

26. Forestier G, Riffaud L, Jannin P. Automatic phase prediction from low-level surgical activities. *Int J Comput Assist Radiol Surg.* 2015;10:833-841.

27. Quellec G, Lamard M, Cochener B, Cazuguel G. Real-time segmentation and recognition of surgical tasks in cataract surgery videos. *IEEE Trans Med Imaging.* 2014;33:2352-2360.

28. Charriere K, Quellec G, Lamard M, et al. Real-time multilevel sequencing of cataract surgery videos. In: *2016 14th International Workshop on Content-Based Multimedia Indexing (CBMI).* IEEE; 2016:1-6.

29. Charrière K, Quellec G, Lamard M, et al. Automated surgical step recognition in normalized cataract surgery videos. *Annu Int Conf IEEE Eng Med Biol Soc.* 2014;2014:4647-4650.

30. Volkov M, Hashimoto DA, Rosman G, Meireles OR, Rus D. Machine learning and coresets for automated real-time video segmentation of laparoscopic and robot-assisted surgery. Accessed October 5, 2020. https://ieeexplore.ieee.org/document/7989093.

31. Quellec G, Lamard M, Cochener B, Cazuguel G. Real-time task recognition in cataract surgery videos using adaptive spatiotemporal polynomials. *IEEE Trans Med Imaging.* 2015;34:877-887.

32. Tran DT, Sakurai R, Yamazoe H, Lee JH. Phase segmentation methods for an automatic surgical workflow analysis. *Int J Biomed Imaging.* 2017;2017:1985796.

33. Twinanda AP, Shehata S, Mutter D, et al. EndoNet: a deep architecture for recognition tasks on laparoscopic videos. *IEEE Trans Med Imaging.* 2017;36:86-97.

34. Hashimoto DA, et al. Computer vision analysis of intraoperative video: automated recognition of operative steps in laparoscopic sleeve gastrectomy. *Ann Surg.* 2019;270:414-421.

ARTIFICIAL INTELLIGENCE FOR SURGICAL EDUCATION AND INTRAOPERATIVE ANALYSIS

7

Babak Namazi, Venkat Devarajan, and Ganesh Sankaranarayanan

HIGHLIGHTS

- Three major areas of surgical training in which artificial intelligence is being explored include intraoperative feedback, postoperative analysis, and simulation training.

- The use of artificial intelligence for surgical training attempts to overcome limitations of manual assessment, namely that manual assessment can be very time consuming and expensive and that manual assessment is inherently subjective because it relies on raters observing and evaluating performance.

- Automated assessment can be performed by replicating well-validated manual scoring systems and then augmenting those systems with quantitative metrics of performance captured by sensors.

INTRODUCTION

Surgery is a complex task that involves both technical and decision-making skills. Acquiring surgical competence is critical for ensuring an optimal outcome. A systematic review of the incidence of adverse events during surgery has shown it to be over 14.4%, and 14% of these adverse events were either fatal or severe. Preventable adverse events were present in 5.2% of the cases, highlighting the role of surgical expertise in reducing the potentially avoidable harm to patients' health.[1]

Gaining surgical competence is a lengthy, multifaceted process that takes many years to complete.[2] Surgical residency programs in North America, of which the current model was originally inspired by Halsted and later Churchill as a structured apprenticeship model, involve immersing surgical trainees in a clinical environment under graduated supervision. Over time, the training methodology has evolved to include simulation-based training,[3] establishment of skills laboratories in residency programs, and the development of a national skills curriculum jointly by the American College of Surgeons (ACS) and the Association for Program Directors in Surgery (APDS). The ACS/APDS curriculum consists of 3 phases: (1) basic/core skills and tasks, (2) advanced procedures, and (3) team-based training.[4] Surgical education has benefited tremendously from recent advances in technology, such as artificial intelligence (AI), computer vision, and virtual/augmented reality. Some of the most common applications of this technology in surgical training include the following:

- Intraoperative feedback: As one of the most powerful teaching tools, objective feedback during the operation can significantly help the residents learn the technical skills through real-time performance assessment.
- Postoperative analysis: Recorded videos from the operation can be a valuable educational resource.
- Simulation training: Skills can be developed by training on various types of simulators such as benchtop part-task trainers, full procedural simulators on a cadaver, or virtual reality–based surgical trainers.

To take full advantage of any of these methods, the performance of the trainee needs to be evaluated based on some proficiency criteria.[5] For this purpose, several scoring systems have been developed for assessment. For instance, the Objective Structured Assessment of Technical Skills (OSATS)[6] is a widely used evaluation tool and has been extensively studied and validated for the manual grading of surgical skills in the operating room for different procedures.[7] The OSATS global rating scale is based on the cumulative performance score on 7 domains using a 5-point Likert scale: (1) respect for tissue, (2) time and motion, (3) instrument handling, (4) knowledge of instruments, (5) the flow of operation, (6) use of assistants, and (7) knowledge of the specific procedure. Although the maximum possible global rating is 35 points, there is no validated score for minimum competency. Rather, this score is used to compare performance across groups of individuals (eg, novice vs experienced trainees) and forms the bedrock for much of the literature in surgical education. However, use of OSATS requires trained observers to monitor and evaluate trainees in their performance, either live or by video. Related scoring systems have also been developed for specific subdomains of minimally invasive surgery, including the Global Operative Assessment of Laparoscopic Skills (GOALS), the Global Evaluative Assessment of Robotic Skills (GEARS), and the Global Assessment of Gastrointestinal Endoscopic Skills (GAGES).

Despite the effectiveness of such scoring systems in surgical education, there are several limitations with manual assessment, namely cost and bias. The manual assessment can be very time consuming and expensive because it needs experts' supervision during the process. In addition, these evaluations are, even with rater training, ultimately subjective, and the results from multiple surgeons need to be aggregated to provide a sense of performance.

Recent advances in AI have revolutionized the areas of computer vision, robotics, and automation, and work is underway to apply such advances to surgical education.[8,9] The main perceived advantage of using AI-based methods in surgical education is the potential for reduced time and monetary costs compared to manually scored methods. Once fully developed, an intelligent system could be used either automatically or semi-automatically at any time without the need for human experts to be present for every performance evaluation. Furthermore, an AI-based system could be developed to consider primarily objectively collected metrics over more subjective ones.

Automated assessment can be performed by using a general scoring system that is applicable to any type of surgery or by using a grading method that is geared toward specific types of surgeries. For instance, OSATS can be very well applied to various kinds of operations, whereas the Prostatectomy Assessment and Competence Evaluation (PACE)[10] was designed for robot-assisted radical prostatectomy skill assessment.

Another way of developing an automated system for surgical performance assessment is to use the structured format of a procedure to evaluate the training process at different levels of granularity. For example, a laparoscopic cholecystectomy can be evaluated at each phase, such as Calot's triangle dissection, and each phase can consist of various tasks, such as cystic duct dissection. To accomplish this objective, each process needs to be segmented into phases, tasks, and subtasks. The subtasks can be further analyzed at even more fundamental levels, often called "surgemes," which are the shortest surgical motion units with semantic sense. Detecting the phases of an operation and the tools being used in an operation, along with a thorough understanding of the surgical scene (ie, semantics) and anatomy, are the critical elements of an automated surgical education system.

This chapter provides an overview of applications in surgical education of some of the methodologies covered in earlier chapters of the book. To date, few papers have described the direct use of AI for assessment. The majority of work has centered around lower-level analyses, such as detecting surgical tools or detecting surgical phases, that can be used in both automated and manual assessment systems, and most of the recent works on AI in surgical education are based on deep-learning techniques, such as convolutional neural networks (CNNs) and recurrent neural networks (RNNs). The applications of 3 types of data are reviewed to provide a framework for understanding applications in surgical education: (1) operative videos alone, which are typically available in laparoscopic and endoscopic procedures; (2) operative videos and kinematic data, which are derived from robot-assisted surgeries; and (3) performance data from surgical simulators.

▌LAPAROSCOPIC SURGERY

In laparoscopic surgery, a form of minimally invasive surgery (MIS), the size of incisions is smaller compared to traditional open surgeries, due to the use of fiberoptic cameras and specially designed instruments inserted into the body through trocars. As a result of avoiding large open incisions, patients often benefit from less pain and blood loss, shorter hospital stay and recovery time, and a significant reduction in the risk of surgical site infections. However, the lack of sensible touch during the manipulation of the instruments within the body cavity (particularly in robotic surgery, which lacks haptic feedback) and a 2-dimensional (2D) view of the operative field create challenges in the learning curve of surgical trainees. Thus, quite a bit of research in the field has looked specifically at improving acquisition of skill in laparoscopic surgery, including development of curricula, simulators, and other techniques to overcome the learning curve. As previously introduced, however, assessing performance in MIS often requires review of the video, which is a time-consuming task and requires expertise. Therefore, automated systems will be essential for future applications in surgical education.

The most crucial factor in developing an automated system based on deep-learning techniques is the availability of the right amount and quality data since the critical patterns for performing a specific task need to be directly extracted from data itself. Unfortunately, the high cost of collecting and annotating laparoscopic videos as well as patient privacy-related concerns have limited the number of widely available data sets for research. There are only a few data sets that have been used as a benchmark for validating AI algorithms. For example, cholec80 from Institut de Recherche contre les Cancers de l'Appareil Digestif (IRCAD) in Strasbourg, France, contains 80 videos from laparoscopic cholecystectomy with labels for surgical tools and phases.[11] Smaller publicly available data sets are from the 2016 M2CAI tool detection and workflow recognition challenges (see http://camma.u-strasbg.fr/m2cai2016/index.php/program-challenge/). Otherwise, many projects are conducted at the institutional level using proprietary data sets.

In this section, we review vision-based methods for analyzing laparoscopic procedures using the videos. Some examples of such analyses include surgical workflow recognition, tool usage monitoring, surgical key-frame extraction, surgical shot classifications, surgical rating, and skill assessment.[12] Table 7-1 summarizes some of the key works that are discussed in this section.

Phase Detection

Automatic detection of surgical steps or phases is essential for analyzing the workflow of the operation. Given a recorded surgical video, the phases, tasks, and subtasks can be extracted using deep-learning algorithms and other techniques, allowing the video to be more easily analyzed and assessed with task-specific performance criteria. Furthermore, a well-organized database of automatically indexed videos can be used for different forms of education without the use of AI.

In the field of surgical phase recognition, frames of a video are classified into an operation's component phases or steps. As described in Chapter 6, video contains both visual information within frames and temporal information across frames. EndoNet[11] is perhaps one of the best known machine learning networks to use the high-level visual features in each frame of a laparoscopic video with a CNN architecture similar to AlexNet.[13] In their work, the CNN was trained to simultaneously identify surgical tools and phases. The tools were first detected, and the output was concatenated with the extracted features from the last layer of the CNN. By adding another fully connected layer, the phases were recognized based on the visual features and the tools that were present in a frame. In the next step, the outputs from the feature extractor CNN were sent as the input to a hierarchical hidden Markov model (HHMM) to incorporate the temporal dependencies between different frames. This resulted in 87% accuracy in detecting phases of laparoscopic cholecystectomy and 81%

Table 7-1   SUMMARY OF THE MOST IMPORTANT PAPERS FOR AI-BASED ANALYSIS OF LAPAROSCOPIC SURGERIES USING RECORDED VIDEOS

Method	Year	Task	Data Set	Highlights
EndoNet[11]	2017	Phase detection Tool detection	Cholec80	• First deep-learning framework • Multitask learning
Jin et al[16]	2018	Phase detection	Cholec80	• End-to-end CNN-RNN training
SPD[17]	2018	Phase detection	Cholec80	• Timestamping frames • Long-term LSTM training
Yi and Jiang[18]	2019	Phase detection	Cholec80 M2CAI16	• Considering hard frames
Bodenstedt et al[19]	2019	Phase detection Tool detection	Cholec80	• Active learning
Namazi et al[21]	2019	Phase boundaries	Cholec80	• Sequence to sequence modeling • Attention Mechanism
Yengera et al[20]	2018	Phase detection Remaining time	Cholec120	• Self-supervised learning
Mishra et al[24]	2017	Tool detection	M2CAI16	• End-to-end CNN-RNN training
Al Hajj et al[28]	2018	Tool detection	Cholec80	• Gradient boosting • Ensemble learning
Wang et al[25]	2019	Tool detection	Cholec80 M2CAI16	• Temporal modeling with 3D CNN and graph convolutional network
LapTool-Net[29]	2019	Tool detection	Cholec80 M2CAI16	• Tools co-occurrence consideration • Multitask multilabel training • Long-term RNN training
Jin et al[31]	2018	Tool localization Skill assessment	M2CAI16	• Localizing tools with bounding boxes • GOALS assessment
Nwoye et al[34]	2019	Tool localization Tool tracking	Cholec80	• Weakly supervised learning • Temporal considerations
Fuentes-Hurtado et al[35]	2019	Tool segmentation	EndoVis2015[a]	• Weakly labeling
MTRCNet-CL[37]	2020	Tool detection Phase detection	Cholec80	• Multitask learning • Correlation-aware loss function

[a]MICCAI 2015: Endovis 2015 Instrument Segmentation and Tracking. Accessed September 30, 2020. https://endovissub-instrument.grand-challenge.org/.

3D, 3-dimensional; AI, artificial intelligence; CNN, convolutional neural network; GOALS, Global Operative Assessment of Laparoscopic Skills; LSTM, long short-term memory; RNN, recurrent neural network; SPD, surgical phase detection.

accuracy in detecting tools such as graspers, clip appliers, and monopolar cautery hooks.

Although hidden Markov models (HMMs) are excellent tools for pattern recognition in sequential data, RNNs are usually preferred when a large training set is available. RNNs benefit from hidden states, which work as memory cells and enable them to learn sequential correlations from previous elements. Therefore, Twinanda et al[14] replaced the HHMM with an RNN architecture called long short-term memory (LSTM).[15] LSTM was developed to tackle the issue of long-term memory in regular RNNs caused by a phenomenon called vanishing gradients during training. Using LSTM, sequences with a length of up to a few hundred units can theoretically be processed. In these methods, the spatial feature extraction and the temporal features are performed by the CNN and then the HMM or LSTM in sequential order. Alternatively, CNNs and RNNs can be trained in an end-to-end fashion, a core concept of deep-learning algorithms. In end-to-end training, different parts of the model (typically neural networks) are simultaneously trained as a unified input-output mapping. For instance, in an end-to-end CNN-RNN architecture, the spatial and temporal (spatiotemporal) features are jointly learned.

To train a CNN with LSTM in an end-to-end fashion, Jin et al[16] took successive frames from operative video to simultaneously train a CNN and an LSTM. To consider the long-term structure of the phases, they introduced a probabilistic method called prior knowledge inference, which took the probability of the previous frames as input and updated the predictions according to the previously known ordering of the surgical phases in the videos (eg, step B necessarily follows step A). Using this technique, they reached state-of-the-art results in detecting the workflow from cholecystectomy data sets.

In another method called surgical phase detection (SPD) using a deep-learning system,[17] 2 architectures for real-time (ie, "online") and offline modes were designed. In both architectures, in addition to the visual features, the frame number was added as a separate feature before the fully connected layer of the frame-level classification. The experimental results showed that adding the actual position of the frame with respect to the other frames of the video, which they called timestamping, improved the performance of their CNN. In the offline model, a temporal median filter was applied to a short window of frames to smooth the predictions. The outputs of both architectures were sent to a separate LSTM network for the final decision making on the phase detection. The block diagram of the SPD is shown in Figure 7-1.

Because a surgical phase typically consists of frames that do not contain distinguishable information, given a single image or a short video

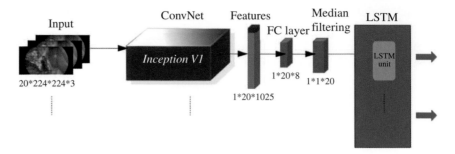

Figure 7-1 • The block diagram of surgical phase detector for identifying the laparoscopic phases in offline mode.[17] The extracted features with the Inception V1[82] convolutional neural network (ConvNet) are augmented by the frame numbers (the red block). The predictions are smoothened using a median filter, and the outputs for all the frames of a videos are sent to a long short-term memory (LSTM) to generate the phase classification's output.

snippet, it might be hard to detect the current phase from a small number of frames alone. Yi and Jiang[18] considered these "hard frames" in detecting the phases in laparoscopic cholecystectomy videos. The training set in their work is first cleansed using a K-fold validation method based on the predictions of a CNN classifier. The hard samples are then assigned a separate label and included in the training phase. The hard frames are finally mapped to their corresponding phase by combining the predictions of a CNN and an LSTM branch.

The works that were described earlier required the model to have the correct output, also known as ground truth, for training. This training strategy is called supervised learning, which aims at mapping a set of inputs to a known output. Due to the high cost of annotating surgical videos, other approaches have been explored to identify the surgical phases using laparoscopic videos.

In the paper by Bodenstedt et al,[19] the first active learning method based on a deep Bayesian network was proposed to analyze the workflow of cholecystectomy. The goal of active learning techniques is to use experts' annotations only when they are needed to reduce the expense of labeling. In their work, a recurrent Bayesian network based on a CNN-LSTM architecture captured the uncertainty based on the spatiotemporal features to select further data for annotation by human experts. They validated their solution on phase and tool detection tasks and demonstrated the effectiveness of their Bayesian-based active learning approach. In a different approach that uses pretrained networks, Yengera et al[20] proposed using self-supervised learning to predict the remaining time of the surgery. As a form of unsupervised learning, in self-supervised learning, the ground truth is determined based on an auxiliary task that does not need an additional annotation. The auxiliary task can be used in the pretraining of the feature extractor. For instance, the pretrained CNN-LSTM model in Yengera et al[20] was used as the initial step for learning the phases of the surgery. Their results showed that better phase recognition performance could be obtained with fewer manually labeled videos using their pretrained model.

The methods we have described earlier for analyzing the workflow of a laparoscopic procedure rely on a multiclass classification for all the frames, which does not explicitly find the transition time between 2 consecutive phases. In other words, the approaches we have described thus far work to classify, for example, frame 15 into phase A and frame 45 into phase B. However, these approaches do not specifically look for which frames correspond to phase A becoming phase B. Unless we have 100% accuracy for the classification of every frame, this might result in multiple chunks of frames identified for each phase. Under these circumstances, detecting the boundaries of each phase is an alternative solution for video segmentation because it could better allow identification of transitions from one phase to another.

Despite the distinctive features of each phase of a laparoscopic procedure, the identification of the boundaries of a phase using a deep-learning technique is a challenging problem. Namazi et al[21] adopted a sequence-to-sequence (seq2seq) architecture[22] to map the entire length of a video to a sequence of the first and last frame numbers of all the phases. The block diagram of this deep-learning model is shown in Figure 7-2. Introduced for natural language translation, a seq2seq model consists of an encoder for processing a variable-length sequence as input and a decoder for generating the output sequence (usually of variable length too) in an autoregression fashion. However, seq2seq lacks long-term memory, which is problematic in long laparoscopic videos. To address this limitation, the authors adopted the attention mechanism.[23] In a deep-learning context, attention is defined as the impact of each of the elements of input in making a particular prediction. In other words, with the aid of an alignment vector, which is typically connected to all the input elements, the locations where the model needs to pay more attention to each output class are determined. Besides tackling the long-term memory issue, the alignment vectors in Namazi et al[21] were used to find the probability of each frame belonging to the beginning or end of each phase. The boundaries are chosen from the input sequence according to the attention vectors with a classification loss function.

Tool Detection

Tracking surgical tools is another main component in the assessment and rating of the laparoscopic videos. In the EndoNet paper,[11] the first

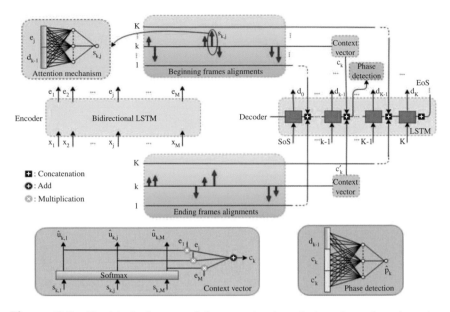

Figure 7-2 • The block diagram of the attention-based phase boundary detection (APBD) method.[21] Given the vector X of extracted visual features, the attention block is responsible for finding the alignments between the encoder outputs containing spatio-temporal features and the decoder states, which are the phase numbers. The alignment vectors are used to calculate the probability of each frame of a video being the beginning (or ending) of a phase k. The probability of the presence of the phase is calculated at phase detection block. LSTM, long short-term memory.

deep-learning model was designed for detecting the presence of surgical instruments. Inspired by this work, other researchers have used various CNN architectures for classifying the frames based on surgical tools.

Mishra et al[24] were the first to apply an LSTM to a short sequence of frames to simultaneously extract spatiotemporal patterns for detecting the presence of the tools by an end-to-end training strategy. Wang et al[25] used a graph convolutional network (GCN), a powerful tool for processing graphs,[26] for detecting the presence of surgical tools. The GCN was applied to a short snippet of video after the visual features were extracted with an inflated DenseNet (a CNN architecture that consists of densely connected layers to tackle the vanishing gradient issue in deep neural networks[27]). A temporal pooling layer was finally added to combine the features along the time dimension.

Due to hardware constraints, the end-to-end training of a deep CNN and an RNN has been accomplished with only a few consecutive frames (between 5 and 20 images). This limitation hinders the extraction of the long-term temporal features in lengthy surgical videos. To address this issue, in Al Hajj et al,[28] a gradient boosting machine (GBM) was used to combine different CNNs and RNNs. The goal of a GBM is to combine multiple "weak" learners in order to form a strong classifier. For this purpose, the CNN and RNN were progressively improved by training different CNN/RNN architectures. They achieved state-of-the-art results with their proposed ensemble learning technique.

LapTool-Net[29] was another context-aware tool detector in laparoscopic cholecystectomy videos that exploited the pattern in the co-occurrence of surgical tools. To this end, a decision layer was added on top of a multilabel classifier based on a CNN-RNN architecture. The role of the decision layer was to map the output of the multilabel classifier to a multiclass classifier based on the combinations of multiple tools while considering the most frequent combinations. The decision model and the multilabel classifier were jointly trained as a multitask learning algorithm. The advantage of this approach was that the prediction of the model was made based on the local features of single tools and the global context of the tools' co-occurrence. Another contribution of the work was the undersampling approach based on tool combinations by finding the smallest training set without losing accuracy to avoid overfitting caused by the high correlation among the neighboring frames of a video (algorithms can "assume" that frames adjacent to a known frame are likely to belong to the same phase, and such an assumption can lead to overfitting of data). After the training was completed, the outputs were further smoothed by training a separate RNN over the entire video's length to take into account the long-term ordering of the presence of different tools, which follows the same structured pattern in the workflow of the surgery.

Besides the presence of the instruments, their locations need to be identified to track the instruments' movements and trajectories. In the literature, there exist a plethora of solutions for object localization in still images and videos.[30] For laparoscopic videos, for instance, Jin et al[31] were the first to apply the Faster R-CNN architecture[32] for tool localization, after labeling the data set with bounding boxes containing the surgical tools. In addition to localization, they also reported the results of the presence of the tools and showed that including the locations of the tools in training could improve the performance, even while using fewer labeled images.

Although fully supervised learning has shown promise in automated extraction of the usage of the tools, the performance is typically bounded by the quality and the amount of annotated data. To address this issue, weakly supervised learning has been studied in surgical video analysis. Weak supervision refers to the use of imprecise or noisy sources to provide training data, and its use in developing algorithms for surgical video analysis has been growing due to the cost of well-annotated data sets. For example, Vardazaryan et al[33] proposed a weakly supervised tool localization model based on CNN. Nwoye et al[34] extended the previous work by considering both spatial and temporal correlations for localizing and motion tracking in laparoscopic videos. They used convolutional LSTM instead of the conventional LSTM to process the last layers feature maps, which is a multidimensional array. In the paper by Fuentes-Hurtado et al,[35] a new method was introduced for weak labeling of the laparoscopic video frames for segmenting surgical instruments. The proposed annotation method draws rigid lines, which they called "stripes," for foreground objects (tools) along their longitudinal dimensions that are then fed into a fully convolutional network. Using this technique, they were able to perform weakly supervised learning with similar accuracy to a fully supervised method.

Due to the structure of a typical operation, there is often a high correlation between the tasks and the tools. For example, a Maryland grasper is a tool commonly used to perform dissection, and shears are used to cut. By leveraging such correlation between tools and phases, a deep-learning model can be trained to perform multiple tasks at the same time, a process also known as multitask learning.[36] In the pioneering work of EndoNet, such an approach led to improved accuracy of tool and phase detection. Jin et al[37] presented a multitask recurrent convolutional network with correlation loss (MTRCNet-CL) (Figure 7-3), which boosted the performances of the 2 tasks by sharing the earlier features and introducing a correlation loss. The purpose of the correlation loss function was to ensure the consistency between the outputs of the tool and phase detectors. The results from experiments on the multitask learning approach demonstrated significant improvement over single-task models.

Beyond providing information on surgical phases, tools and the way the tools are manipulated by the surgeons can reflect a surgeon's level of expertise. To validate the effectiveness of the information about the usage of laparoscopic tools, Jin et al[31] validated the correlation between the video ratings by experts and ones calculated solely from a tool detection system. They used GOALS,[38] which is a widely studied assessment tool for grading overall surgical skills in laparoscopic surgery. The scoring system consists of 5 domains: depth perception, bimanual dexterity, efficiency, tissue handling, and autonomy; the score for each domain ranges from

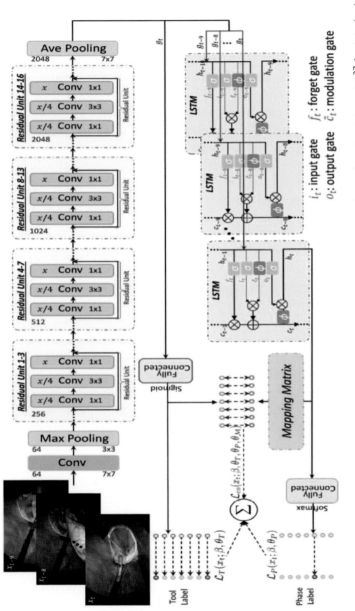

Figure 7-3 • The block diagram of the multitask recurrent convolutional network with correlation loss (MTRCNet-CL)[37] for jointly detection of tools and phases in laparoscopic videos. The tool branch consists of a convolutional neural network, whereas for the phase branch, a recurrent neural network block is added to take into account the temporal features. The correlation loss function extracts the tool-phase correlation and is added to the overall multitask loss function. LSTM, long short-term memory.

1 to 5. The results of their study demonstrated that quantitative objective metrics derived from deep learning—the time tools were used and total distance traveled by the instruments—correlated with GOALS scores.

▌ROBOT-ASSISTED SURGERY

Robot-assisted surgery is becoming increasingly popular because it provides enhanced control and precision during the operation with a better view of the surgical site (see Chapter 12). Currently, more than 1 million procedures are performed each year worldwide using the Intuitive da Vinci Surgical System (Intuitive, Sunnyvale, CA),[39] a minimally invasive robotic surgical system with wristed instruments and a 3-dimensional (3D) stereoscopic view.

Many studies have been devoted to objective assessment in robotic surgeries.[40] Most scoring methods are modified versions of OSATS or GOALS to incorporate the requirements of robotic surgeries. For instance, R-OSATS[41] is used to assess performance on 5 robotic surgery drills. Another standard tool is the GEARS, which measures the skills in six 5-point domains: depth perception, bimanual dexterity, efficiency, force sensitivity, robotic control, and autonomy.[42] Similar to laparoscopic procedures, an automated evaluation system that extracts critical features such as tools and tasks could be extremely beneficial in robot-assisted surgeries.

In addition to recorded videos in minimally invasive procedures, in robot-assisted surgeries, the collected data can be augmented with the kinematics or other sensor-based data such as force or vibration. For instance, using the da Vinci Research API (Intuitive Surgical, Sunnyvale, CA), an additional set of motion data, such as position and velocity, joint angles, torque, and even the instrument changes, is available. Other platforms provide access to different kinematic data as well.[39]

Although most da Vinci–based platforms have data storage capabilities, collecting a large annotated data set that can be used in clinical assessment is not a trivial task due to the size of such data sets and concerns around legal and regulatory requirements for storing such data. For this purpose, the JHU–ISI Gesture and Skill Assessment Working Set (JIGSAWS) was developed by the Laboratory for Computational Sensing and Robotics (LCSR) lab at Johns Hopkins University (JHU) and Intuitive Surgical Inc. (ISI).[43] The publicly available data set contains kinematic data such as Cartesian positions, orientations, velocities, angular velocities, and gripper angles along with the stereo videos captured during the operation and is manually assessed with different expertise levels. The annotated data are available from 8 subjects for 3 general

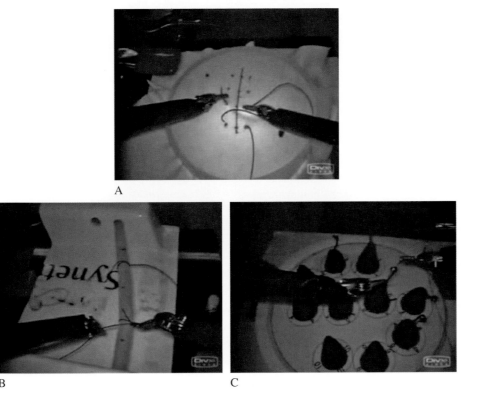

Figure 7-4 • An example of the frames for the tasks in the JIGSAWS data set. (**A**) Suturing, (**B**) knot tying, and (**C**) needle parsing. (Reproduced, with permission, from CIRL Lab (LCSR), Johns Hopkins University, Baltimore, MD. Accessed October 7, 2020. https://cirl.lcsr.jhu.edu/research/hmm/datasets/jigsaws_release/.)

tasks: suturing, knot tying, and needle passing. Another key feature of the JIGSAWS is the manual annotation data of 15 atomic surgical activities (surgemes) called "gestures." Three examples of the annotated tasks in the JIGSAWS data set are shown in Figure 7-4.

In this section, we discuss different deep-learning algorithms that have been recently used for various tasks in robot-assisted education. Table 7-2 summarizes the most important breakthroughs in activity recognition, tool detection and segmentation, and surgical skill assessment. The types of data that are used in the algorithm (kinematics or videos) are included in the table.

Activity Recognition

Automatic recognition of activities is essential in understanding surgical workflow and is the first step in a manual or automated skill assessment routine. The availability of the kinematic data in robotic surgery can

Table 7-2   SUMMARY OF THE MOST IMPORTANT PAPERS FOR AI-BASED ANALYSIS OF ROBOT-ASSISTED SURGERIES

Method	Year	Task	Data Set	Data	Highlights
Dipietro et al[48]	2016	Gesture recognition	JIGSAWS MISTIC-SL	Kinematics	• First RNN for kinematics
TCN[50]	2016	Gesture recognition	JIGSAWS	Kinematics Videos	• Temporal convolutional network
Liu and Jiang[51]	2018	Gesture recognition	JIGSAWS	Kinematics Videos	• Deep reinforcement learning for handling oversegmentation
Sarikaya et al[52]	2018	Task recognition Gesture recognition	JIGSAWS	Videos	• Multitask learning • Multimodel (RGB + flow)
Sarikaya and Jannin[53]	2019	Task recognition	JIGSAWS	Videos	• Motion features (dense optical flow) using CNN
Van Amsterdam et al[55]	2019	Gesture recognition	JIGSAWS	Kinematics	• Weakly supervised labeling
Zia et al[58]	2019	Phase detection	Radical prostatectomy	Videos	• CNN-LSTM for phase detection
ToolNet[64]	2017	Tool segmentation	EndoVis 2017	Videos	• Fully convolutional semantic segmentation • Cascaded feature fusion
Mohammed et al[67]	2019	Scene segmentation	EndoVis 2017	Videos	• Multiview segmentation • 2 encoders, 1 decoder
Da et al[70]	2019	Tool segmentation	STRAS robot[70] data	Videos Kinematics	• Self-supervised learning
Ross et al[72]	2018	Tool segmentation	EndoVis 2017	Videos	• Self-supervised learning • Using recolorization as an auxiliary task
Du et al[68]	2018	Tool pose estimation	EndoVis 2017	Videos	• Multi-instrument parsing • Joint localization
FSNet[69]	2019	Tool pose estimation	EndoVis 2017	Videos	• Key points localization
Fawaz et al[76]	2019	Skill assessment	JIGSAWS	Kinematics	• Multitask learning

(continued)

Table 7-2 SUMMARY OF THE MOST IMPORTANT PAPERS FOR AI-BASED ANALYSIS OF ROBOT-ASSISTED SURGERIES (CONTINUED)

Method	Year	Task	Data Set	Data	Highlights
Doughty et al[79]	2018	Skill assessment	JIGSAWS	Videos	• Pairwise ranking • 2-stream network (Siamese)
Oğul et al[78]	2019	Skill assessment	JIGSAWS	Kinematics	• 2-stream network (Siamese)

AI, artificial intelligence; CNN, convolutional neural network; JIGSAWS, JHU–ISI Gesture and Skill Assessment Working Set; LSTM, long short-term memory; MISTIC-SL, Minimally Invasive Surgical Training and Innovation Center–Science of Learning; RGB, red, green, and blue; RNN, recurrent neural network; TCN, temporal convolutional network.

potentially improve the performance of computer vision methods described earlier by adding to the video analysis. Thus, task segmentation and gesture recognition have widely been studied after the release of the JIGSAWS data set because it provided a well-annotated, accessible data set.[44]

Lea et al[45] presented the Latent Convolutional Skip Chain Conditional Random Field (LC-SC-CRF) using time series data from JIGSAWS to learn the action primitives for gesture recognition. The primitives were captured using convolutional filters, and the temporal segmentation was performed with the Skip Chain Conditional Random Field.[46] In their other work,[47] they used a CNN for capturing the spatiotemporal features. These approaches allowed them to use kinematic data to further understand the relationship between actions (via measurement of the robotic instruments' position in space and the tasks being performed by the instruments) and the phase of the surgical task. Despite their superior performance over traditional graphical models, their method lacked the end-to-end training paradigm in modern deep-learning architectures.

DiPietro et al[48] were the first to use RNNs in processing the kinematic for segmenting and classifying the fine-grained activities in JIGSAWS and the Minimally Invasive Surgical Training and Innovation Center–Science of Learning (MISTIC-SL) data sets. In another work, DiPietro et al[49] applied 4 bidirectional RNN architectures and obtained state-of-the-art results by exploring the optimal hyperparameters. A bidirectional RNN consists of 2 RNNs for the forward and backward sequences, where the backward sequence is the inverse of the sequence. The outputs of the 2 RNNs are concatenated and connected to the output through a fully connected layer. The performance was measured at the higher-level maneuvers as well as the more granular gestures.

In the paper by Lea et al,[50] the authors introduce an end-to-end framework for segmenting the videos into the fine-grained activities. The model called temporal convolutional network (TCN) replaced RNNs in previous designs with a 1-dimensional CNN that simultaneously captures the spatial and temporal features. The model consists of multiple layers of "temporal convolutions" to consider the low-level, mid-level, and high-level spatiotemporal patterns in a hierarchical way. Using an encoder-decoder architecture, the input videos were mapped to the corresponding frame-level gesture classes. The model was evaluated on the JIGSAWS data set and separately for sensors data and videos, showing the superiority of CNN and encoder-decoder architecture over RNN.

Liu et al[51] replaced the graphical models, such as HMM and conditional random field (CRF), and RNNs with a reinforcement learning-based model to deal with the oversegmentation issue that causes the videos to be divided into too many segments. To this end, the problem was modeled as a sequential decision-making process, and an intelligent agent was trained with reinforcement learning using the extracted spatiotemporal features. The rewarding methods included both frame-level accuracy and the edit score. They reported their results for vision-based and sensor-based models and showed minor improvement over the TCN model.

In the paper by Sarikaya et al,[52] a joint surgical gesture and task classification model was proposed based on a multitask and multimodal learning paradigm. In addition to the videos, motion (optical flow) representation was extracted from the videos and included as part of the input of the model. Their experiments showed that training a single model for jointly learning the tasks and gestures is superior to training separate models for the 2 tasks. The work was later extended[53] to use dense optical flow as the only input for training the task recognition model. The optical flow was calculated using the convolutional network proposed in Simonyan and Zisserman.[54]

To mitigate the cost of labeling, Van Amsterdam et al[55] proposed a weakly supervised learning method that uses a minimum of 1 expert to generate the ground truth. The labels were used as the initialization of an unsupervised gesture recognition method based on Gaussian mixture models (GMMs). They used kinematic data for validating their method.

The collected data from robotic surgeries can also be used to identify the surgical steps (similar to phase detection in laparoscopic videos) using the data from the entire operation. Zia et al[56] presented an automated model to identify the steps in robot-assisted radical prostatectomy on a large data set from 100 completed operations. They experimented on several data modalities such as the surgeon-side console (SSC), the patient-side cart (SI), and surgical system event data (EVT), all collected from the da Vinci surgical system and multiple deep-learning architectures including LSTM and 3D CNN, and a modified version of Inception V3[57] was the best performer. They later improved their results using a CNN-LSTM architecture.[58]

Tool Detection

To track surgical instruments in robotic surgeries, a team at Intuitive Surgical manually annotated data from porcine robot-assisted nephrectomy procedures using da Vinci Xi systems and started the 2017 Robotic Instrument Segmentation Challenge (see https://endovissub2017-roboticinstrumentsegmentation.grand-challenge.org/). The data set contains labels for pixel-level classification of surgical tools and their articulating parts. In 2018, the team released a larger data set with annotation of several tissue types and some additional instruments (see https://endovissub2018-roboticscenesegmentation.grand-challenge.org/).

For pixel-wise semantic segmentation, the most successful deep-learning architectures are based on fully convolutional networks (FCNs).[59,60] The improved version called U-Net[61] benefits from skip connections[62] and an encoder-decoder architecture and has been widely applied to many medical imaging problems. Some variations of these models have also been successfully adopted for generating the output masks for surgical instrument segmentation.[63] For example, ToolNet[64] was a real-time tool segmentation model based on "holistically nested" CNN architecture, and Hasan and Linte[65] introduced U-NetPlus, which modified the U-Net architecture for semantic and instance segmentation of robotic surgical instruments. A slightly different approach was proposed in LWANet,[66] an attention-guided lightweight segmentation model. In this work, the conventional convolutional layers at the decoder were replaced by depth-wise separable convolutions, and transposed convolution was used for up-sampling. The attention blocks were introduced to fuse the high-level and low-level features. Their experiments showed their superior performance over the existing works with lower computational costs and faster run time.

In the paper by Mohammed et al,[67] the authors presented a new model that took stereo video frames (the robotic system has a left and right camera to recreate stereoscopic vision) as input and produced the output mask for segmenting surgical instruments. To accomplish this objective, the model (called StreoScenNet) consisted of 2 encoders for left and right camera frames with 1 decoder to generate the output. Using a pretrained model on a larger data set, they obtained better results compared with the single-view models.

Du et al[68] proposed a fully convolutional detection and regression method for articulated multi-instrument 2D pose estimation without using the kinematic data. After detecting the joints and the association between joint pairs, the maximum bipartite matching method is used to estimate the pose of the instruments. In another work,[69] the detection of surgical tools was accomplished by localizing key points in the images using a new architecture called Feature Stacked Network (FSNet). Five key points (the handle end, the rigid shaft, the articulated head, and the left and right claspers) were manually labeled for 6 tools. The bounding boxes were regressed for tool localization after the low-level and high-level feature fusion using a pyramid network. Similarly, the locations of the key points were found to estimate the pose of the instruments.

Annotation for tool detection in surgery has similarly high costs to phase detection in surgery, although in the case of tools, expert surgeons may not be necessary for all annotation tasks. To mitigate against cost of annotation, efforts have been made to investigate semi- and self-supervised learning in robotic tool detection as well. A self-supervised approach for surgical tool segmentation based on the kinematic data was tested in Da et al[70] and used kinematic data to generate the labels for training a fully convolutional network on the images. The experimental results on a data set collected with the STRAS robotic system[71] were on par with supervised semantic segmentation models. As an example of semi-supervised learning for laparoscopic tool segmentation, Ross et al[72] designed a new model to leverage the information present in unlabeled data in a self-supervised fashion. For this purpose, an auxiliary task was defined for the recolorization of surgical images. The pretrained model was then fine-tuned by the labeled videos. The recolorization was performed by a conditional generative adversarial network (c-GAN), which is a modified version of the generative adversarial network (GAN).[73] In a typical GAN, 2 competing subnetworks, namely generator and discriminator, are jointly trained. The role of a generator is to generate "fake" output, whereas the discriminator determines whether the generated output is real or not. The U-Net architecture[61] was used in the proposed c-GAN model, which outperformed the existing supervised learning models.

Skill Assessment

Skill assessment using kinematic data is an area of interest to engineers, clinicians, and educators alike. Work on automated skill assessment using kinematic data especially increased after the introduction of the JIGSAWS skill assessment data set. The data set has annotations for technical performance for 3 robotic surgical tasks performed by 8 participants based on 3 categories: (1) self-proclaimed, which has 3 skill levels (novice, intermediate, and expert) based on the time spent on the system; (2) modified-OSATS, which has 6 criteria (additional criteria for suturing) on a scale of 1 to 5; and (3) Global Rating Score (GRS), which is the sum of the modified-OSATS scores.[74]

Using only the kinematics, Fawaz et al[75] designed a CNN architecture for classifying the data based on the skill levels. They extended their work to perform modified-OSATS scores by adding a separate regression layer to the previous design.[76] They further visualized the attention of their model to find the parts of the videos that influenced the skill assessment the most. With additional development, their explainable model could very well be used in a feedback generation system.

While some papers used conventional video classification methods, such as 3D Convolution in Funke et al,[77] the problem of surgical skill assessment was formulated as a pairwise ranking task in Oğul et al.[78] This allowed for direct comparison of performance between individuals rather than against a set standard. Given the kinematics data, a Siamese (2-stream) architecture was adopted to compare 2 streams of input. The models in the proposed Siamese architectures are LSTMs. The pairwise ranking has also been proposed for skill assessment using videos.[79] The inputs to the 2-stream architecture were videos, and the temporal segment network (TSN)[80] was adopted to capture the spatial and temporal information. Numerous experiments have shown the superiority of this approach over the existing single-stream models.

▌ CONCLUSION

Surgical data science has been gaining more attention over the past few years.[81] In this chapter, we reviewed some of the most important papers in applying AI in surgical education. We limited the scope of this survey to laparoscopic surgery due to its increasing popularity and clinical benefits. The research papers were chosen based on the contributions of their work to nonrobotic, robot-assisted, and simulation-based education and the novelty of the methodologies. In addition, we focused our survey on deep-learning methods and neural network–based models, which are the state-of-the-art solutions for surgical video analysis. Therefore, we did not cover traditional computer vision techniques for feature extraction and machine learning techniques, such as support vector machine and HMM, although these techniques are just as important and effective in the field and should not be summarily dismissed. See Table 7-3 for a glossary of the terms used in this chapter.

Table 7-3 GLOSSARY	
Terms	**Description**
Active learning	A learning algorithm for interactively annotating data by the users and only when necessary during training
Attention	A vector of importance weighting showing how strongly each element of input is correlated to the output
Bayesian neural network	A type of neural network that assigns a probability distribution to all the weights instead of a single point and is therefore suitable for estimating uncertainty in predictions
Conditional random field (CRF)	A type of discriminative probabilistic graphical model used for encoding known correlation in sequential data
Convolutional neural network (CNN)	A type of neural network that consists of convolutional kernels for processing data in the form of single or multidimensional arrays such as images
Ensemble learning	Combining multiple learning algorithms to obtain better predictive performance
Gated recurrent unit (GRU)	A type of recurrent neural network that consists of multiple logical gates to capture long-term correlation in sequential data
Gaussian mixture model (GMM)	A probabilistic model used for clustering
Generative adversarial network (GAN)	A generative model that consists of 2 subnetworks competing with each other to generate new data with the same statistics as the training set
Gradient boosting machine (GBM)	A method for training several models to convert weak learners into a strong classifier
Graph convolutional network (GCN)	A type of neural network that operates on data in the form of graphs
Hidden Markov model (HMM)	A statistical Markov model useful for temporal pattern recognition

(continued)

Table 7-3 GLOSSARY (CONTINUED)	
Terms	**Description**
Long short-term memory (LSTM)	An RNN architecture that consists of several gates for learning long-term correlation in sequential data
Loss function	The measure of error for the optimization process of a neural network
Prior knowledge inference (PKI)	A probabilistic approach for using the knowledge about previous frames for estimating the current surgical phase during the model inference
Recurrent neural network (RNN)	A type of neural network that benefits from hidden states and weight sharing for processing sequential data
Self-supervised learning	Learning representations through automatically labeling the data with the help of auxiliary tasks
Sequence to sequence (seq2seq)	A neural network–based architecture for mapping a variable-length sequence to another variable-length sequence
Siamese architecture	A neural network–based architecture that consists of 2 networks with shared weights
Skip chain conditional random field	A type of CRF that explicitly models dependencies of not-neighboring and long-term elements of a sequence
Supervised learning	A machine learning that is trained by inferring from labeled data
Unsupervised learning	Learning to perform tasks that do not require correct labels
Vanishing gradients	A difficulty in training deep neural networks with gradient-based methods, which prevents weights from being updated after some iterations
Weakly supervised learning	Learning from lower-quality data or higher-level supervision

AI is applicable to a wide range of tasks in surgical education, including:

- Tracking surgical instruments by identifying the presence, location, or pose of the tools from still images, video streams, and kinematic data
- Organizing the videos or kinematic data into different phases, tasks/subtasks, and gestures and classifying the surgical parts
- Segmenting the surgical scene by localizing the anatomic structures and surgical instruments and parts
- Rating based on performance for short snippets of tasks or entire operation length using the standard criteria such as OSATS, GOALS, and GEARS

The methods that have been adopted include most of the conventional techniques from fully supervised learning to unsupervised and reinforcement learning. Several solutions have been proposed based on semi-supervised, weakly supervised, self-supervised, and active learning.

As for the deep-learning components that have been used for surgical education applications, we found CNNs to be the most popular one. Modern 2D architectures such as ResNet[62] have been widely used for capturing the visual representation, whereas the 1-dimensional CNNs have been adopted for temporal feature learning, and spatiotemporal feature extraction was performed by 3D CNNs. Similar to CNNs, RNNs have been developed for time series data, especially in robot-assisted surgeries, with LSTM and gated recurrent unit being the most popular choices.

The trend in surgical data science is to favor using methods that minimize the degree of necessary supervision, because the process of collecting and annotating data is expensive and time consuming. To this end, methods for weakly supervised learning and semi-supervised learning, which do not need large, manually annotated data sets, are attracting more attention. Furthermore, with the aid of self-supervised pretraining, the unlabeled portion of a data set can be used to capture the general features that could be used as the initial state for training a deep-learning–based model.

For robot-assisted surgeries, the availability of data from different sensors is crucial in designing an AI-based system. Such data contain complementary information that can potentially be used to provide additional annotation for the unlabeled or weakly labeled data or augment the performance in a multimodal deep-learning model. Finally, multi-task learning strategies have been rising in popularity in order to take advantage of the correlation among different tasks and the large amount of information present in each surgical record. Thus, a model may consist of multiple fully supervised outputs, a combination of fully and self-supervised tasks, or multiple intermediate tasks.

As research in the field of AI continues to mature, surgeons and educators will need to develop and validate performance assessments on which AI technologies can be trained. In addition, techniques in AI, such as computer vision, may provide surgical education with more quantitative measures of performance across a wide range of procedures, measures that can be incorporated into new performance assessment systems.

REFERENCES

1. Anderson O, Davis R, Hanna GB, Vincent CA. Surgical adverse events: a systematic review. *Am J Surg*. 2013;206(2):253-262.
2. Tsuda S, Scott D, Doyle J, Jones DB. Surgical skills training and simulation. *Curr Prob Surg*. 2009;46:271-370.
3. Ujiki M, Zhao JC. Simulation training in surgery. *Dis Mon*. 2011;57:789-801.
4. Scott DJ, Dunnington GL. The new ACS/APDS skills curriculum: moving the learning curve out of the operating room. *J Gastrointest Surg*. 2008;12:213-221.
5. Gallagher AG. Metric-based simulation training to proficiency in medical education: what it is and how to do it. *Ulster Med J*. 2012;81(3):107-113.
6. Martin JA, Regehr G, Reznick R, et al. Objective structured assessment of technical skill (OSATS) for surgical residents. *Br J Surg*. 1997;84:273-278.
7. Niitsu H, Hirabayashi N, Yoshimitsu M, et al. Using the Objective Structured Assessment of Technical Skills (OSATS) global rating scale to evaluate the skills of surgical trainees in the operating room. *Surg Today*. 2013;43:271-275.
8. LeCun Y, Bengio Y, Hinton G. Deep learning. *Nature*. 2015;521:436-444.
9. Litjens G, Kooi T, Bejnordi BE, et al. A survey on deep learning in medical image analysis. *Med Image Anal*. 2017;42:60-88.
10. Hussein AA, Ghani KR, Peabody J, et al. Development and validation of an objective scoring tool for robot-assisted radical prostatectomy: prostatectomy assessment and competency evaluation. *J Urol*. 2017;197:1237-1244.
11. Twinanda AP, Shehata S, Mutter D, Marescaux J, De Mathelin M, Padoy N. EndoNet: a deep architecture for recognition tasks on laparoscopic videos. *IEEE Trans Med Imaging*. 2017;36:86-97.
12. Loukas C. Video content analysis of surgical procedures. *Surg Endosc*. 2018;32:553-568.
13. Krizhevsky A, Sutskever I, Hinton GE. ImageNet Classification with deep convolutional neural networks. *Adv Neural Inform Process Syst*. 2012:1-9. Accessed October 6, 2020. https://papers.nips.cc/paper/4824-imagenet-classification-with-deep-convolutional-neural-networks.pdf.

14. Twinanda AP, Padoy N, Troccaz MJ, Hager G. Vision-based approaches for surgical activity recognition using laparoscopic and RBGD videos. 2017. Accessed October 6, 2020. https://tel.archives-ouvertes.fr/tel-01557522/document.

15. Hochreiter S, Schmidhuber JU. Long short-term memory. *Neural Comput.* 1997;9:1735-1780.

16. Jin Y, Dou Q, Chen H, et al. SV-RCNet: workflow recognition from surgical videos using recurrent convolutional network. *IEEE Trans Med Imaging.* 2018;37:1114-1126.

17. Namazi B, Sankaranarayanan G, Devarajan V. Automatic detection of surgical phases in laparoscopic videos. *Proceedings on the International Conference in Artificial Intelligence (ICAI)*, 2018.

18. Yi F, Jiang T. Hard frame detection and online mapping for surgical phase recognition. International Conference on Medical Image Computing and Computer-Assisted Intervention (MICCAI) 2019. Accessed October 6, 2020. https://link.springer.com/chapter/10.1007%2F978-3-030-32254-0_50.

19. Bodenstedt S, Rivoir D, Jenke A, et al. Active learning using deep Bayesian networks for surgical workflow analysis. *Int J Comput Assist Radiol Surg.* 2019;14:1079-1087.

20. Yengera G, Mutter D, Marescaux J, Padoy N. Less is more: surgical phase recognition with less annotations through self-supervised pre-training of CNN-LSTM networks, arXiv:1805.08569. Accessed October 6, 2020. https://arxiv.org/pdf/1805.08569.pdf.

21. Namazi B, Sankaranarayanan G, Devarajan V. Attention-based surgical phase boundaries detection in laparoscopic videos. Presented at the 6th Annual Conference on Computational Science and Computational Intelligenece CSCI, Las Vegas, NV, 2019.

22. Sutskever I, Vinyals O, Le QV. Sequence to sequence learning with neural networks. Advances in Neural Information Processing Systems 2014. Accessed October 6, 2020. https://papers.nips.cc/paper/5346-sequence-to-sequence-learning-with-neural-networks.pdf.

23. Luong MT, Pham H, Manning CD. Effective approaches to attention-based neural machine translation. arXiv:1508.04025. Accessed October 6, 2020. https://arxiv.org/abs/1508.04025.

24. Mishra K, Sathish R, Sheet D. Learning latent temporal connectionism of deep residual visual abstractions for identifying surgical tools in laparoscopy procedures. 2017 IEEE Conference on Computer Vision and Pattern Recognition Workshops (CVPRW). Accessed October 6, 2020. https://openaccess.thecvf.com/content_cvpr_2017_workshops/w37/papers/Mishra_Learning_Latent_Temporal_CVPR_2017_paper.pdf.

25. Wang S, Xu Z, Yan C, Huang J. Graph convolutional nets for tool presence detection in surgical videos. Lecture Notes in Computer Science (including subseries Lecture Notes in Artificial Intelligence and Lecture Notes in Bioinformatics), 2019. Accessed October 6, 2020. https://link.springer.com/chapter/10.1007/978-3-030-20351-1_36.

26. Zhang S, Tong H, Xu J, Maciejewski R. Graph convolutional networks: a comprehensive review. *Comput Social Netw.* 2019;6:1-12.

27. Huang G, Liu Z, Van Der Maaten L, Weinberger KQ. Densely connected convolutional networks. Proceedings of the 30th IEEE Conference on Computer Vision and Pattern Recognition, 2017. Accessed October 6, 2020. https://arxiv.org/abs/1608.06993.

28. Al Hajj H, Lamard M, Conze P-H, Cochener B, Quellec G. Monitoring tool usage in surgery videos using boosted convolutional and recurrent neural networks. *Med Image Anal.* 2018;47:203-218.

29. Namazi B, Sankaranarayanan G, Devarajan V. LapTool-Net: a contextual detector of surgical tools in laparoscopic videos based on recurrent convolutional neural networks. Accessed October 6, 2020. https://arxiv.org/pdf/1905.08983v1.pdf.

30. Zou Z, Shi Z, Guo Y, Ye J, Member S. Object detection in 20 years: a survey. arXiv:1905.05055. Accessed October 6, 2020. https://www.arxiv-vanity.com/papers/1905.05055/.

31. Jin A, Yeung S, Jopling J, et al. Tool detection and operative skill assessment in surgical videos using region-based convolutional neural networks. 2018 IEEE Winter Conference on Applications of Computer Vision (WACV). Accessed October 6, 2020. https://ieeexplore.ieee.org/document/8354185.

32. Ren S, He K, Girshick R, Sun J. Faster R-CNN: towards real-time object detection with region proposal networks. Accessed October 6, 2020. https://arxiv.org/pdf/1506.01497.pdf.

33. Vardazaryan A, Mutter D, Marescaux J, Padoy N. Weakly-supervised learning for tool localization in laparoscopic videos. Lecture Notes in Computer Science (including subseries Lecture Notes in Artificial Intelligence and Lecture Notes in Bioinformatics), 2018. Accessed October 6, 2020. https://link.springer.com/chapter/10.1007/978-3-030-01364-6_19.

34. Nwoye CI, Mutter D, Marescaux J, Padoy N. Weakly supervised convolutional LSTM approach for tool tracking in laparoscopic videos. *Int J Comput Assist Radiol Surg.* 2019;14:1059-1067.

35. Fuentes-Hurtado F, Kadkhodamohammadi A, Flouty E, Barbarisi S, Luengo I, Stoyanov D. EasyLabels: weak labels for scene segmentation in laparoscopic videos. *Int J Comput Assist Radiol Surg.* 2019;14(7):1247-1257.

36. Subhra S, Rachana M, Sheet DS. Multitask learning of temporal connectionism in convolutional networks using a joint distribution loss function to simultaneously identify tools and phase in surgical videos. arXiv:1905.08315. Accessed October 6, 2020. https://arxiv.org/pdf/1905.08315.pdf.

37. Jin Y, Li H, Dou Q, et al. Multi-task recurrent convolutional network with correlation loss for surgical video analysis. *Med Image Anal.* 2020;59:101572.

38. Vassiliou MC, Feldman LS, Andrew CG, et al. A global assessment tool for evaluation of intraoperative laparoscopic skills. *Am J Surg.* 2005;190:107-113.

39. Elek RN, Haidegger T. Robot-assisted minimally invasive surgical skill assessment-manual and automated platforms, 2019. Accessed October 6, 2020. http://acta.uni-obuda.hu/Nagyne-Elek_Haidegger_95.pdf.

40. Chen J, Cheng N, Cacciamani G, et al. *Objective Assessment of Robotic Surgical Technical Skill: A Systematic Review,* vol. 201. Lippincott Williams and Wilkins; 2019:461-469.

41. Siddiqui NY, Galloway ML, Geller EJ, et al. Validity and reliability of the robotic objective structured assessment of technical skills. *Obstet Gynecol.* 2014;123:1193-1199.

42. Goh AC, Goldfarb DW, Sander JC, Miles BJ, Dunkin BJ. Global evaluative assessment of robotic skills: validation of a clinical assessment tool to measure robotic surgical skills. *J Urol.* 2012;187:247-252.

43. Gao Y, Swaroop Vedula S, Reiley CE, et al. JHU-ISI Gesture and Skill Assessment Working Set (JIGSAWS): a surgical activity dataset for human motion modeling. MICCAI Workshop: M2CAI, 2014. Accessed October 6, 2020. https://cirl.lcsr.jhu.edu/research/hmm/datasets/jigsaws_release/.

44. Ahmidi N, Tao L, Sefati S, et al. A dataset and benchmarks for segmentation and recognition of gestures in robotic surgery. *IEEE Trans Biomed Eng.* 2017;64:2025-2041.

45. Lea C, Vidal R, Hager GD. Learning convolutional action primitives for fine-grained action recognition. Proceedings of the IEEE International Conference on Robotics and Automation, 2016. Accessed October 6, 2020. http://colinlea.com/docs/pdf/2016_ICRA_CLea.pdf.

46. Lea C, Hager GD, Vidal R. An improved model for segmentation and recognition of fine-grained activities with application to surgical training tasks. Proceedings of the 2015 IEEE Winter Conference on Applications of Computer Vision. Accessed October 6, 2020. https://ieeexplore.ieee.org/document/7046008.

47. Lea C, Reiter A, Vidal R, Hager GD. Segmental spatiotemporal CNNs for fine-grained action segmentation. Lecture Notes in Computer Science (including subseries Lecture Notes in Artificial Intelligence and Lecture Notes in Bioinformatics) European Conference on Computer Vision ECCV, 2016. Accessed October 6, 2020. https://arxiv.org/abs/1602.02995.

48. Dipietro R, Lea C, Malpani A, et al. Recognizing surgical activities with recurrent neural networks. International Conference on Medical Image Computing and Computer-Assisted Intervention MICCAI, 2016. Accessed October 6, 2020. https://arxiv.org/abs/1606.06329.

49. DiPietro R, Ahmidi N, Malpani A, et al. Segmenting and classifying activities in robot-assisted surgery with recurrent neural networks. *Int J Comput Assist Radiol Surg.* 2019;14:2005-2020.

50. Lea C, Vidal R, Reiter A, Hager GD. Temporal convolutional networks: a unified approach to action segmentation. European Conference on Computer Vision ECCV Workshops, 2016. Accessed October 6, 2020. https://arxiv.org/abs/1608.08242.

51. Liu D, Jiang T. Deep reinforcement learning for surgical gesture segmentation and classification. Medical Image Computing and Computer Assisted Intervention, MICCAI, 2018. Accessed October 6, 2020. https://arxiv.org/abs/1806.08089.

52. Sarikaya D, Guru KA, Corso JJ. Joint surgical gesture and task classification with multi-task and multimodal learning. arXiv:1805.00721. Accessed October 6, 2020. https://arxiv.org/abs/1805.00721.

53. Sarikaya D, Jannin P. Surgical gesture recognition with optical flow only. arXiv:1904.01143. Accessed October 6, 2020. https://deepai.org/publication/surgical-gesture-recognition-with-optical-flow-only.

54. Simonyan K, Zisserman A. Two-stream convolutional networks for action recognition in videos. Proceedings of the 27th International Conference on Neural Information Processing Systems, Volume 1, 2014. Accessed October 6, 2020. https://papers.nips.cc/paper/5353-two-stream-convolutional-networks-for-action-recognition-in-videos.pdf.

55. Van Amsterdam B, Nakawala H, De Momi E, Stoyanov D. Weakly supervised recognition of surgical gestures. arXiv:1907.10993. Accessed October 6, 2020. https://arxiv.org/pdf/1907.10993.pdf.

56. Zia A, Hung A, Essa I, Jarc A. Surgical activity recognition in robot-assisted radical prostatectomy using deep learning. International Conference on Medical Image Computing and Computer-Assisted Intervention MICCAI, 2018. Accessed October 6, 2020. https://arxiv.org/abs/1806.00466v1.

57. Szegedy C, Vanhoucke V, Ioffe S, Shlens J, Wojna Z. Rethinking the inception architecture for computer vision. 2016 IEEE Conference on Computer Vision and Pattern Recognition (CVPR). Accessed October 6, 2020. https://arxiv.org/abs/1512.00567.

58. Zia A, Guo L, Zhou L, Essa I, Jarc A. Novel evaluation of surgical activity recognition models using task-based efficiency metrics. *Int J Comput Assist Radiol Surg.* 2019;14:2155-2163.

59. Shelhamer E, Long J, Darrell T. Fully convolutional networks for semantic segmentation. *IEEE Trans Pattern Anal Mach Intell.* 2017;39(4):640-651.

60. Badrinarayanan V, Kendall A, Cipolla R. SegNet: a deep convolutional encoder-decoder architecture for image segmentation. *IEEE Trans Pattern Anal Mach Intell.* 2017;39:2481-2495.

61. Ronneberger O, Fischer P, Brox T. U-net: convolutional networks for biomedical image segmentation. Lecture Notes in Computer Science (including subseries Lecture Notes in Artificial Intelligence and Lecture Notes in Bioinformatics), 2015. Accessed October 7, 2020. https://arxiv.org/abs/1505.04597.

62. He K, Zhang X, Ren S, Sun J. Deep residual learning for image recognition. 2016 IEEE Conference on Computer Vision and Pattern Recognition (CVPR). Accessed October 7, 2020. https://arxiv.org/abs/1512.03385.

63. Allan M, Shvets A, Kurmann T, et al. 2017 Robotic Instrument Segmentation Challenge. arXiv:1902.06426. Accessed October 7, 2020. https://arxiv.org/pdf/1902.06426.pdf.

64. Garcia-Peraza-Herrera LC, Li W, Fidon L, et al. ToolNet: holistically-nested real-time segmentation of robotic surgical tools. IEEE International Conference on Intelligent Robots and Systems, 2017. Accessed October 7, 2020. https://ieeexplore.ieee.org/document/8206462.

65. Hasan SMK, Linte CA. U-NetPlus: a modified encoder-decoder U-Net architecture for semantic and instance segmentation of surgical instrument. arXiv:1902.08994. Accessed October 7, 2020. https://arxiv.org/abs/1902.08994.

66. Ni Z-L, Bian G-B, Hou Z-G, Zhou X-H, Xie X-L, Li Z. Attention-guided lightweight network for real-time segmentation of robotic surgical instruments. arXiv:1910.11109. Accessed October 7, 2020. https://arxiv.org/pdf/1910.11109v1.pdf.

67. Mohammed A, Yildirim S, Farup I, Pedersen M, Hovde Ø. StreoScenNet: surgical stereo robotic scene segmentation. SPIE 10951, Medical Imaging 2019: Image-Guided Procedures, Robotic Interventions, and Modeling, 2019. Accessed October 7, 2020. https://ntnuopen.ntnu.no/ntnu-xmlui/handle/11250/2630676.

68. Du X, Kurmann T, Chang PL, et al. Articulated multi-instrument 2-D pose estimation using fully convolutional networks. *IEEE Trans Med Imaging*. 2018;37(5):1276-1287.

69. Chu Y, Yang X, Ding Y, et al. FSNet: pose estimation of endoscopic surgical tools using feature stacked network. In Proceedings of the 9th International Workshop on Computer Science and Engineering, Hong Kong, June 15-17, 2019.

70. Da C, Rocha C, Padoy N, Rosa B. Self-supervised surgical tool segmentation using kinematic information. arXiv:1902.04810. Accessed October 7, 2020. https://arxiv.org/abs/1902.04810.

71. De Donno A, Zorn L, Zanne P, Nageotte F, De Mathelin M. Introducing STRAS: a new flexible robotic system for minimally invasive surgery. Proceedings of the IEEE International Conference on Robotics and Automation, 2013. Accessed October 7, 2020. https://ieeexplore.ieee.org/document/6630726.

72. Ross T, Zimmerer D, Vemuri A, et al. Exploiting the potential of unlabeled endoscopic video data with self-supervised learning. *Int J Comput Assist Radiol Surg*. 2018;13:925-933.

73. Goodfellow IJ, Pouget-Abadie J, Mirza M, et al. Generative adversarial nets. Advances in Neural Information Processing Systems 27 (NIPS 2014), 2014. Accessed October 7, 2020. https://papers.nips.cc/paper/5423-generative-adversarial-nets.pdf.

74. Zia A, Essa I. Automated surgical skill assessment in RMIS training. *Int J Comput Assist Radiol Surg*. 2018;13:731-739.

75. Ismail Fawaz H, Forestier G, Weber J, Idoumghar L, Muller PA. Evaluating surgical skills from kinematic data using convolutional neural networks. Lecture Notes in Computer Science (including subseries Lecture Notes in Artificial Intelligence and Lecture Notes in Bioinformatics), 2018. Accessed October 7, 2020. https://link.springer.com/chapter/10.1007/978-3-030-00937-3_25.

76. Ismail Fawaz H, Forestier G, Weber J, Idoumghar L, Muller PA. Accurate and interpretable evaluation of surgical skills from kinematic data using fully convolutional neural networks. *Int J Comput Assist Radiol Surg*. 2019;14:1611-1617.

77. Funke I, Mees ST, Weitz J, Speidel S. Video-based surgical skill assessment using 3D convolutional neural networks. *Int J Comput Assist Radiol Surg*. 2019;14:1217-1225.

78. Oğul BB, Gilgien MF, Şahin PD. Ranking robot-assisted surgery skills using kinematic sensors. In: Chatzigiannakis I, De Ruyter B, Mavrommati I, eds. *Ambient Intelligence.* Springer; 2019:330-336.

79. Doughty H, Damen D, Mayol-Cuevas W. Who's better? Who's best? Pairwise deep ranking for skill determination. Proceedings of the IEEE Computer Society Conference on Computer Vision and Pattern Recognition, 2018. Accessed October 7, 2020. https://arxiv.org/abs/1703.09913.

80. Wang L, Xiong Y, Wang Z, et al. Temporal segment networks: towards good practices for deep action recognition. In European Conference on Computer Vision ECCV, 2016. Accessed October 7, 2020. https://link.springer.com/chapter/10.1007/978-3-319-46484-8_2.

81. Maier-Hein L, Vedula SS, Speidel S, et al. Surgical data science for next-generation interventions. *Nat Biomed Eng*. 2017;1:691-696.

82. Szegedy C, Liu W, Jia Y, et al. Going deeper with convolutions. In Proceedings of the IEEE Computer Society Conference on Computer Vision and Pattern Recognition, 2015. Accessed October 7, 2020. https://arxiv.org/abs/1409.4842.

AUTOMATED SURGICAL COACHING FOR INDIVIDUAL IMPROVEMENT

8

Anand Malpani

HIGHLIGHTS

- Surgical coaching is gaining popularity and meets the needs of current limitations in surgical training and assessment as well as continuous professional development for practicing clinicians.
- There is evidence supporting feasibility and effectiveness of surgical coaching.
- Limitations to surgical coaching include limited availability and time of coaches and coachees, affecting both scheduling and frequency of coaching sessions.
- Automated surgical coaching could alleviate some limitations via automated skill assessment, automated video chaptering/indexing for quicker review, and automated targeted and actionable feedback or individualized learning plans.

SURGICAL COACHING

Coaching is a common term used in sports, performing arts, and scholastic competitions; however, until recently, coaching was an alien concept to the profession of surgery. Unlike professional athletes who have a coach throughout their career, surgeons are their own masters once they "go pro" (ie, complete training and become independent practitioners). This does not mean, however, that surgeons are done mastering their skills once they enter independent practice. On the contrary, surgeons may find that more structured forms of engagement and continuous learning are needed once in practice because they may no longer have access to the constant supervision of a more senior surgeon.

In surgery, coaching has largely been defined by differentiating it from teaching, mentoring, and training.[*] For example, a coach may not be an expert in the field of the learner, whereas a mentor typically is. Coaching is not focused on imparting skills and knowledge, as is the case in teaching and training. In sports terminology, coaching is about taking your game to the next level. How do surgeons who have finished training and are (assumed) competent to perform their job become masters and then continuously develop their mastery? This question becomes even more important as research has shown correlations between the skill of attending surgeons and their patient outcomes.[2] As lifelong learning and deliberate practice have gained importance as evidence-based strategies to improve performance, many studies have found a positive impact on performance from coaching in surgery.[3]

In this chapter, we will describe surgical coaching from an individual learning perspective (ie, a trainee's or practicing surgeon's skill development around procedures) and how advances in artificial intelligence (AI) could make coaching more accessible. Although coaching can be applied to team training and has been studied for broader surgical and medical care, we will focus on coaching for technical and nontechnical skills and automated coaching in the context of technical skills.

The Need for Surgical Coaching

Coaching in surgery is relevant to all stakeholders involved in the surgical care process, but patient outcome is one of the leading factors driving efforts in surgical coaching. Although a causal relationship has not been validated between coaching and patient outcomes, there is evidence demonstrating associations between coaching and skill acquisition/improvement[4] and between operator skill level and patient outcomes.[2] From the surgeon's perspective, attaining the best possible patient outcome is key, but surgeons are also invested in the development of their trainees as well. A trainee is focused on improving their competency at various surgical skills; thus, coaching creates an opportunity for them to engage in deliberate practice, a well-documented method to improve skill.[5,6] Other stakeholders beyond surgery stand to benefit from the implementation of surgical coaching. For example, hospital administrators, invested in improving health care processes, must carefully consider patient outcomes and operating room (OR) efficiency. Insurance providers may benefit from well-organized

[*]Surgical Coaching [Internet]. American College of Surgeons. [cited 2020 Jan 7]. Available from: https://www.facs.org/education/division-of-education/publications/rise/articles/surg-coaching.

coaching of surgeons due to coaching's role in improving skill and decreasing costly complications that lead to readmissions and reoperations.

Components of Coaching

Across different industries, many models of coaching have been developed. In surgery, the Wisconsin Surgical Coaching Program (WSCP)[7] has been adopted by multiple groups, including the American Hernia Surgery Quality Collaborative and the Michigan Bariatric Surgery Collaborative (Figure 8-1). In WSCP, the activities of a coach have been grouped into the following categories: (1) set goals, (2) encourage/motivate, and (3) develop/guide. The activities under "set goals" relate to assessing a surgeon's skill, identifying progress milestones, and recommending practice plans. Activities like active listening, promoting, and inspiring fall under "encourage/motivate." The activities grouped under "develop/guide" revolve around the process of providing targeted and actionable feedback. The WSCP applies its model differentially to technical skills and cognitive skills, allowing trainees to focus on one component or another based on

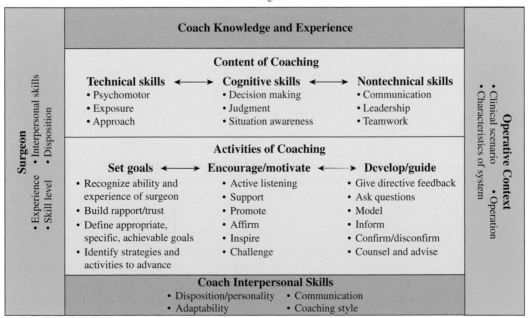

Figure 8-1 • Modified schematic of the Wisconsin Surgical Coaching Program framework.[7]

their needs. A similar coaching model, focused on technical skills only, was proposed by Stefanidis et al[8] and consisted of 5 steps: (1) assessing skills through video, (2) identifying areas of growth, (3) group and individual coaching sessions, (4) deliberate practice with coaching, and (5) monitor patient outcomes. The similarity between the 2 models was the video-based assessment of performance from the OR to identify deficits in skill. Similarly, surgical coaching studies have used other models such as GROW[9] and PRACTICE,[10] which have similar coaching components of identifying skill deficits and setting up goals, followed by recommendations for improvement, and wrapping up by evaluating skill development in a measurable way.

Existing Evidence

The initial papers in the field of surgical coaching were qualitative analyses regarding the structure of surgical coaching as described earlier regarding the WSCP.[7,8] Next, there were observational studies on surgical coaching. Hu et al[1] described, using thematic analysis, the topics of sessions where 4 study participants were engaged in an expert-based coaching system. They provided examples of coaching techniques (surgeon-driven vs coach-driven) and conversational content (operative technique, teaching, and value of such postgame analysis). Similarly, Hu et al[11] presented a comparison of teaching and coaching in 2 scenarios: intraoperatively and during a dedicated coaching session. They demonstrated the following advantages of a dedicated coaching session: more teaching points per unit time, more resident-centered teaching, and more learning goals set.

Mathur et al[12] reported lack of formal training in coaching within staff surgeons at 2 academic hospitals. They conducted a workshop on the WSCP with residents and faculty to increase awareness about formal surgical coaching concepts and showed that the number of goals set for learning in a surgeon-resident dyad was higher after the workshop. Mutabdzic et al[13] presented challenges facing surgical coaching based on a semi-structured interview-style observational study. The 3 main categories of challenges that emerged from their analysis were (1) the lack of perceived value of technical improvement (patient outcomes depend on a large numbers of factors and technical skills play only a small role; promotions and leadership positions do not evaluate one's technical skills), (2) concern of image (other surgical team members may perceive a surgeon to be incompetent and not respect their authority in the OR if a coach is present), and (3) loss of self-regulatory control (losing autonomy in the OR and coaching on trivial matters like choice of suture).

More recent papers have described randomized controlled trials (RCTs) studying surgical coaching and measured coaching's effect on both technical skills and nontechnical skills, with positive results for groups of participants receiving some form of surgical coaching. Yule et al[14] compared nontechnical skills coaching with self-reflection in surgery residents and demonstrated that surgical coaching improves trainees' nontechnical skills. In a systematic review on surgical coaching studies, Min et al[3] presented all studies related to surgical coaching prior to November 2013, including both observational studies and RCTs investigating technical and nontechnical skills as outcomes of the coaching intervention. They observed that surgical coaching showed a positive impact on the learner's technical and nontechnical skills. For example, Bonrath et al[10] showed improved skill scores for residents who were provided comprehensive surgical coaching with performance analysis, debriefing, feedback, and behavior modeling versus residents who underwent conventional training. Similarly, Singh et al[9] observed that residents who received video-based coaching by a surgeon scored more highly on laparoscopic technical skills compared to residents who viewed surgical lectures on the web. Gagnon and Abbasi[4] concluded in their systematic review that all 5 RCTs on surgical coaching have shown improved technical performance after coaching with high learner satisfaction.

Known Limitations of Surgeon-Led Surgical Coaching

As seen in the various studies comparing surgical coaching with routine learning, there are definite benefits to coaching, including measured improvements in skills for the learner (coachee). There is evidence that supports the feasibility of surgical coaching by the success of the coaching programs within the WSCP, Michigan Bariatric Surgery Collaborative, and Americas Hernia Society Quality Collaborative. The work led by Dr. Caprice Greenberg at the WSCP has produced resources on how to train and develop effective surgical coaches. This effort has been translated into the Academy for Surgical Coaching (https://surgicalcoaching.org/) to build, host, train, and orient the surgical community into the coaching mindset. Although coaching as a concept has been gaining popularity among surgical educators, the implementation of coaching has many challenges.

The most significant challenge is the time needed to engage in a 1-on-1 coaching relationship. Time is a scarce resource for both practicing and trainee surgeons. Time spent in activities outside of clinical care is time that surgeons are unavailable to see additional patients, with the negative effect of loss of clinical revenue for the hospital enterprise. Additionally, finding a common time for the coachee and coach can be challenging given the limited time available within their schedules. This is, perhaps, the major reason why surgical coaching has not become routine within residency programs, despite the growing evidence of its effectiveness in improving performance.

Existing surgical coaching programs have set up quarterly coaching sessions to coincide with other events, such as a clinical society meeting. During such quarterly sessions, the coach and coachee typically share a video recording of the performance and focus their 1-on-1 time on a coaching relationship centered around the video. This is the second important challenge facing surgical coaching—long intervals between coaching sessions. Although there has yet to be a study in surgery analyzing the effect of coaching intervals, lessons can be learned from another industry where coaching is prevalent—sports. A professional coach in sports is available for each performance (before, during, and after), enabling the coach and coachee to frequently reflect on performance and then identify and set goals for improvement. This more readily fits the framework of deliberate practice and expert performance described by K. Anders Ericsson. One potential solution to address the limitation of time for coaching might be the use of nonsurgeon coaches or retired surgeon coaches who may have more availability to provide coaching on a routine basis similar to other professions.

Another challenge that was identified by the findings of Mutabdzic et al[13] was a perceived loss of autonomy and control of learning by the coachee (ie, feeling as though there was little choice in the topics upon which the coach would provide coaching). Greenberg et al,[15] in the WSCP, suggested educating coaches about the differences between coaching and mentoring, advising, or instructing, emphasizing the shared decision-making approach to coaching to ensure coachees felt respected and empowered.

▌AUTOMATED SURGICAL COACHING

What Can Automation Bring?

Although existing challenges can limit the use of coaching in surgery, the potential advantages of coaching in surgical training and in the professional development of practicing surgeons merit close inspection of possible alternative strategies to in-person coaching. This is where AI in surgery may play a useful role in transforming the way learning, improvement, and retention of surgical skills are conducted.

Imagine if a trainee surgeon arrives at the simulation lab and logs on to their account. They are shown a learning plan for surgical skills charted out for them, with specific recommendations on which skills they need to practice and improve, which skills they have mastered sufficiently for the time being, what is lacking in their performance of said skills, how to improve them, and what an expert surgeon would do differently than them. Their learning plan would then be updated every day after every practice of every skill. Even if a few pieces of information from this example were available, the learning of surgical skills for a trainee might be significantly enhanced. Likewise, imagine that a practicing surgeon logs on to their computer on the day of surgery to see their performance dashboard about the particular procedure they are to perform. They are informed about steps during the procedure where they may be below par in terms of proficiency as well as areas that may lead to overall lower OR efficiency. They are recommended a simulation-based warm-up routine that fits their current skill level and matches the procedure they will be performing. Their learning plan is updated by monitoring every case and every step within a case throughout each operative day to identify whether any specific skills should be worked on to advance their skill above their current level of mastery. Additionally, in academic programs, they could be updated about the competence of the trainee who will be assisting them in the OR. They can identify what steps of the procedure the trainee is competent to assist with and perform, as well as what steps may be beyond their current expertise. All of these interesting scenarios could be enabled via automated surgical coaching by the use of machine learning methods and AI frameworks. Malpani[16] presented an automated virtual coach for surgical training that addressed these types of coaching activities and tied into the existing coaching models proposed in surgery.[7-10]

An automated virtual coach (VC) can be developed to address existing limitations and challenges in surgical coaching that were described earlier. If a framework powered by machine learning algorithms can assess skill, identify deficits, demonstrate expert-like performance, recommend practice/set goals, and monitor progress toward set goals, it can provide more regular and frequent virtual coaching sessions to augment the intermittent coaching delivered by an expert surgeon. A VC could further empower both the coachee and the coach with rich information about the skill development that occurs between 1-on-1 human coaching sessions (Figure 8-2). In addition, a VC could function as an objective coach to protect the privacy of patients, surgeons, and trainees, if needed.

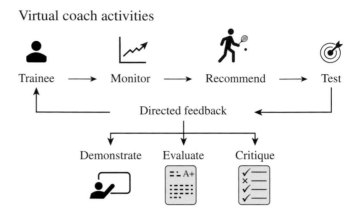

Figure 8-2 • A hypothetical automated virtual coaching cycle for learning and developing surgical skills.

It can enable closed-loop training and learning wherein assessment of performance from the simulation lab determines participation in the OR. Performance assessment from the OR determines practice sessions in the simulation lab, and the cycle continues. The VC can identify learning trajectories for individuals and cater learning curricula based on other previously observed learning trajectories. It could direct learners onto a fast-track versus slow-track curriculum that is best suited for their learning style. Overall, a VC could enable active learning, deliberate practice, and individualized feedback and possibly make surgical training efficient and effective.

So, how would a VC work? In what learning settings can such a VC be feasible? Do we have the technology and methods available to realize this vision? What are the underlying computer modeling problems that a machine learning method needs to solve? What kind of data would be used to power this VC? Let us take a deeper dive into these questions.

Data for Automated Surgical Coaching

There are various senses used to perceive an activity. We use vision to see what action is being done, how it is performed (movement), and its effect. We use touch to feel and measure how it is being done (force) and to what effect. Activities that involve, for example, application of electrical current can also involve hearing (the sound of either the instrument or the tissue during coagulation) or smelling (the result of fulguration). If we want to quantify these, then we use sensors of different types that can measure direct or indirect signals. A camera is a simple example of a sensor that approximates sight. Motion sensors of different types can measure position, orientation, acceleration, and angular velocity of the object to which they are attached. Microphones capture sound, and force and pressure sensors can capture partially the effect of touch. Electromyography can provide a measure of muscle activity of the operator. Galvanic skin response sensors can measure emotional stress and cognitive load. Sophisticated cameras using different sources of light can capture eye gaze (where is someone looking) and measure the depth (distance) at which different objects may appear in the visual scene. All of these sensors and their corresponding measurements have been used in studies on surgical skill assessment.[17,18]

Video images captured using a camera, such as an endoscope, provide details about the surgical process. By looking at a video, surgeons are able to judge the skill of the operator reliably and accurately.[19–21] It provides the context of the task, such as anatomy, instrument, other surgical objects, hands, and events like irrigation, suction, smoke, and bleeding. It contains information about interactions between these objects. Position and orientation sensors (eg, electromagnetic sensors) can provide precise measurements of hand and instrument motion that may not be as easily obtained from video images. Similarly, accelerometers and gyroscopes deliver a precise capture of surgical motion. These can provide a proxy for efficiency in performance and surgical planning and have been shown to capture information about underlying surgical skill. Force and pressure sensors provide a direct measure of the interaction between the objects in the surgical scene. For example, a force sensor attached to the instrument could measure the amount of force that is being applied by the instrument on the surgical workspace. Eye gaze tracking sensors provide an accurate measure of the region of interest where surgical care is being delivered within the entire video image. Each of these measurements maps to various items such as respect for tissue or force sensitivity, economy of motion, or efficiency that are part of multi-item global rating scales for surgical skill assessment, such as Objective Structured Assessment of Technical Skill[22] or Global Operative Assessment of Laparoscopic Skills.[23] In summary, video images could possibly capture all the information needed to enable coaching. However, surgical AI is not yet advanced enough to comprehend different dimensions of the performance using video only. Thus, complementary signals measured by the other sensors mentioned earlier can aid a machine to extract context from a video image that is relevant for the surgical coaching task.

What to Automate: Machine Learning Problems Relevant to Surgical Coaching

It is popularly said that an image is worth a thousand words. Extending that thought, a video is worth a lot more, especially considering videos are composed of 24 images (or more) per second. Analyzing the video using machine learning (ie, computer vision; see Chapter 6) could thus deliver a lot of value to educators, learners, and researchers alike. Malpani[16] describes 5 activities for a VC: demonstrate, evaluate, critique, recommend, and monitor. To perform these coaching interventions, a machine should be able to extract different pieces of information from the performance.

Evaluation or assessment of skill is by far the most researched topic in surgical data science[24] that is relevant to coaching. Various review articles have summarized findings on data and methods used to predict and measure surgical skill of the performer using sensor data.[17,18,25,26] Most of this literature has focused on assessment of skill in simulation settings with limited examples of algorithms that predict skill in the OR. Even these methods have been limited to predict surgical skill as a binary variable (ie, classify a performance as expert or novice) or, in some cases, to classify skill into 3 categories (expert, intermediate, and novice). Ahmidi et al[27] presented a method to classify performances into expert and novice for septoplasty procedures using electromagnetic motion tracking. Azari et al[28] show that motion tracking using overhead video cameras can predict skill scores like fluidity of motion, motion economy, and tissue handling.

What is common in these and other works is that global measures of skill were predicted or measured in an automated way. However, something that is essential for successful coaching is the breakdown of performance and identification of where technique was good or bad relative to expert performance. This is where an understanding of the underlying activity sequence in a performance is useful. This is referred to as activity recognition in the computer vision community with several variations such as activity segmentation and activity classification (see Chapter 7).

Moving to the "critique" activity for the VC, the goal is to support an assessment with a relevant explanation of why a particular assessment was made. Even in a 1-on-1 setting, this is often done verbally and qualitatively, not via a checklist or a score card that can be analyzed quantitatively, which makes it even harder to automate. Thus, there is no publicly disclosed work on automation on this topic. To deliver a reasoning behind scoring of a performance, AI would need a method to know (1) whether a performance was above or below par, (2) what segment(s) of the performance was above or below par, and (3) what sequence of actions or single action led to the ultimate classification as above or below par. Next, for the VC to recommend a deliberate practice session to the coachee, it would need a performance history consisting of the outputs of the "evaluate" and "critique" components so that the appropriate practice tasks could be assigned. The goal of deliberate practice is to focus the attention of the learner on a specific subskill until they develop mastery that contributes to an overall improvement in performance. A VC would thus be dependent on activity recognition and skill assessment to deliver this intervention. Similarly, the monitor activity of the VC relies on skill assessment and activity recognition.

Finally, for the demonstrate activity, the VC should be able to show expert behavior to model and teach to the coachee. There has been work on automated demonstration of expert behavior and feedback on deviation from such behavior using virtual and augmented reality.[16,29-31] Another mechanism for demonstration is to show a video of correct and incorrect performance relevant to the learning scenario. In this case, the machine should be able to compute the similarity between 2 videos, one of them being the current performance for which demonstration is needed and the other being a previously recorded performance that is part of a library. This is referred to as video retrieval in the machine learning community. A couple of papers have shown the feasibility of doing this in bench-top simulation.[32,33] The problem of video retrieval also relies on activity recognition indirectly and would require skill assessment to find videos (demonstrations) of a specific skill appropriate to the level of the learner. Overall, what we can see is that the VC relies heavily upon activity recognition and skill assessment to perform coaching activities. Thus, automated surgical activity recognition and automated surgical skill assessment are 2 main areas that need to be addressed to achieve automated surgical coaching.

Automated Activity Recognition

The topic of automated activity recognition in surgery is covered in greater depth in Chapter 7. Automated activity recognition is an important component of automated surgical coaching because it provides context for the skills being performed (ie, are the right skills being performed at the right time?).

Automated Skill Assessment

Automated skill assessment has been an active area of research since the early 2000s. As shown in Figure 8-3, work on this exists for various surgical settings from simulation to the OR. Vedula et al[17] provide a great overview of all the work on this topic prior to 2016. Dias et al[34] provide

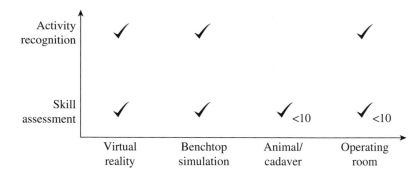

Figure 8-3 • Current state of work on automation of problems required to power automated surgical coaching. In the figure, "<10" indicates that fewer than 10 publications exist in the literature attempting those problem scenarios.

a broader review of machine learning applied for physician competence (not limited to surgery and surgical specialties). Although a large number of studies have been conducted to develop and test machine learning models for skill assessment, a detailed view of the surgical tasks that were assessed is highly limited, with the majority of studies focusing on suturing and knot-tying skills. The skill assessment in the majority of the works has focused on classification of experts and novices, rather than on providing feedback to the learner.

Unlike classification of novice/expert performance, automated score prediction on a surgical task provides more directed feedback as the learner can gain insight into whether their performance is improving. The majority of the prior work in skill assessment has been on performances in the simulation lab using bench-top or dry lab models. In the case of an expert/novice skill classification for bench-top suturing and knot tying skills, the accuracy of machine learning models has been shown to reach the high 90s and 100 in some cases. Most of the work has focused on global (task-level) skill assessment with the exception of the work by Malpani et al,[35] which developed methods to assess and score segment-level performance within the task of interrupted suturing.

Automated assessment of skills at the segment level is key to addressing many of the coaching activities. Such segment-level assessment can occur at different levels of granularity. For example, it can provide assessment for each individual step within a procedure such as wound closure or suturing, and more granularly, it can include the assessment of each individual surgical knot. Recent works on automated skill assessment of intraoperative performance of the procedural steps of cataract surgery[36] and robot-assisted radical cystectomy[37] have described ways to deliver targeted feedback. This can direct trainees to focus their learning in the simulation lab on skills related to the steps where they were assessed to be less proficient, thereby enabling deliberate practice.

How Would an Automated Coach Function?

The VC engages in multiple coaching interventions, relying on automated activity recognition and skill assessment methods. Figure 8-2 depicts a possible workflow for the VC. A coachee aiming to learn or develop a skill engages in coaching with the VC. First, the VC gives a test exercise with known difficulty and performance benchmarks. The performance data of the coachee are recorded and analyzed over multiple repetitions to build a performance history. Here, the VC evaluates and critiques the multiple performances and logs them. The VC uses an algorithm to monitor such assessment and identifies the competency level of the coachee on the given exercise and skill. Based on this estimated competency, it determines whether the coachee should be given a practice session on a subset of skills (not competent) or whether the coachee should progress to a more complex exercise for the same skill (competent). This cycle of assessment, feedback, and skill progression continues until the VC determines that the coachee has reached the highest level of competency for the basic skill. At this point, the coachee "graduates" from the skill and continues on to the next skill they want to develop.

However, although automation may not replace human coaches (HCs), it could augment their coaching (Figure 8-4). As shown in this figure, green indicates human coaching, whereas blue indicates automated coaching. A coachee's performance is observed by the HC, and certain recommendations are made and goals are set. These are transferred over to the VC's profile for the coachee, and thereafter, the VC presents

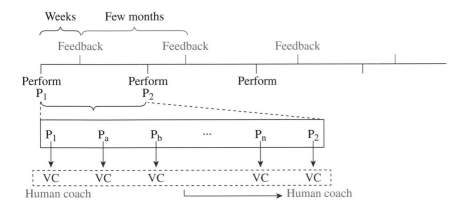

Figure 8-4 • A sketch depicting augmentation of human coaching (shown in green) by data and coaching delivered by the automated virtual coach (VC; shown in blue).

exercises and coaching relevant to the HC's recommendations using the cycle described in the previous paragraph. After a set period of time, the coachee engages with the HC again. This time, the HC is equipped with all the coaching data from the VC since the last time the HC had a coaching session with the coachee. Thus, the HC's coaching is powered by a rich set of information on the day-to-day training of the coachee on the recommended skills. In return, the coachee receives more frequent coaching from the VC that results in their skill development. If the coachee was a trainee surgeon, attending surgeons feel more trust in the trainee surgeon's improved proficiency to allow more case participation in the OR. If the coachee is a practicing surgeon, then the coachee's improved proficiency reflects in overall improved patient care delivery and OR efficiency that could be measured through patient outcomes and operative time.

FUTURE DIRECTIONS

Delivery Mechanism for Automated Coaching

Although a coach may have a lot of information about the coachee and the skill, delivering effective coaching interventions is what makes coaching an art and a skill. Similarly, the VC would require a well-designed user interface and user design to deliver effective and efficient learning. The underlying machine learning methods that would power a VC are still under development, and the human factors engineering behind designing the VC's front end (ie, the user-facing side) is similarly a work in progress, although design thinking has undergone a resurgence in the past decade. A lot of learning environments outside of surgery are being developed in the virtual reality and augmented reality worlds, and some of these are now being translated to surgical training. Many questions remain, however. What sensors will be used to measure performance? How would a VC be packaged? Would it be an ecosystem that exists on virtual reality headsets, laptops, and mobile devices? Will it be a virtual assistant like Alexa (Amazon, Seattle, WA) to which the coachee could talk? There is a possibility that a VC can become an integral part of the surgical education system as the coaching partner for medical students, surgical residents, fellows, and practicing surgeons from day 1. However, care must be taken to ensure that evidence-based and cost-effective principles are incorporated into any VC to ensure the most efficient delivery of education.

Data Sets

As seen in previous chapters, data sets are integral to machine learning. The machine needs previously captured data to model the underlying problem and identify its best quantitative representation. For the VC, a large variety of data will be needed to deliver the various coaching interventions. Although the performance data would be similar, the labels assigned to the performances would be the most interesting and challenging part of the data set building. For example, there is no standardized way to deliver constructive feedback in surgical training, and thus, generating appropriate training data sets for a machine learning algorithm would require building these standards.

Another challenge would be capturing longitudinal data to power the monitoring and recommendation interventions. Performance samples collected on a routine basis would be needed to deliver accurate monitoring of skill. Like most AI and health care discussions, multi-institutional data sets would be needed to extend the framework beyond a single learning center. All these issues present severe challenges given the sensitive nature of these data. Today, in the surgical data science community, the largest public data sets are on the order of 120 to 200 performance samples compared to millions of samples in the general computer vision community. Efforts at the national and international levels with the support of societies and colleges would be needed to put such data sets in place.

Competency-Based Education

Automated coaching has an increasingly important role to play as the surgical education community gears up to embrace competency-based education and entrustable professional activities (EPAs). The burden on educators to assess the skill, competency, and entrustability of learners is going to be massive. These quantities are reliable if measured frequently. For example, a competency assessment of a resident is not meaningful if it is based on a handful of observations during the year. Assessment of skill at the procedure level and at the subtask level on each episode of intraoperative performance by the resident will be needed. Coaching activities will need to be aligned with the competencies and EPAs set up by entities such as the Association of American Medical Colleges, the American Board of Surgery, and the Accreditation Council for Graduate Medical Education; otherwise, the coaching provided to trainee surgeons will not be aligned with the final assessments that will determine their graduation. Similarly, lifelong learning and continuous professional development for practicing surgeons will need to be aligned with maintenance of certification requirements.

Automated coaching may become an essential part of development for both trainees and practicing surgeons as each individual works to attain the next level of mastery and deliver better patient care with each operation he or she performs.

▌REFERENCES

1. Hu Y-Y, Peyre SE, Arriaga AF, et al. Postgame analysis: using video-based coaching for continuous professional development. *J Am Coll Surg*. 2012;214(1):115-124.
2. Fecso AB, Szasz P, Kerezov G, Grantcharov TP. The effect of technical performance on patient outcomes in surgery: a systematic review. *Ann Surg*. 2017;265(3):492-501.
3. Min H, Morales DR, Orgill D, Smink DS, Yule S. Systematic review of coaching to enhance surgeons' operative performance. *Surgery*. 2015;158(5):1168-1191.
4. Gagnon L-H, Abbasi N. Systematic review of randomized controlled trials on the role of coaching in surgery to improve learner outcomes. *Am J Surg*. 2018;216(1):140-146.
5. Palter VN, Grantcharov TP. Individualized deliberate practice on a virtual reality simulator improves technical performance of surgical novices in the operating room: a randomized controlled trial. *Ann Surg*. 2014;259(3):443-448.
6. Hashimoto DA, Sirimanna P, Gomez ED, et al. Deliberate practice enhances quality of laparoscopic surgical performance in a randomized controlled trial: from arrested development to expert performance. *Surg Endosc*. 2015;29(11):3154-3162.
7. Greenberg CC, Ghousseini HN, Pavuluri Quamme SR, Beasley HL, Wiegmann DA. Surgical coaching for individual performance improvement. *Ann Surg*. 2015;261(1):32-34.
8. Stefanidis D, Anderson-Montoya B, Higgins RV, et al. Developing a coaching mechanism for practicing surgeons. *Surgery*. 2016;160(3):536-545.
9. Singh P, Aggarwal R, Tahir M, Pucher PH, Darzi A. A randomized controlled study to evaluate the role of video-based coaching in training laparoscopic skills. *Ann Surg*. 2015;261(5):862-869.
10. Bonrath EM, Dedy NJ, Gordon LE, Grantcharov TP. Comprehensive surgical coaching enhances surgical skill in the operating room: a randomized controlled trial. *Ann Surg*. 2015;262(2):205-212.
11. Hu Y-Y, Mazer LM, Yule SJ, et al. Complementing operating room teaching with video-based coaching. *JAMA Surg*. 2017;152(4):318-325.
12. Mathur S, Cherniak R, Bodley J, Farrugia M. Surgical coaching in obstetrics and gynecology: a multi-centre pilot project. *J Obstet Gynaecol Can*. 2019;41(5):724-725.
13. Mutabdzic D, Mylopoulos M, Murnaghan ML, et al. Coaching surgeons: is culture limiting our ability to improve? *Ann Surg*. 2015;262(2):213-216.
14. Yule S, Parker SH, Wilkinson J, et al. Coaching non-technical skills improves surgical residents' performance in a simulated operating room. *J Surg Educ*. 2015;72(6):1124-1130.
15. Greenberg CC, Dombrowski J, Dimick JB. Video-based surgical coaching: an emerging approach to performance improvement. *JAMA Surg*. 2016;151(3): 282-283.
16. Malpani A. Automated virtual coach for surgical training. 2017. Accessed October 5, 2020. https://jscholarship.library.jhu.edu/handle/1774.2/59327.

17. Vedula SS, Ishii M, Hager GD. Objective assessment of surgical technical skill and competency in the operating room. *Annu Rev Biomed Eng*. 2017;19:301-325.

18. Shackelford S, Bowyer M. Modern metrics for evaluating surgical technical skills. *Curr Surg Rep*. 2017;5(10):24.

19. Grenda TR, Pradarelli JC, Dimick JB. Using surgical video to improve technique and skill. *Ann Surg*. 2016;264(1):32-33.

20. Dimick JB, Varban OA. Surgical video analysis: an emerging tool for improving surgeon performance. *BMJ Qual Saf*. 2015;24(8):490-491.

21. McQueen S, McKinnon V, VanderBeek L, McCarthy C, Sonnadara R. Video-based assessment in surgical education: a scoping review. *J Surg Educ*. 2019;76(6):1645-1654.

22. Martin JA, Regehr G, Reznick R, et al. Objective structured assessment of technical skill (OSATS) for surgical residents. *Br J Surg*. 1997;84(2):273-278.

23. Vassiliou MC, Feldman LS, Andrew CG, et al. A global assessment tool for evaluation of intraoperative laparoscopic skills. *Am J Surg*. 2005;190(1):107-113.

24. Maier-Hein L, Vedula SS, Speidel S, et al. Surgical data science for next-generation interventions. *Nat Biomed Eng*. 2017;1(9):691-696.

25. Van Hove PD, Tuijthof GJM, Verdaasdonk EGG, Stassen LPS, Dankelman J. Objective assessment of technical surgical skills. *Br J Surg*. 2010;97(7):972-987.

26. Oropesa I, Sánchez-González P, Lamata P, et al. Methods and tools for objective assessment of psychomotor skills in laparoscopic surgery. *J Surg Res*. 2011;171(1):e81-e95.

27. Ahmidi N, Poddar P, Jones JD, et al. Automated objective surgical skill assessment in the operating room from unstructured tool motion in septoplasty. *Int J Comput Assist Radiol Surg*. 2015;10(6):981-991.

28. Azari DP, Frasier LL, Quamme SRP, et al. Modeling surgical technical skill using expert assessment for automated computer rating. *Ann Surg*. 2019;269(3):574-581.

29. Malpani A, Swaroop Vedula S, Lin HC, Hager GD, Taylor RH. Real-time teaching cues for automated surgical coaching. Accessed October 3, 2020. http://arxiv.org/abs/1704.07436.

30. Wijewickrema S, Piromchai P, Zhou Y, et al. Developing effective automated feedback in temporal bone surgery simulation. *Otolaryngol Head Neck Surg*. 2015;152(6):1082-1088.

31. Zhou Y, Bailey J, Ioannou I, Wijewickrema S, Kennedy G, O'Leary S. Constructive real time feedback for a temporal bone simulator. *Med Image Comput Comput Assist Interv*. 2013;16(Pt 3):315-322.

32. Chen L, Zhang Q, Zhang P, Li B. Instructive video retrieval for surgical skill coaching using attribute learning. In: *2015 IEEE International Conference on Multimedia and Expo (ICME)*. IEEE; 2015:1-6.

33. Gao Y, Vedula SS, Lee GI, Lee MR, Khudanpur S, Hager GD. Query-by-example surgical activity detection. *Int J Comput Assist Radiol Surg*. 2016;11(6):987-996.

34. Dias RD, Gupta A, Yule SJ. Using machine learning to assess physician competence: a systematic review. *Acad Med*. 2019;94(3):427-439.

35. Malpani A, Vedula SS, Chen CCG, Hager GD. A study of crowdsourced segment-level surgical skill assessment using pairwise rankings. *Int J Comput Assist Radiol Surg*. 2015;10(9):1435-1447.

36. Kim TS, O'Brien M, Zafar S, Hager GD, Sikder S, Vedula SS. Objective assessment of intraoperative technical skill in capsulorhexis using videos of cataract surgery. *Int J Comput Assist Radiol Surg*. 2019;14(6):1097-1105.

37. Baghdadi A, Hussein AA, Ahmed Y, Cavuoto LA, Guru KA. A computer vision technique for automated assessment of surgical performance using surgeons' console-feed videos. *Int J Comput Assist Radiol Surg*. 2019;14(4):697-707.

PREOPERATIVE RISK STRATIFICATION

9

Majed W. El Hechi, Samer A. Nour Eddine, and
Haytham M.A. Kaafarani

HIGHLIGHTS

- Preoperative risk stratification allows surgeons to set patient and family expectations for postoperative outcomes.
- Artificial intelligence (AI) allows risk stratification calculators to accurately capture the complex interactions of preoperative risk factors in surgical patients.
- Newly developed preoperative risk calculators use different technologies within AI, each with its own unique set of capabilities.
- Although AI improves the accuracy of preoperative risk stratification, surgeons should remain aware of the technology's limitations and pitfalls.

INTRODUCTION

Picture a 45-year-old gentleman with known moderate cirrhosis presenting to the emergency department with acute cholecystitis. On evaluation, the patient appears frail and fatigued, complaining of fever and abdominal pain. Should the surgeon book the patient for an emergent cholecystectomy? Will the patient survive the postoperative course? Would percutaneous cholecystostomy be a more appropriate temporizing measure while the patient is clinically optimized for surgery? How should the risks, benefits, and alternatives to surgery be explained to the patient and his family?

Clinical scenarios that carry a significant risk of postoperative complications, like the one just described, are common. *Primum non nocere*[1] is a philosophy embodied in the Hippocratic oath made by doctors worldwide. The maxim is intuitive and theoretically unproblematic. However, contemporary medical practice is complex, and despite best intentions, some patients are inadvertently harmed. The Institute of Medicine estimates that almost 98,000 people die every year from medical errors.[2]

The world of surgery is no exception to this reality: errors happen. Even when a surgeon's decision to operate was sound and a technically safe procedure was performed, postoperative adverse events and complications are still common. Postoperative complications occur in 15% of the 19 million surgeries performed yearly in the United States,[3] incurring a total cost of 31.35 billion dollars.[4] As such, many preoperative risk stratification systems have been created over the past 2 decades to support surgeon experience and gestalt in estimating a patient's postoperative course. Throughout the years, these systems have proved to be invaluable, allowing providers to set patient and family expectations and to guide preoperative decision making.

This chapter tackles the introduction of artificial intelligence (AI) into preoperative risk stratification by providing an overview of the AI technologies used in state-of-the-art preoperative surgical risk calculators. The chapter also addresses the limitations and pitfalls of AI in risk stratification, shedding light on the future of preoperative risk stratification using AI methodologies.

▍BACKGROUND ON LINEAR RISK STRATIFICATION

Prior to delving into the world of AI, some background knowledge of existing non-AI risk stratification models can help readers better understand the advances offered by this new technology.

One of the earliest non-AI preoperative risk stratification tools that is still in use today is the American Society of Anesthesiologists (ASA) Physical Classification System. Originally conceived in 1941, the scale allows the simple albeit subjective classification of preoperative patients into 1 of 5 risk classes, each representing a qualitative measure of illness severity. For example, class I describes healthy patients, class III describes patients who have a severe disease that limits activity, and class V describes moribund patients who are not expected to survive 24 hours with or without an operation. Patients in the more severe groups have been shown to have less favorable postoperative outcomes.[5]

In contrast to the subjectivity of the ASA system, the Physiological and Operative Severity Score for the Enumeration of Mortality and Morbidity (POSSUM) was designed to be objective and comprehensive. This 18-item score was developed in 1991 to assess quality of care and to provide a scoring system for benchmarking general surgery.[6] Additionally, in the same decade, comprehensive preoperative risk stratification models were developed catering to specific surgery types. For instance, a mortality risk score was developed for cardiac surgery candidates by the

Society of Thoracic Surgeons.[7] This tool uses over 40 clinical parameters to calculate a postoperative mortality figure, making it comprehensive yet cumbersome.

In 2013, the American College of Surgeons (ACS) National Surgical Quality Improvement Program (NSQIP) Surgical Risk Calculator (SRC) was created. Developed using clinical data from nearly 400 US hospitals, this web-based tool allows surgeons to predict 30-day patient outcomes; namely, mortality, morbidity, and 18 individual complications common to most surgical procedures. In addition, the SRC is also capable of predicting procedure-specific complications (eg, risk of bladder fistula in hysterectomy procedures and risk of anastomotic leaks in colectomy procedures).[8]

Because the NSQIP database consists mostly of patients undergoing elective surgery, there was a concern that the SRC is less accurate in predicting risk in patients undergoing emergency operations,[9,10] necessitating a dedicated calculator for that subpopulation. To address this concern, the Emergency Surgery Score (ESS) was conceived by training the model on patients identified as having undergone emergency surgery in the NSQIP database. The validated ESS model indeed achieved better predictive and discriminatory power for predicting mortality and morbidity in emergency surgery.

Similarly, in 2014, the Surgical Outcome Risk Tool (SORT) web calculator was created using multi-institutional data from nearly 330 hospitals in the United Kingdom.[11] SORT predicts 30-day mortality after inpatient nonneurologic and noncardiac surgery in adults. The performance of the original model was comparable to that of the SRC with respect to mortality prediction and was later upgraded to predict postoperative morbidity with modest accuracy.[12]

All of these models have been updated since their creation, resulting in improvements in accuracy,[5,13,14] measured by the area under the receiver operating characteristic (ROC) curve. The area under the curve (AUC) or c-statistic represents the goodness of fit of a model to its intended outcomes and has values that range from 0.5 to 1, where 0.5 denotes no predictive power and 1 denotes perfect prediction.[15-17] For instance, validating the ESS on the NSQIP database yielded mortality and morbidity AUCs of 0.86 and 0.78, respectively.[13]

UNMET NEED

Although these models and calculators are undoubtedly useful and have respectable AUCs, they share a common inherent characteristic: they assume that the variables in their models interact in a linear and additive fashion.[18] In other words, when applied to different patients, the same variables have the same weight in predicting the outcome every time. In medical reality, however, the interaction between existing comorbidities and illness severity is not linear.[19] Some variables will weigh more (or less) toward an outcome based on the presence (or absence) of another variable.

We use 2 hypothetical examples to illustrate 2 important concepts relevant to preoperative risk stratification models: the concept of linearity versus nonlinearity and the trade-off between predictive accuracy and interpretability.

To demonstrate the distinction between linear and nonlinear models, consider patients undergoing heart valve replacement surgery. Three independent risk factors that predict poor long-term postoperative outcomes are increased age, heart failure with reduced ejection fraction (HFrEF), and chronic obstructive pulmonary disease (COPD).[20] In a linear predictive model, each of these variables is marked as "present" or "absent" and given fixed weights, regardless of the presence of the other variables. Hypothetically, however, in a patient older than age 65 years, it might be possible for COPD to play a role while HFrEF does not, whereas in patients younger than age 65, HFrEF impacts outcome but COPD does not. Nonlinear models allow variables such as HFrEF and COPD to impact the outcome to a variable degree depending on the value of another variable (ie, age in this case). Linear models do not have this flexibility.

To illustrate the trade-off between predictive accuracy and interpretability, consider this fictional linear regression model that predicts preoperative mortality risk based only on age and presence of diabetes:

$$\text{Mortality risk} = (0.04 * \text{age}) + (2 * \text{diabetic}) - 1.5$$

In a 50-year-old patient without diabetes (ie, age = 50 and diabetic = 0), one can calculate a mortality risk of 0.5%. Because the input variables in this model combine linearly and contribute to the outcome independently of one another, the mortality risk is readily interpretable in terms of the input variables. For example, the presence of diabetes will add 2% to the mortality risk estimate independently of the age of the patient, so it is easy to interpret diabetes as a risk factor. However, the determinants of surgical risk are not actually independent of one another.[19] For example, the presence of diabetes might be expected to make a greater contribution to the mortality risk estimate in an older patient compared to a younger one. Although its linearity makes the model more interpretable, it sacrifices important nonlinear patterns in the data.[18] Even if the fictional linear model were extended to include more variables (eg, international normalized ratio, potassium level), those would still combine linearly to compute the outcome. A different kind of model is needed to capture nonlinear patterns in the data.

One solution to this problem is to artificially combine the variables in nonlinear ways. For example, one could add the term $(age^2 * diabetic)$ to the model and train it again to produce a new equation:

Mortality risk = $(0.04 * age) + (2 * diabetic) + (0.0003 * age^2 * diabetic) - 1.5$

Age and diabetes can now interact, allowing the model to capture nonlinear patterns between the variables: in the absence of diabetes (ie, diabetic = 0), an age of 50 contributes 0.5% toward the outcome; in the presence of diabetes (ie, diabetic = 1), age now contributes a different value, 1.25%. However, this comes at a cost in interpretability because the variables are no longer contributing independently to the mortality risk outcome. Moreover, as more variables are added to the model (eg, hypertension, hematocrit), the model becomes difficult to train: the number of new terms increases exponentially, and the number of interactions to account for becomes intractably large. Fortunately, the formal study of models and their training algorithms, a subfield of AI commonly known as machine learning (ML), has yielded a plethora of methods that can tackle these issues.

Nonlinear ML models can be applied to essentially any domain where pattern recognition is useful. They have been widely used in areas as diverse as image classification, fraud detection, and structure discovery in complex data sets. In the context of medicine, ML has found fruitful applications in diagnosis, prognosis, and risk stratification. For example, nonlinear models have attained expert-level performance on image-based diagnosis of skin cancer, pneumonia, and diabetic retinopathy.[21] Nonlinear models for prognosis trained on clinical and gene expression data have also been successful, achieving high accuracy on survival prediction in breast, lung, and oral cancer, for example.[22]

The artificial neural network is an example of a widely used nonlinear model. Rather than search the whole space of possible variable combinations (which expands explosively with more input variables), a neural network quickly learns complex but relevant features during its training (see Chapter 4). Most of the features it learns are too complicated to be readily interpretable. However, this confers the flexibility needed to capture nonlinear relationships in large data sets while retaining the ability to generalize to data outside the training set. A neural network can handle heterogeneous data (eg, continuous, categorical), and its performance often improves if it is trained on larger data sets. After it is trained, one could write down a big equation that represents exactly how a neural network is using the input variables to compute the output, but because this equation involves many variables interacting in nonlinear ways, it does not provide any underlying insight about the patterns it is capturing. In other words, if a surgeon wishes to understand why a neural network predictive model estimated a 3% mortality risk for her patient, the model cannot be probed for an answer. Viewing an output without having the ability to decipher the internal workings of the model that produced that output is what is known as the *black box* dilemma of AI. Although advances in explainable AI are improving the interpretability problem, current AI-based surgical risk calculators are largely grounded in black box models, as we describe later in this chapter.

EXAMPLES OF AI-BASED PREOPERATIVE RISK STRATIFICATION MODELS

Mortality Risk Prediction With Random Forest and Neural Network: RheSCORE

RheSCORE was created by the University of Sao Paulo Medical Center to predict mortality risk for candidates who require valve surgery secondary to rheumatic heart disease.[23] The team collected data prospectively from 2919 patients, from which they developed 13 different models. Using the AUC metric, the models were then compared to each other and to benchmark scoring systems that are based on linear models (ie, Bernstein-Parsonnet, EuroSCORE II) using the AUC metric. The top 2 performing models were neural network and random forest, with AUC values of 0.973 and 0.981, respectively. The neural network RheSCORE model had a sensitivity of 0.286 and a specificity of 0.994, whereas the random forest model had a sensitivity of 0.591 and a specificity of 1.0. Both models outperformed all the benchmark models, the top 2 of which are Bernstein-Parsonnet and EuroSCORE II, with AUC scores of 0.876 and 0.857, respectively.

Despite its great performance, the score produced by the RheSCORE risk calculator is uninterpretable in terms of the input variables (eg, age, left atrial size, high creatinine) because it is based on black box random forest models. *Random forest* is so named because of the many decision trees it comprises: every individual decision tree can be thought of as an interpretable flow chart (a series of if-then statements that end with an outcome prediction) that was trained on a random subset of the data. For example, one of the decision trees might be trained on the age, ejection fraction, and left atrial size subset of the whole data set, whereas another might be trained only on age, pulmonary hypertension, and the presence of high creatinine. When presented with a new input (ie, a patient), each of the decision trees of the random forest makes a yes or no mortality prediction; the most popular prediction is selected as the final output of the random forest (see Chapter 3). Because every decision tree assigns a unique profile of importance to the different variables, it is difficult to assess the overall contribution of any one variable to the final mortality prediction, thus resulting in a black box.

Anastomotic Leak Prediction With Kernel Methods

Innovative nonlinear models have also been developed to predict the risk of particular complications. Soguero-Ruiz et al[24] used kernel methods to train a model on data combined from heterogeneous sources. They trained the classification model on data from 402 patients admitted for colorectal cancer surgery, 31 of whom developed anastomotic leak. Three types of predictor variables were used: free text, blood tests, and vital signs. Free text was extracted from all the available documentation related to inpatient and outpatient visits and was analyzed according to the presence or absence of certain words (eg, coloanal, air). Nine different blood tests were included, encompassing measures of blood chemistry and cell count. The model's performance greatly improved when the model was trained on all 3 data types simultaneously (median AUC_{all} = 0.96) compared to when it was trained on each data type individually (median AUC_{text} = 0.83, AUC_{blood} = 0.74, AUC_{vitals} = 0.65). Although the model was not developed as a publicly available risk estimation tool, it represents a powerful proof of concept that ML methods can use structured and unstructured data to boost the performance of surgical risk estimators.

Decision Tree Models

We have described risk prediction tools based on linear models, where the surgical risk estimate is interpretable in terms of the input variables at the expense of missing important nonlinear patterns in the data. We then discussed powerful black box models that sacrifice interpretability but efficiently capture nonlinear patterns in a large data set and provide more accurate risk estimates than traditional prediction tools, namely, neural networks, random forest models, and nonlinear kernel methods. However, there is nothing inherent in the nature of nonlinear models that makes them uninterpretable.[25] In this section, we describe decision trees, which embody the best of both worlds by being faithful to the nonlinear structure in the data without losing interpretability.[26]

In our discussion of random forest models, we alluded to the fact that the output of an individual classification decision tree is fully interpretable

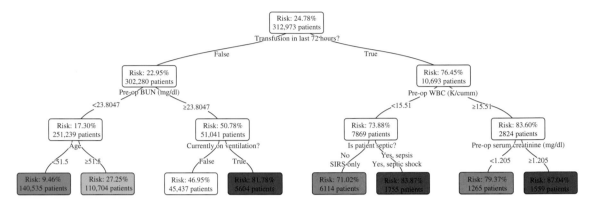

Figure 9-1 • An illustrative example of a segment of a decision-tree to predict any complication (including mortality). SIRS, systemic inflammatory response syndrome. (Reproduced, with permission, from Bertsimas D, Dunn J, Velmahos GC, Kaafarani HMA. Surgical risk is not linear: derivation and validation of a novel, user-friendly, and machine-learning-based Predictive OpTimal Trees in Emergency Surgery Risk (POTTER) Calculator. *Ann Surg.* 2018;268(4):574-583.)

in terms of the input variables. This is best demonstrated by walking through an example (Figure 9-1). Assume a surgeon wants to use a decision tree model to assess the mortality risk of a recently transfused nonseptic patient whose leukocyte count is 8000. The only relevant variable at the first node of the tree is whether the patient received a transfusion in the past 72 hours. The right branch of the tree is followed to the next node, and the relevant variable at this node is whether the patient's preoperative leukocyte count is less than 15,510, which leads to the left branch of the tree. The most important variable at the next level is whether the patient is septic. Following the left branch of the tree again (because the patient is not septic), there are no further splits possible that would provide finer information about risk. The tree now makes a final mortality prediction of 71% (surgical intervention is very risky), and the decision tree model is transparent about why this is the case.

Optimal Classification Trees: POTTER

Most classification decision trees (eg, Classification and Regression Trees [CART], C4.5) are learned using a top-down approach, where the optimal split at a given node is determined independently of downstream splits. For example, the first split is determined by solving an optimization problem at the first node, without considering the optimization problem that will have to be solved at each of the 2 newly created nodes. The optimal classification tree (OCT) method overcomes this issue by learning the whole decision tree in one step; because the split at each level is determined with the knowledge of all the other splits in the tree, OCT learns the best possible tree structure for the training data. When used to predict a yes or no outcome, as is the case in preoperative risk assessment (eg, mortality prediction), the performance of OCT parallels that of the black box random forest models and exceeds that of CART.[26]

The ability of OCTs to capture nonlinear patterns in big data sets at an accuracy level on par with random forests while remaining interpretable renders this model ideal for preoperative risk assessment. A user-friendly tool based on this technology was implemented in a smartphone app, the Predictive Optimization Trees in Emergency Surgery Risk (POTTER) calculator.[18] A separate OCT model was trained to predict each of the following 20 outcomes: 30-day postoperative mortality and morbidity and each of the 18 postoperative complications assessed by ACS-NSQIP. After restricting the 2007 to 2014 ACS-NSQIP data set to patients who underwent emergency surgery, model training was carried out on the 2007 to 2013 subset, and testing and validation were performed on the 2014 subset. POTTER attained a mortality c-statistic of 0.9199, surpassing that of the ASA system (0.8743) and ESS (0.8979); POTTER also surpassed the performance of ASA and ESS in predicting 30-day postoperative morbidity (ie, the development of any complication), attaining a c-statistic of 0.8414 compared to 0.7842 (ASA) and 0.7768 (ESS). The c-statistic for the 18 individual complications ranged from 0.6808 to 0.9338 (Table 9-1), confirming that POTTER can provide risk estimates superior in accuracy to traditional risk calculators.[18]

The phone application is intuitive to use. It first prompts the user to select the outcome of interest. By answering a series of brief questions about a patient, the provider navigates the branches of the decision tree to the final risk prediction. Figure 9-2 presents 2 screenshots, where different answers to the starting questions take the user down different paths in the decision tree toward a final risk estimate. Figure 9-3 presents screenshots of the calculator being used to calculate the risk of different postoperative complications (renal failure vs myocardial infarction). Every individual complication has an independent decision tree, each with a different set of questions and variables.

Interestingly, the calculator does not always ask the user about the type of emergency procedure being performed. This is the case because, during model testing, *forcing* the type of surgery into the algorithm did not change the accuracy of the final risk prediction. Although it is difficult to accept that the type of procedure being performed does not always influence outcome, the authors report that the type of surgery manifests itself through the answers to the algorithm's questions. For example, an elderly patient requiring an emergent colectomy for perforated diverticulitis will

Table 9-1 THE PERFORMANCE OF OPTIMAL CLASSIFICATION TREES IN PREDICTING 30-DAY POSTOPERATIVE MORTALITY	
Outcome	AUC
30-day mortality	0.916
30-day morbidity	0.841
Superficial SSI	0.681
Deep incisional SSI	0.754
Pulmonary embolism	0.733
Organ space SSI	0.786
Sepsis	0.845
Wound disruption	0.779
Urinary tract infection	0.740
DVT/thrombophlebitis	0.789
Progressive renal insufficiency	0.819
Myocardial infarction	0.824
Pneumonia	0.847
Unplanned intubation	0.849
Stroke/CVA	0.834
Cardiac arrest requiring CPR	0.888
Septic shock	0.934
Bleeding requiring transfusions	0.903
Acute renal failure	0.913
On ventilator >48 hours	0.925

have a significantly more deranged physiologic profile as compared to a healthy, young patient undergoing an uncomplicated appendectomy.

The POTTER mortality decision tree requires the user to answer 4 to a maximum of 11 questions to reach the final risk estimate, and the number of questions needed to predict any specific complication ranges from as few as 3 to a maximum of 20. This makes POTTER more convenient to use than other risk calculators. Contrast this, for example, with the ACS-NSQIP calculator, which requires the user to enter 19 values to

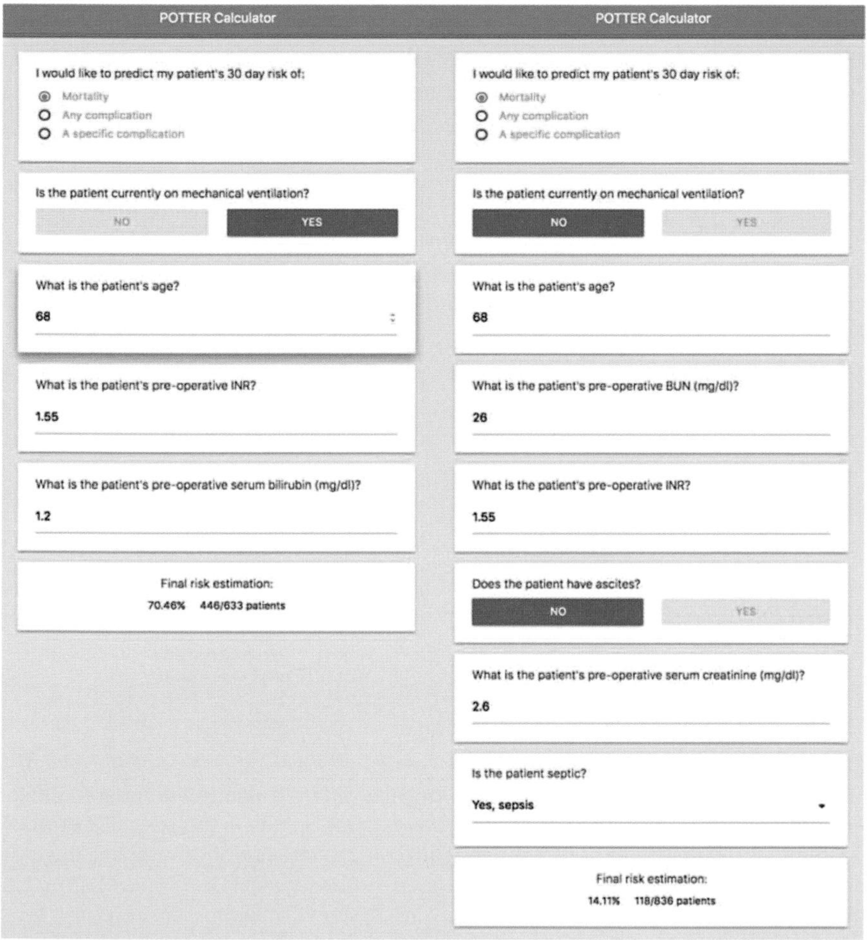

Figure 9-2 • An example illustrating how Predictive Optimization Trees in Emergency Surgery Risk (POTTER) is interactive and how the answer to a question dictates the next question. In this specific example, depending on whether the provider answers yes or no to the question regarding mechanical ventilation, the algorithm and questions take a different direction. BUN, blood urea nitrogen; INR, international normalized ratio. (Reproduced, with permission, from Bertsimas D, Dunn J, Velmahos GC, Kaafarani HMA. Surgical risk is not linear: derivation and validation of a novel, user-friendly, and machine-learning-based Predictive OpTimal Trees in Emergency Surgery Risk (POTTER) Calculator. *Ann Surg.* 2018;268(4):574-583.)

compute a risk estimate. Furthermore, as determined through user testing, less than 1 minute was required to reach the final risk estimate for any of the POTTER outcomes. In summary, POTTER is an ML-based tool that the provider can use at the bedside to calculate an interpretable, highly accurate risk estimate for each of the 20 outcomes by ACS-NSQIP in an emergency surgery setting.

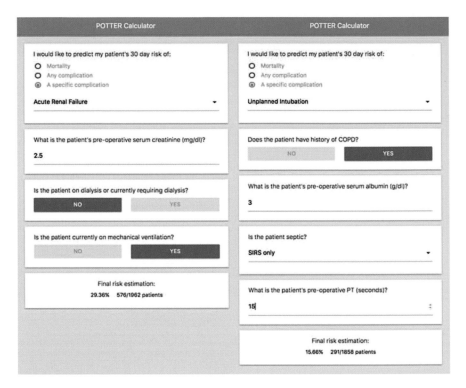

Figure 9-3 • An example illustrating how Predictive Optimization Trees in Emergency Surgery Risk (POTTER) interactively uses completely different algorithms and thus different questions to predict different postoperative complications. In this specific example, we see that different questions are needed to predict the risk of developing postoperative acute renal failure versus an unplanned intubation. COPD, chronic obstructive pulmonary disease; PT, prothrombin time; SIRS, systemic inflammatory response syndrome. (Reproduced, with permission, from Bertsimas D, Dunn J, Velmahos GC, Kaafarani HMA. Surgical risk is not linear: derivation and validation of a novel, user-friendly, and machine-learning-based Predictive OpTimal Trees in Emergency Surgery Risk (POTTER) Calculator. *Ann Surg.* 2018;268(4):574-583.)

Integration of AI Surgical Risk Predictors Into Hospital Electronic Health Records

MySurgeryRisk

Integrating a postoperative risk calculator with a hospital's electronic health record (EHR) is a formidable task. Calculators are optimized to work with certain variables whose values occupy a certain range and are represented in a certain format; a patient's EHR could be missing data or contain errors or outliers, and certain values might be represented in a format incompatible with the calculator (see Chapter 2). At the

University of Florida, Bihorac et al[27] tackled this challenge by developing MySurgeryRisk, an analytics platform that allows these systems to talk to one another. The workflow in the system is as follows: raw data are continuously pulled from the patient's EHR and transformed into a format for which the risk calculator has been optimized, and the resulting risk estimates are displayed for the provider in a simple graph (Figure 9-4). Errors and outliers are removed in a data preprocessing step. If a continuous variable is missing, its mean value is passed to the calculator; missing categorical variables are replaced with a distinct "missing" category.

The operations internal to the calculator are quite involved. MySurgeryRisk uses a model stacking approach: a nonlinear model (generalized additive model) predicts the risk of developing 8 postoperative complications and then passes those 8 risk estimates to another nonlinear

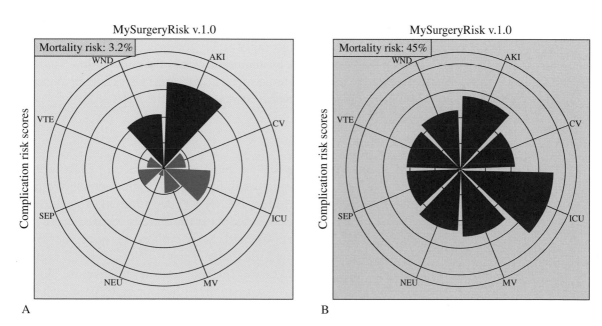

Figure 9-4 • MySurgeryRisk output. The sample output for subjects with (**A**) low mortality risk and (**B**) high mortality risk. The figure shows the predicted risks for 8 postoperative complications for the given patient in 8 equal-sized pies. The calculated cutoff values for AKI, ICU, MV, WND, CV, NEU, SEP, and VTE were 0.35, 0.35, 0.13, 0.1, 0.07, 0.07, 0.06, and 0.03, respectively. Subjects are classified as high risk for a complication if the calculated risk score exceeds the respective cutoff and the respective pie is marked as red (or green if not at high risk). The size of the pie represents the proportion of the risk, scaled based on the cutoff for each complication. Green background color represents low mortality risk (**A**), whereas red background color shows high mortality risk (**B**). AKI, acute kidney injury; CV, cardiovascular complications; ICU, intensive care unit admission >48 hours; MV, mechanical ventilation >48 hours; NEU, neurologic complications; SEP, sepsis; VTE, venous thromboembolism; WND, wound complications. (Reproduced, with permission, from Bihorac A, Ozrazgat-Baslanti T, Ebadi A, et al. MySurgeryRisk: development and validation of a machine-learning risk algorithm for major complications and death after surgery. *Ann Surg.* 2019;269(4):652-662.)

model (random forest) to predict mortality risk. The 8 postoperative complications are sepsis, acute kidney injury, wound complications (mechanical and infectious), intensive care unit admission >48 hours, mechanical ventilation >48 hours, cardiovascular complications, venous thromboembolism, and neurologic complications.

The authors derived predictive features from 285 variables encompassing clinical, pharmacy, and laboratory information as well as socioeconomic and demographic measures. A nonlinear generalized additive model was trained on these features to estimate the probability that a patient will develop each of the 8 postoperative complications listed earlier. The 8 AUC values attained by the model range between 0.82 (wound complication) and 0.94 (mechanical ventilation >48 hours), indicating excellent predictive performance. The authors paired these complication probabilities together with mortality data to train random forest models in predicting mortality at 1, 3, 6, 12, and 24 months after the index surgery. The resulting models had AUC values ranging between 0.77 and 0.83, corresponding to mortality at 24 months and 1 month, respectively. Because the relevant risk estimates are computed and displayed as soon as the necessary data become available, MySurgeryRisk effectively embeds accurate preoperative risk assessment within the EHR.

Pythia

Another example where ML has been used to create an EHR integrated postoperative complication predictive model (Pythia) comes from Duke University in North Carolina. Nearly 100,000 surgical procedures from the institutional EHR were used to train models to predict any of 14 outcomes (30-day mortality and 13 complication outcome groups). Three models were trained for that purpose—1 linear and 2 nonlinear. The linear model selected was the one with least absolute shrinkage and selection operator (lasso) penalized logistic regression, which is a variant of logistic regression that better accounts for highly correlated predictors than standard logistic regression. Among the 2 nonlinear models used, one was a random forest model—similar to the model used to develop RheSCORE—and the other was composed of extreme gradient boosted decision trees, a model that resembles the random forest.[28]

Upon validation on out-of-sample test data, the lasso penalized model was found to be high performing and comparable to the 2 nonlinear models, with outcome prediction AUC values ranging between 0.780 and 0.924 (Figure 9-5). The lasso model was also linear, as opposed to random forests and extreme gradient boosted decision trees. As such, it

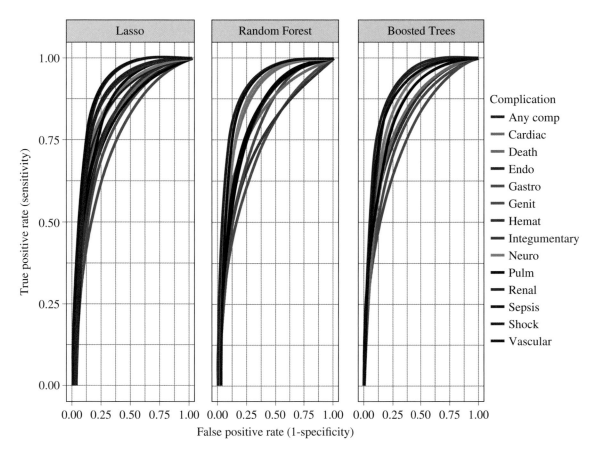

Figure 9-5 • Graphs displaying the resulting receiver operator characteristic curves for each modeling method across all 14 complications. Comp, complication; Endo, endocrine; Gastro, gastrointestinal; Genit, genitourinary; Hemat, hematologic; Lasso, least absolute shrinkage and selection operator; Neuro, neurologic; Pulm, pulmonary. (Reproduced, with permission, from Corey KM, Kashyap S, Lorenzi E, et al. Development and validation of machine learning models to identify high-risk surgical patients using automatically curated electronic health record data (Pythia): a retrospective, single-site study. *PLoS Med.* 2018;15(11):e1002701.)

was also more interpretable, prompting the developers to adopt it as the model to predict the 14 outcomes in the 9-item web calculator. This demonstrates that, in certain circumstances, linear models can perform comparably to nonlinear models and might be preferably chosen because of their increased interpretability. The performance of the pilot calculator was then compared to the ACS-NSQIP SRC by predicting 30-day mortality outcomes for 75 randomly selected hospital patients not in the Pythia model training set. On that subpopulation, Pythia's lasso model outperformed the SRC with respect to sensitivity, specificity, positive predictive value, and AUC (0.79 vs 0.67).[28]

LIMITATIONS OF AI IN PREOPERATIVE RISK STRATIFICATION

With the current hype surrounding the capabilities of AI in predictive modeling, it is the surgeon's responsibility to be mindful of the technology's limitations.[29] For example, one model that had excellent performance measures in predicting mortality and 30-day readmission for patients with pneumonia reached an odd conclusion. The model deemed a history of asthma to be a protective factor against mortality from pneumonia.[30] Investigation of this anomaly revealed that despite the pattern truly being in the data, it was due to the fact that, in the data set used, asthmatic patients who developed pneumonia were directly admitted to the intensive care unit (ICU) as opposed to a regular floor bed. Therefore, as a result of high-acuity care, those patients had better mortality outcomes than the general population of pneumonia patients. The actual protective factor was admission to ICU, but the ML algorithm picked up a correlated variable—asthma—and deemed it to be a protective factor against mortality. This example demonstrates that despite their performance, ML algorithms are blind to confounders that are not directly encoded in the data set on which they were trained. Moreover, this example highlights the importance of using clinical context to critically evaluate model predictions.[31]

An important concern with AI algorithms revolves around their interpretability.[32] Although major strides are being taken to make predictive models more interpretable, such as OCT technology, most AI models remain largely uninterpretable at this time. Developers and users have limited ability to dissect how or why a given pattern was recognized, so the model cannot be held accountable if a patient's outcome is significantly different than what the model predicted.[33] This represents a trust barrier that prevents the widespread adoption of AI tools.[34,35]

Additionally, it is important for physicians to be wary of systematic biases in data collection that may affect the way AI generates predictions.[36,37] In particular, because of the long-standing underrepresentation of racial minorities in clinical trial and patient registry populations, using a model trained on these data sets to predict outcomes for these patients may be misleading (see Chapter 14).[31]

Another pitfall is physician overreliance on AI tools. For example, in a subgroup analysis of radiologists given access to a US Food and Drug Administration–approved computer-aided detection (CAD) system to aid with mammogram interpretation, it was found that the same radiologists had lower sensitivity in cancer detection when using CAD as compared to screening without computer aid.[38] To avoid similar situations among surgeons, it is important to emphasize that, up until now, the primary purpose of these predictive models was to facilitate patient and family discussions, with a secondary goal of supporting a surgeon's decision making.

FUTURE PROSPECTS FOR AI IN PREOPERATIVE RISK STRATIFICATION

In this era of big data, the creation of large data sets containing standardized information on millions of patients is becoming increasingly common. Existing models will continue to exploit the constant stream of data to make more accurate predictions. As data sets in different subfields of surgery become available, it is expected that models will be created to risk stratify patients across those disciplines. Surgeons are in a unique position to contribute to this growth by providing clinical input to the development of accountable and interpretable algorithms.[31]

Another promising feature of these models is potential integration into a hospital's electronic health record (EHR). The impact of integration is 2-fold. First, preoperative risk will be automatically generated using the patient variables in the EHR, allowing prediction to merge seamlessly into the physician workflow without the need of manual data entry. The merger can be performed with confidence as studies have demonstrated that models extracting EHR data automatically and those that require manual data entry perform comparably.[39,40]

Examples of nonlinear ML models that have been integrated into an EHR include MySurgeryRisk from the University of Florida and Pythia from Duke University in North Carolina. Additionally, at the Massachusetts General Hospital, plans for integration of the POTTER calculator into the EHR are in place. This is a crucial advantage for these models moving forward, as these calculators are still in their infancy and prospective validation of their algorithms through integration is essential in determining whether they will truly impact and elevate the standard of care.

Second, integration will ensure closed-loop learning, whereby models will have access to a patient's postoperative outcome and can continuously learn to improve prediction accuracy. A learning cycle can be achieved by programming the prediction software to periodically incorporate EHR records and retrain its algorithms on the new data. This will remove the need to manually update a data set every time new data become available.

Moving ahead with risk prediction, the next step will be identifying variables in the preoperative period that can be targeted by clinicians as "breakpoints" to improve a patient's postoperative outcome. A recently developed ML methodology, named Optimal Prescriptive Trees (OPT), promises to do just that.[41] The goal is to identify (prescribe) personalized interventions for each patient that will alter their postoperative outcome. These interventions will identify actionable variables that directly impact patient outcomes, not merely surrogate markers of disease severity.

Furthermore, as per a tutorial published by the World Federation of Societies of Anesthesiologists, the ideal preoperative scoring system should use routinely available patient characteristics and variables, be easily accessible, be extensively validated in different populations, and be applicable to patient populations across different demographics. Finally, the model should be able to accurately predict postoperative outcomes. Although no preoperative risk prediction system currently satisfies all of these criteria, the continuous advent of big data and AI holds promise for achieving this goal in the near future.[42] This goal will potentially be surpassed when the subtle patterns in data detected by ML inspire new scientific questions and hypotheses,[43,44] leading to a better understanding of surgical pathology and treatment.

CONCLUSION

AI is increasing the accuracy of our preoperative risk stratification models. With patients' lives on the line, the expectations for the various models to augment care delivery are high. Achieving needed interpretability as well as a user-friendly interface are crucial for significant AI dissemination in the bedside clinical practice of decision making and perioperative counseling of patients and families. Nevertheless, the surgeon remains the ultimate decision maker and communicator with the patient. In that capacity, the surgeon also carries the responsibility of understanding the capabilities and limitations of these calculators for appropriate use of AI-generated predictions.

REFERENCES

1. Gifford RW Jr. Primum non nocere. *JAMA*. 1977;238(7):589-590.
2. Havens DH, Boroughs L. "To err is human": a report from the Institute of Medicine. *J Pediatr Health Care*. 2000;14(2):77-80.
3. Inpatient vs. outpatient surgeries in U.S. hospitals. Healthcare Cost and Utilization Project. Accessed October 5, 2020. https://www.hcup-us.ahrq.gov/reports/infographics/inpt_outpt.jsp.
4. Desebbe O, Lanz T, Kain Z, Cannesson M. The perioperative surgical home: an innovative, patient-centred and cost-effective perioperative care model. *Anaesth Crit Care Pain Med*. 2016;35(1):59-66.

5. Wolters U, Wolf T, Stutzer H, Schroder T. ASA classification and peri-operative variables as predictors of postoperative outcome. *Br J Anaesth.* 1996;77(2):217-222.

6. Copeland GP, Jones D, Walters M. POSSUM: a scoring system for surgical audit. *Br J Surg.* 1991;78(3):355-360.

7. Anderson RP. First publications from the Society of Thoracic Surgeons National Database. *Ann Thorac Surg.* 1994;57(1):6-7.

8. Bilimoria KY, Liu Y, Paruch JL, et al. Development and evaluation of the universal ACS NSQIP surgical risk calculator: a decision aid and informed consent tool for patients and surgeons. *J Am Coll Surg.* 2013;217(5):833-842.e1-3.

9. Hyder JA, Reznor G, Wakeam E, et al. Risk prediction accuracy differs for emergency versus elective cases in the ACS-NSQIP. *Ann Surg.* 2016;264(6):959-965.

10. Bohnen JD, Ramly EP, Sangji NF, et al. Perioperative risk factors impact outcomes in emergency versus nonemergency surgery differently: time to separate our national risk-adjustment models? *J Trauma Acute Care Surg.* 2016;81(1):122-130.

11. Protopapa KL, Simpson JC, Smith NC, Moonesinghe SR. Development and validation of the Surgical Outcome Risk Tool (SORT). *Br J Surg.* 2014;101(13):1774-1783.

12. Wong DJN, Oliver CM, Moonesinghe SR. Predicting postoperative morbidity in adult elective surgical patients using the Surgical Outcome Risk Tool (SORT). *Br J Anaesth.* 2017;119(1):95-105.

13. Peponis T, Bohnen JD, Sangji NF, et al. Does the emergency surgery score accurately predict outcomes in emergent laparotomies? *Surgery.* 2017;162(2):445-452.

14. Mercer S, Guha A, Ramesh V. The P-POSSUM scoring systems for predicting the mortality of neurosurgical patients undergoing craniotomy: further validation of usefulness and application across healthcare systems. *Indian J Anaesth.* 2013;57(6):587-591.

15. Sangji NF, Bohnen JD, Ramly EP, et al. Derivation and validation of a novel Physiological Emergency Surgery Acuity Score (PESAS). *World J Surg.* 2017;41(7):1782-1789.

16. Ladha KS, Zhao K, Quraishi SA, et al. The Deyo-Charlson and Elixhauser-van Walraven Comorbidity Indices as predictors of mortality in critically ill patients. *BMJ Open.* 2015;5(9):e008990.

17. Hanley JA, McNeil BJ. The meaning and use of the area under a receiver operating characteristic (ROC) curve. *Radiology.* 1982;143(1):29-36.

18. Bertsimas D, Dunn J, Velmahos GC, Kaafarani HMA. Surgical risk is not linear: derivation and validation of a novel, user-friendly, and machine-learning-based Predictive OpTimal Trees in Emergency Surgery Risk (POTTER) calculator. *Ann Surg.* 2018;268(4):574-583.

19. Chen JH, Asch SM. Machine learning and prediction in medicine: beyond the peak of inflated expectations. *N Engl J Med.* 2017;376(26):2507-2509.

20. Toumpoulis IK, Chamogeorgakis TP, Angouras DC, et al. Independent predictors for early and long-term mortality after heart valve surgery. *J Heart Valve Dis.* 2008;17(5):548-556.

21. Watson DS, Krutzinna J, Bruce IN, et al. Clinical applications of machine learning algorithms: beyond the black box. *BMJ.* 2019;364:l886.

22. Kourou K, Exarchos TP, Exarchos KP, Karamouzis MV, Fotiadis DI. Machine learning applications in cancer prognosis and prediction. *Comput Struct Biotechnol J.* 2015;13:8-17.

23. Mejia OAV, Antunes MJ, Goncharov M, et al. Predictive performance of six mortality risk scores and the development of a novel model in a prospective cohort of patients undergoing valve surgery secondary to rheumatic fever. *PLoS One.* 2018;13(7):e0199277.

24. Soguero-Ruiz C, Hindberg K, Mora-Jimenez I, et al. Predicting colorectal surgical complications using heterogeneous clinical data and kernel methods. *J Biomed Inform.* 2016;61:87-96.

25. Rudin C. Please stop explaining black box models for high stakes decision. 32nd Conference on Neural Information Processing Systems (NIPS 2018), Workshop on Critiquing and Correcting Trends in Machine Learning 2018. Accessed October 5, 2020. https://www.arxiv-vanity.com/papers/1811.10154/.

26. Bertsimas D, Dunn J. Optimal classification trees. *Machine Learn.* 2017;106:1039-1082.

27. Bihorac A, Ozrazgat-Baslanti T, Ebadi A, et al. MySurgeryRisk: development and validation of a machine-learning risk algorithm for major complications and death after surgery. *Ann Surg.* 2019;269(4):652-662.

28. Corey KM, Kashyap S, Lorenzi E, et al. Development and validation of machine learning models to identify high-risk surgical patients using automatically curated electronic health record data (Pythia): a retrospective, single-site study. *PLoS Med.* 2018;15(11):e1002701.

29. Emanuel EJ, Emanuel LL. Four models of the physician-patient relationship. *JAMA.* 1992;267(16):2221-2226.

30. Caruana R, Lou Y, Gehrke J, Koch P, Sturm M, Elhadad N. Intelligible models for healthcare: predicting pneumonia risk and hospital 30-day readmission. Proceedings of the 21th ACM SIGKDD International Conference on Knowledge Discovery and Data Mining. Accessed October 5, 2020. http://people.dbmi.columbia.edu/noemie/papers/15kdd.pdf.

31. Hashimoto DA, Rosman G, Rus D, Meireles OR. Artificial intelligence in surgery: promises and perils. *Ann Surg.* 2018;268(1):70-76.

32. Ribeiro MT, Singh S, Guestrin C. Why should I trust you? Explaining the predictions of any classifier. In: Proceedings of the 22nd ACM SIGKDD International Conference on Knowledge Discovery and Data Mining 2016. Accessed October 5, 2020. https://arxiv.org/pdf/1602.04938.pdf.

33. Cabitza F, Rasoini R, Gensini GF. Unintended consequences of machine learning in medicine. *JAMA.* 2017;318(6):517-518.

34. Tan S, Sim KC, Gales M. Improving the interpretability of deep neural networks with stimulated learning. In: *Automatic Speech Recognition and Understanding (ASRU).* IEEE; 2015:617-623.

35. Sturm I, Lapuschkin S, Samek W, Muller KR. Interpretable deep neural networks for single-trial EEG classification. *J Neurosci Methods.* 2016;274:141-145.

36. Hopewell S, Loudon K, Clarke MJ, Oxman AD, Dickersin K. Publication bias in clinical trials due to statistical significance or direction of trial results. *Cochrane Database Syst Rev.* 2009;1:MR000006.

37. Juni P, Altman DG, Egger M. Systematic reviews in health care: assessing the quality of controlled clinical trials. *BMJ.* 2001;323(7303):42-46.

38. Lehman CD, Wellman RD, Buist DS, et al. Diagnostic accuracy of digital screening mammography with and without computer-aided detection. *JAMA Intern Med.* 2015;175(11):1828-1837.

39. Amrock LG, Neuman MD, Lin HM, Deiner S. Can routine preoperative data predict adverse outcomes in the elderly? Development and validation of a simple risk model incorporating a chart-derived frailty score. *J Am Coll Surg.* 2014;219(4):684-694.

40. Anderson JE, Chang DC. Using electronic health records for surgical quality improvement in the era of big data. *JAMA Surg.* 2015(150):24-29.

41. Bertsimas D, Dunn J, Mundru N. Optimal prescriptive trees. Under review. Accessed October 5, 2020. https://nmundru.github.io/files/Optimal%20Prescriptive%20Trees.pdf.

42. Watson X, Chereshneva M. Perioperative risk prediction scores: Anaesthesia Tutorial of the Week; 2016 [03/02/2019]. Accessed October 5, 2020. https://www.wfsahq.org/components/com_virtual_library/media/09a3a98aa6c774ae5f03c6ca5713e0c8-343-Periop-risk-scoring.pdf.

43. National Research Council. *Frontiers in Massive Data Analysis.* National Academies Press; 2013.

44. Rudin C. Discovery with data: leveraging statistics with computer science to transform science and society. American Statistical Association White Paper 2014. Accessed October 5, 2020. https://www.amstat.org/asa/files/pdfs/POL-BigDataStatisticsJune2014.pdf.

THE OR BLACK BOX SYSTEM 10

Marc Levin, Mitchell G. Goldenberg, and Teodor P. Grantcharov

HIGHLIGHTS

- The operating room (OR) Black Box simultaneously captures audiovisual data, physiologic data from the patient and members of the surgical team, and data from instrumentation and sensors.
- During enhanced morbidity and mortality conferences, the OR Black Box can provide objective, quantifiable data from the OR to stakeholders to not only ensure they present accurate and granular data to attendees, but also so they can perform detailed root-cause analyses to identify often opaque or overlooked intraoperative factors that may have impacted the clinical outcome.

INTRODUCTION

In the mid-1950s, the United Kingdom airline de Havilland Comet was involved in multiple airplane crashes. David Warren, an Australian inventor, recognized that something had to be changed. He subsequently created a device that could record pilots' voices as well as cockpit instrument usage. Warren posited that by collecting such data, explanations for why planes were crashing could be quantified. Furthermore, with such information, airlines could better predict and prevent planes from crashing in the future.[1] Warren's airplane black box has become a hallmark of aviation cockpit safety, allowing airlines to learn from mistakes and saving the lives of many.

Similar to aviation, safety in the operating room (OR) is essential. Despite this, errors occur regularly in the OR.[2] Surgical errors such as miscommunication and tension between surgical team members, equipment being used incorrectly or failing, breaks in sterility, and most devastatingly, wrong-sided surgeries are not uncommon.[3,4] The surgical community needed a way to adequately record data in the OR to identify errors in an objective way, learn from these errors, and improve. Analogous to Warren's black box in aviation, the OR Black Box (Surgical Safety Technologies, Toronto, Canada) is an all-encompassing data collection platform for the intraoperative phase of care in surgery.[5] The OR Black Box system simultaneously records audiovisual data, physiologic data from the patient and members of the surgical team, and data from instrumentation and sensors. Video data are captured from both the wide-angle room camera and the laparoscopic/robot camera. The implications of the OR Black Box platform include improving patient safety, surgical training, quality, and surgical efficiency. This chapter will focus on how the OR Black Box captures data and uses novel technology to make these data meaningful for surgeons, surgical trainees, and patients alike.

MEASURES OF PERFORMANCE AND QUALITY

Surgical data science is an emerging and innovative field.[6] In ORs around the world, different modalities of data collection are used, such as safety checklists and procedural records. Despite the frequency and necessity of effective data collection in the OR, the current methods used can be subjective, inefficient, and lacking important data.[7]

From an education perspective, gathering surgical trainees' OR data is imperative to provide effective feedback and promote improvement. Many surgical training programs use the Objective Structured Assessment of Technical Skills (OSATS) to evaluate surgical technical skill.[8] Although the OSATS is validated across different surgical specialties and environments,[9] it requires human observers, making it resource intensive. With recent literature supporting an array of automated methods to evaluate technical skill in surgery, the OR Black Box has the potential to harness such techniques to evaluate trainees' skill in a more objective way.[10] The Non-Technical Skills for Surgeons (NOTSS) score has been described to evaluate nontechnical skills of surgeons and trainees in the OR. Similar to the OSATS, the NOTSS requires human observers, which can inherently introduce bias into the evaluation and requires valuable time and resources.[11,12]

From an OR human factors approach, the Systems Engineering Intervention in Patient Safety (SEIPS) model has been used to evaluate a multitude of different elements in the OR that contribute to patient care and safety outcomes.[13] Although this model places importance on the evaluation of all parts of the OR system (eg, surgeon ergonomics, communication, room layout), this model and others like it rely on human evaluators and manual recording/coding of OR data. As such, its ability to efficiently and effectively capture data to improve patient safety across a multitude of surgical institutions across the world is limited.

The ability of surgical team members to recognize surgical errors and events both during surgery and retrospectively is important in promoting future prevention of such surgical errors. Currently described techniques to evaluate surgical errors and events include the Generic Error Rating Tool (GERT), which uses surgical experts to evaluate unedited operative video recordings to identify surgical error.[14]

▌APPLICATIONS OF DATA

It is important to understand how data captured by the OR Black Box can be used to gain insight into surgical team member behaviors, errors, and adverse events as well as contribute to surgical education. The OR Black Box audiovisual capture system can be used to identify near misses of adverse events in the OR. A near miss is defined as a potential adverse event that did not reach the patient due to random chance or recovery from other processes.[15] Identifying near misses and learning from them are imperative to improve patient safety in the OR by preventing future adverse events.[16] Because the OR Black Box data are digitalized and do not require human observers for collection, the automatic implementation of machine learning and artificial intelligence (AI) to the data sets is possible.[5] This allows for more efficient data analysis and turnaround time between surgical events and practice changes that surgical team members can implement.

The OR Black Box also allows for much-needed innovation in surgical education. Surgical coaching can be effective at improving both technical and nontechnical skills among surgical trainees.[17-19] Despite this, the classic apprentice model of surgical coaching is variable and time consuming. The OR Black Box is able to harness automated methods of skill analysis in surgery, providing surgical trainees with objective, timely, and consistent feedback and coaching.

Surgical team training is imperative to the improvement of surgical processes and reduction of team-related communication errors in the OR.[20,21] The OR Black Box data collection techniques provide a unique way for the whole surgical team to be evaluated outside of the OR. The OR Black Box allows structured feedback to be given to all members of the surgical team in a formative learning environment, rather than in the high-pressure environment of the operating room where the focus should be patient care.

APPLICATIONS IN RESEARCH

Recent research has examined the utility of the OR Black Box for evaluating surgical safety. For example, the OR Black Box was used to evaluate how acute mental stress of a surgeon can affect surgical performance.[22] Capturing biometric data from the surgical team members as an additional parameter in the OR Black Box analysis enabled the ability to determine that there is an association between increased mental stress and worse surgical technical performance. In addition, OR Black Box data were used to understand Veress needle injuries during laparoscopic surgery.[23] Veress needle near misses and injuries were recorded from the multiple OR Black Box video cameras. The OR Black Box was able to identify Veress needle injuries and near misses to a much more accurate degree than retrospective chart review. This study demonstrated the utility of the OR Black Box in identifying OR adverse events and injuries with the possibility of reviewing the events, learning from them, and ensuring the reduction of future unsafe events in the OR. The OR Black Box was similarly used to identify device-related interruptions in the OR.[24] A classification system of such interruptions was created from the OR Black Box data. This classification system can now be used for future analysis of adverse interruption events in the OR. An additional study demonstrated the use of the OR Black Box to identify negative technical events in the laparoscopic OR (Figure 10-1).[25] Data from the OR Black Box identified that after negative technical events in the OR, positive nontechnical skills were used by surgical team members. This study demonstrated the utility of the OR Black Box for not only surgeon improvement, but also appraisal of the entire interdisciplinary surgical team. Finally, a 1-year prospective analysis of OR Black Box data confirmed its ability to accurately and efficiently identify intraoperative events and errors, technical skill of surgeons, and environmental distractions.[26]

USE OF ARTIFICIAL INTELLIGENCE

Recent advances in computer science, especially in AI and machine learning, have been driven by the widespread availability of large data sets.[27] As the ability to capture data has improved, the desire to efficiently process these data to decipher their utility has increased. Breakthroughs in machine learning have made it possible to use data captured from sensory devices, such as cameras and audio recorders, and to extract information such as presence and location of objects in an image and classification of different voices in an audio clip.[28] The method that is most commonly

Characterization of device-related interruptions in minimally invasive surgery

Jung, J. J., Kashfi, A., Sharma, S., & Grantcharov, T. (2019) Characterization of device-related interruptions in minimally invasive surgery: need for intraoperative data and effective mitigation strategies. Surgical endoscopy, 1-7.

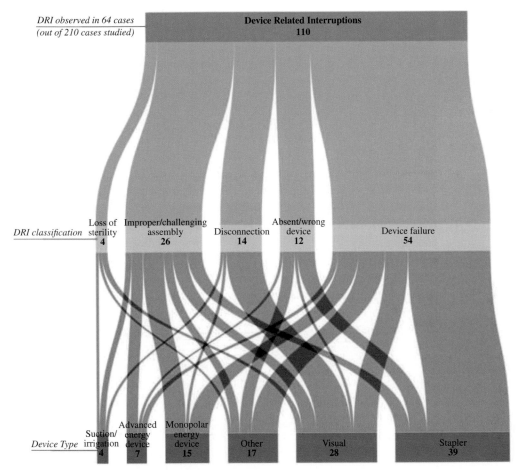

Take Away
Device-related interruptions occurred frequently in the OR and could be characterized into one of the five categories. Understanding the nature of the device-related interruptions can help guide implementation of safety interventions and user training in the future.

Figure 10-1 • Characterization of device-related interruptions in minimally invasive surgery. (Reproduced with permission from Surgical Safety Technologies Inc. © 2019 Surgical Safety Technologies Inc. All rights reserved.)

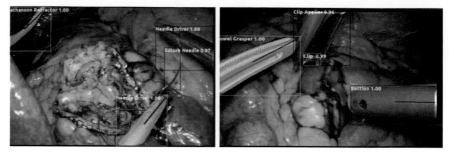

Figure 10-2 • Labels indicating the presence of surgical instruments in images. (Reproduced with permission from Surgical Safety Technologies Inc. © 2019 Surgical Safety Technologies Inc. All rights reserved.)

used for the aforementioned tasks is called *supervised learning* (see Chapter 3). This form of learning requires a set of inputs, a set of labels, and a mathematical model that attempts to find the underlying structure in the provided data.[27] Such a model is predictive because it attempts to generalize the learned representation to future inputs. For example, a model can be trained to predict the presence of surgical instruments in an image (Figure 10-2). To achieve this, the model requires a set of images, with and without the instruments, as inputs and labels indicating the presence of the instruments. The model will then attempt to find correlations between the images and the provided labels and will use them to make predictions about the presence of instruments in images that it has not seen before. Supervised learning thus requires not just large amounts of data but correctly *labeled* data to make effective predictions.

Compared to the staggering progress that has been made in some other fields, the field of health care has seen relatively slow adoption of AI.[27] This can be attributed to the sensitive nature of patient-centric data and the lack of precise labels. For example, to predict the onset of a cardiac episode using anesthesiology data, precise labels are required with timestamps of the exact moment of the onset. This requires clinical expertise and a framework to ensure interanalyst reliability. Furthermore, the cost of an expert clinician's time in annotating such data can be an obstacle.

The data collected by the OR Black Box include, but are not limited to, audiovisual data from the OR and the procedural field, physiologic data, and data from various sensors. The accrual of different types of data streams provides an exciting opportunity to better understand the potential issues that exist in surgical environments. The goal of the OR Black Box AI team has been to experiment with various forms of these data and to pursue approaches that have the greatest potential to provide meaningful insights. Members of the AI team interact with on-site clinical experts to determine how the data should be labeled for modeling purposes so that the models are able to make clinically rationalizable predictions. The team is working on projects that increase the explainability of surgical procedures. This allows the team to provide valuable feedback to hospitals and surgical teams such that they can improve their operations and, by extension, their quality of care. Projects using AI include automated identification and classification of adverse events, deidentification of team members, and evaluation of technical and nontechnical skills.

▌ CURRENT IMPLEMENTATION

The OR Black Box is being implemented across multiple hospitals, health care systems, and countries. Sites that have installed the technology in their hospitals have a shared purpose—to promote patient safety and encourage quality improvement. However, the specific aims of each institution vary from hospital to hospital, and this highlights the variety of ways in which this technology can be implemented.

Human factors research has experienced a recent expansion into the health care space.[29] Defined as the study of how people interact psychologically and physically with their working environment, this field has been used to help describe many aspects of quality and safety in surgery, from the elements in the physical environment that threaten patient safety such as device malfunction and suboptimal operating room design, to the manner in which members of the surgical team mitigate errors and adverse events through vigilance and automation.[30,31] Hospitals that implement the OR Black Box are able to objectively study these issues in their ORs, through the lens of human factors research and engineering. Quantifiable metrics allow for stakeholders to categorize and catalog these threats and resiliency factors in order to measure and improve the way in which health care providers interact with the clinical environment.[13] This research has broad implications for systems-level interventions, such as safety checklists and electronic medical record use, and basic educational interventions, such as team-based training in nontechnical skills. The OR Black Box provides a vantage point from which to appreciate and study the impact that human factors play in determining safe outcomes in surgery.

Sites using the OR Black Box have also harnessed its novel data to enhance existing patient safety interventions. An example of this is the Enhanced Morbidity and Mortality Conference (eMMC) that uses OR

Black Box data to supplement discussion and learning when adverse events occur in surgery. Typical morbidity and mortality conferences are limited by subjectivity and recall bias when recounting safety events in the OR.[32] This leads to misrepresentation of not only the details of the event itself, but also the surrounding and contributory factors that allowed that event to occur. With objective, quantifiable data from the OR, stakeholders can not only ensure they present accurate and granular data to attendees, but also perform detailed root-cause analyses to identify often opaque or overlooked intraoperative factors that may have played a role in iatrogenic harm to a patient.

Finally, other sites implementing the OR Black Box have used its unique data to improve their simulation-based interventions. Simulation requires functional task alignment and high fidelity in order to most benefit trainees' learning.[33] It is important therefore that the scenarios used to assess participants' ability in the simulation environment reflect the environment in which they work and learn. The OR Black Box allows for educators to harness real-world data to create these scenarios. Additionally, OR Black Box–equipped ORs can be used to run in situ simulation exercises, thereby allowing for quality improvement and identification of safety threats to occur without compromising patient safety.

▍ BARRIERS TO IMPLEMENTATION

There are real and perceived barriers that may exist in organizations implementing the OR Black Box. With any disruptive technology, the processes and systems of practice that make up the status quo need to be changed. These primarily relate to confidentiality concerns, medicolegal issues, and ethical dilemmas.[34]

When capturing detailed data in the OR, the issue of patient and provider confidentiality is a central concern. The OR Black Box captures sensitive audiovisual data from throughout the OR environment, including internal and external parts of the patient and surgical team members' faces, voices, and body movements.[35] Although not explicitly captured, it also has the potential to capture written information in the OR environment. To mitigate these threats to confidentiality, the OR Black Box uses computer vision-based built-in face and body deidentification and voice-altering technologies to mask the identities of team members. Furthermore, audiovisual data are quickly converted into numerical, nonidentifiable data and subsequently wiped from servers, thereby further minimizing the likelihood this sensitive information can be used inappropriately.

Many hospitals and health care systems highlight concerns about medicolegal issues that may arise from capturing and evaluating these granular data sources.[36] Litigation brought by patients against physicians and hospitals is a major source of financial strain on health care payers in many parts of the world.[37] The fear among stakeholders is that performance data from the OR could be used as evidence of negligence on the part of the health care team. These concerns are minimized by the manner in which the data is handled and categorized. Much like morbidity and mortality conference proceedings, OR Black Box findings are considered quality improvement data, typically protecting them from legal discovery.[38] As mentioned earlier, readily interpretable data such as audiovisual sources are only kept as raw footage for brief periods of time in order to allow them to be analyzed, additionally reducing the likelihood these data can be used in a persecutory sense.

Finally, seemingly convoluted questions around the ethics of video and audio recording in the clinical environment are often cited when discussing disruptive technologies like the OR Black Box.[34] Patients are at their most vulnerable when in the OR, leaving their care and even lives in the hands of the OR team. This trust is a central tenant of health care practices and must be upheld at all times. The OR Black Box has been engineered in a way that ensures confidentiality for patients while providing surgical teams with invaluable data on how to continuously improve. The ability to harness data to make surgery safer should reassure patients that, as physicians and nurses, we are constantly striving to do better. Furthermore, video recording in the OR adds an additional layer of accountability in the care provided to patients.

▌FUTURE UTILIZATION

The name *OR Black Box* may be a misnomer in itself because the applications of this technology far surpass the walls of the OR. Hugely important and complex aspects of perioperative and nonsurgical patient care environments can be subjected to quality improvement interventions, and the OR Black Box's unique data inputs could be used in these settings in order to better study and improve patient safety.

An immediately apparent part of the hospital where this technology could be readily applied is the trauma bay. Trauma care and resuscitation of the sickest patients is a multidisciplinary activity that usually requires teamwork, communication, and technical mastery.[39]

The aspects of surgical care that are analyzed using the Trauma Black Box platform, such as technical skills, nontechnical skills, and human factors engineering, all play a crucial role in the acute management of traumatically injured patients.[40] Evidence suggests that through the use of educational interventions such as simulation-based assessment, team performance can be improved in the trauma bay for the betterment of patient care.[41-44] The Trauma Black Box system will be invaluable in the collection of performance data for the purposes of quality improvement through multiple means including automation and standardization, simulation, and identification of inefficiencies and threats to patient safety.

Similar to the trauma bay, high-stakes environments such as the intensive care unit (ICU) would benefit from this technology. In the ICU, medical emergencies are frequently encountered and managed.[45] Procedures are often carried out like lumbar puncture, central venous catheter insertion, and intubation. Similar to the OR, these tasks are carried out in a multidisciplinary manner, and the impact on patient safety can be life altering.[45,46] Therefore, it is imperative that health care professionals in these environments strive to improve the quality of care they provide, and this can be facilitated with implementation of the ICU Black Box.

CONCLUSION

Currently used data collection techniques to evaluate technical skill, nontechnical skill, system performance, and error events in the OR exist and have been extensively used and researched. Despite this, these techniques inherently come with human rater–related biases that could influence the data collection and analysis process. In addition, in a health care environment, wherein monetary and personnel resources are in high demand, resources associated with the aforementioned data collection techniques are too intensive for their widespread utilization. Therefore, the implementation of an automated, all-encompassing OR data collection technology is needed to improve upon currently used data collection methods. The OR Black Box fills this need, providing the OR with objective, automated, and effective data collection.

ACKNOWLEDGMENT

We acknowledge Mr. Shuja Khalid for contributing his time and expertise to the writing of this chapter.

❚ REFERENCES

1. Janic M. An assessment of risk and safety in civil aviation. *J Air Transport Manage.* 2000;6:43-50.
2. Jung JJ, Elfassy J, Jüni P, Grantcharov T. Adverse events in the operating room: definitions, prevalence, and characteristics. A systematic review. *World J Surg.* 2019; 43(10):2379-2392.
3. Cuschieri A. Reducing errors in the operating room. *Surg Endosc.* 2005;19(8): 1022-1027.
4. Rassweiler MC, Mamoulakis C, Kenngott HG, Rassweiler J, la Rosette de J, Laguna MP. Classification and detection of errors in minimally invasive surgery. *J Endourol.* 2011;25(11):1713-1721.
5. Goldenberg MG, Jung J, Grantcharov TP. Using data to enhance performance and improve quality and safety in surgery. *JAMA Surg.* 2017;152(10):972-973.
6. Vedula SS, Hager GD. Surgical data science: the new knowledge domain. *Innov Surg Sci.* 2017;2(3):109-121.
7. Noble DJ, Pronovost PJ. Underreporting of patient safety incidents reduces health care's ability to quantify and accurately measure harm reduction. *J Patient Saf.* 2010;6(4):247-250.
8. Martin JA, Regehr G, Reznick R, et al. Objective Structured Assessment of Technical Skill (OSATS) for surgical residents. *Br J Surg.* 1997;84(2):273-278.
9. Hatala R, Cook DA, Brydges R, Hawkins R. Constructing a validity argument for the Objective Structured Assessment of Technical Skills (OSATS): a systematic review of validity evidence. *Adv Health Sci Educ.* 2015;20(5):1-27.
10. Levin M, McKechnie T, Khalid S, Grantcharov TP, Goldenberg MG. Automated methods of technical skill assessment in surgery: a systematic review. *J Surg Educ.* 2019;76(6):1629-1639.
11. Jung JJ, Borkhoff CM, Jüni P, Grantcharov TP. Non-technical skills for surgeons (NOTSS): critical appraisal of its measurement properties. *Am J Surg.* 2018;216(5):990-997.
12. Jung JJ, Yule S, Boet S, Szasz P, Schulthess P, Grantcharov T. Nontechnical skill assessment of the collective surgical team using the non-technical skills for surgeons (NOTSS) system. *Ann Surg.* 2019:1:10.1097/SLA.0000000000003250.
13. Carayon P, Schoofs Hundt A, Karsh BT, et al. Work system design for patient safety: the SEIPS model. *Qual Saf Health Care.* 2006;15(suppl 1):i50-i58.
14. Husslein H, Shirreff L, Shore EM, Lefebvre GG, Grantcharov TP. The generic error rating tool: a novel approach to assessment of performance and surgical education in gynecologic laparoscopy. *J Surg Educ.* 2015;72(6):1259-1265.
15. Hamilton EC, Pham DH, Minzenmayer AN, et al. Are we missing the near misses in the OR? Underreporting of safety incidents in pediatric surgery. *J Surg Res.* 2018;221:336-342.
16. Bonrath EM, Gordon LE. Characterising "near miss" events in complex laparoscopic surgery through video analysis. *BMJ Qual Saf.* 2015;24(8):516-521.
17. Greenberg CC, Dombrowski J, Dimick JB. Video-based surgical coaching: an emerging approach to performance improvement. *JAMA Surg.* 2016;151(3):282-283.

18. Yule S, Parker SH, Wilkinson J, et al. Coaching non-technical skills improves surgical residents' performance in a simulated operating room. *J Surg Educ.* 2015;72(6):1124-1130.

19. Hu Y-Y, Peyre SE, Arriaga AF, et al. Postgame analysis: using video-based coaching for continuous professional development. *J Am Coll Surg.* 2012;214(1):115-124.

20. Armour Forse R, Bramble JD, McQuillan R. Team training can improve operating room performance. *Surgery.* 2011;150(4):771-778.

21. Lee JY, Mucksavage P, Canales C, McDougall EM, Lin S. High fidelity simulation based team training in urology: a preliminary interdisciplinary study of technical and nontechnical skills in laparoscopic complications management. *J Urol.* 2012;187(4):1385-1391.

22. Grantcharov PD, Boillat T, Elkabany S, Wac K, Rivas H. Acute mental stress and surgical performance. *BJS Open.* 2019;3(1):119-125.

23. Jung JJ, Adams-McGavin RC, Grantcharov TP. Underreporting of Veress needle injuries: comparing direct observation and chart review methods. *J Surg Res.* 2019;236:266-270.

24. Jung JJ, Kashfi A, Sharma S, Grantcharov T. Characterization of device-related interruptions in minimally invasive surgery: need for intraoperative data and effective mitigation strategies. *Surg Endosc.* 2019;33(3):717-723.

25. Fecso AB, Kuzulugil SS, Babaoglu C, Bener AB, Grantcharov TP. Relationship between intraoperative non-technical performance and technical events in bariatric surgery. *Br J Surg.* 2018;83:249-257.

26. Jung JJ, Jüni P, Lebovic G, Grantcharov T. First-year analysis of the operating room black box study. *Ann Surg.* 2020;271(1):122-127.

27. Hashimoto DA, Rosman G, Rus D, Meireles OR. Artificial intelligence in surgery. *Ann Surg.* 2018;268(1):70-76.

28. Voulodimos A, Doulamis N, Doulamis A, Protopapadakis E. Deep learning for computer vision: a brief review. *Comput Intell Neurosci.* 2018;2018:1-13.

29. Shouhed D, Gewertz B, Wiegmann D, Catchpole K. Integrating human factors research and surgery: a review. *Arch Surg.* 2012;147(12):1141-1146.

30. Jones M, Howells N, Mitchell S, Burnand H, Mutimer J, Longman R. Human-factors training for surgical trainees. *Clin Teach.* 2014;11(3):165-169.

31. Reason J. Understanding adverse events: human factors. *Qual Health Care.* 1995;4(2):80-89.

32. Alsubaie H, Goldenberg MG, Grantcharov T. Quantifying recall bias in surgical safety: a need for a modern approach to morbidity and mortality reviews. *Can J Surg.* 2019;62(1):39-43.

33. Stefanidis D, Sevdalis N, Paige J, et al. Simulation in surgery: what's needed next? *Ann Surg.* 2015;261(5):846-853.

34. Langerman A, Grantcharov TP. Are we ready for our close-up? Why and how we must embrace video in the OR. *Ann Surg.* 2017;266(6):934-936.

35. Silas MR, Grassia P, Langerman A. Video recording of the operating room: is anonymity possible? *J Surg Res.* 2015;197(2):272-276.

36. Henken KR, Jansen FW, Klein J, Stassen LPS, Dankelman J, van den Dobbelsteen JJ. Implications of the law on video recording in clinical practice. *Surg Endosc*. 2012;26(10):2909-2916.

37. Healthcare Insurance Reciprocal of Canada. Surgical safety in Canada: a 10-year review of CMPA and HIROC medico-legal data. Accessed October 5, 2020. https://www.patientsafetyinstitute.ca/en/toolsResources/Surgical-Safety-in-Canada/Pages/default.aspx.

38. Klein CA. The Patient Safety and Quality Improvement Act of 2005. *Nurse Pract*. 2005;30(12):14.

39. Briggs A, Raja AS, Joyce MF, et al. The role of nontechnical skills in simulated trauma resuscitation. *J Surg Educ*. 2015;72(4):732-739.

40. Capella J, Smith S, Philp A, et al. Teamwork training improves the clinical care of trauma patients. *J Surg Educ*. 2010;67(6):439-443.

41. Miller D, Crandall C, Washington C, McLaughlin S. Improving teamwork and communication in trauma care through in situ simulations. *Acad Emerg Med*. 2012;19(5):608-612.

42. Capella J, Smith S, Philp A, et al. Teamwork training improves the clinical care of trauma patients. *J Surg Educ*. 2010;67(6):439-443.

43. Alken A, Luursema J-M, Weenk M, Yauw S, Fluit C, van Goor H. Integrating technical and non-technical skills coaching in an acute trauma surgery team training: is it too much? *Am J Surg*. 2018;216(2):369-374.

44. Hamilton NA, Kieninger AN, Woodhouse J, Freeman BD, Murray D, Klingensmith ME. Video review using a reliable evaluation metric improves team function in high-fidelity simulated trauma resuscitation. *J Surg Educ*. 2012;69(3):428-431.

45. Gundrosen S, Solligård E, Aadahl P. Team competence among nurses in an intensive care unit: the feasibility of in situ simulation and assessing non-technical skills. *Intensive Crit Care Nurs*. 2014;30(6):312-317.

46. Barsuk JH, McGaghie WC, Cohen ER, O'Leary KJ, Wayne DB. Simulation-based mastery learning reduces complications during central venous catheter insertion in a medical intensive care unit. *Crit Care Med*. 2009;37(10):2697-2701.

APPLICATIONS OF DEEP LEARNING IN SURGERY 11

Quanzheng Li

HIGHLIGHTS

- Applications of deep learning in surgery fit mostly into 3 broad categories: preoperative planning, intraoperative navigation and tracking, and intraoperative control.
- Deep learning for surgery has explored applications including surgical skill assessment, preoperative risk stratification, robotic control of devices, and automation of operative tasks.
- Deep learning could augment surgeons' abilities by further empowering their skills via technologies such as facial tracking for automated control of a laparoscope, estimated force feedback during robotic surgery, or even trajectory planning for the placement of sutures.

▍ INTRODUCTION

Deep-learning (DL) techniques have witnessed great success and achieved performance levels that are almost as good as or even better than human performance in many fields, including computer vision, natural language processing, and control systems (see Chapter 4).[1-9] DL is marked by its computational structure composed of multiple (from tens to thousands) neural layers for feature extraction, probability prediction, and learning optimized representation of data.[9] Because of the different receptive fields in this deep structure, it can learn informative features from training data through a hierarchical level of abstraction that retains information coherence at each level of the hierarchy,[6] hence capturing the distribution of high-dimensional data (eg, an image) with a large number of model parameters.[10]

The advancement of the following elements makes it possible and promising to solve various traditionally difficult challenges in the field of artificial intelligence (AI): (1) DL methods able to take advantage of large training data information; (2) big data technology for storing, transporting, and accessing data of unprecedent sizes; and (3) computing hardware, especially the extensive utilization of graphic processing units (GPUs) for more powerful yet inexpensive computational power.

With reports of various applications of DL in robotic surgery, some hope that DL has the potential to address some of the technological challenges of advancing robot-assisted and computer-integrated surgical systems to a level of targeted autonomy. These hopes are also drawn from advances in the field of medical image analysis, where DL has rapidly become a dominant methodology for applications such as classification, detection, segmentation, registration, and reconstruction.[11] DL's intrinsic capability of automatically learning representative features from data, rather than relying on hand-crafted features based on domain expertise, has proved to be efficient and robust in analyzing medical images of various modalities and diseases.[12]

From the algorithmic perspective, DL is well known for 2 main categories of algorithms: modeling of data and modeling of actions. The algorithms that largely perform modeling of data through hierarchical representation learning (ie, network structure) effectively transform data (eg, images) from their original high-dimensional space (eg, image pixels/voxels) to a lower-dimensional feature and abstract space. The learned features can then be used for further analysis of tasks mainly centered around a logistic regression model (eg, classification). Algorithms that center on modeling of action aim to infer the optimal strategy of interactions between computational agents (ie, robots) and environments (ie, patients) through learning by trial and error or by expert demonstration. This application is mostly known for the recent success of deep reinforcement learning (DRL) methods, which have achieved human expert–level performance in tasks such as the game of Go.[13] Other approaches for learning from a physician's sequence of actions in surgery include recurrent neural networks (RNNs), which capture long-range context of the sequence through long short-term memory mechanism,[14] with applications in learning the control sequence of suturing wounds in robot-assisted surgery.[15]

Current research efforts on applications of DL in surgery can be sorted into the following 3 categories:

- Preoperative planning: A surgical procedure is preplanned by physicians with the assistance of DL algorithms, based on patient information including imaging data, medical records, and laboratory test results.
- Intraoperative navigation and tracking: DL-assisted intraoperative guidance or navigation is provided to surgeons for better

Table 11-1	SUMMARY OF DEEP LEARNING APPLICATIONS FOR SURGERY	
	Modeling of Data	**Modeling of Action**
Planning	Image analysis and computer-aided diagnosis/prognosis[16-20]	Policy inference for clinical decision support[21-26]
Navigation/ tracking	Image/video-guided surgical navigation[27-37]	Surgical training by operation modeling and assessment[38-42]
Control	Surgical interaction[43-49] and operative procedure[50-53]	Surgical control learning and modeling[54-59]

visualization and tracking cues, especially when the operative view is limited (eg, endoscopic surgery).

- Intraoperative control: Increased level of surgical automation is achieved through enhanced representation and modeling of surgical procedures, analyzing the complex operative environment, and optimizing the control sequence through DL.

Based on these categories for DL algorithms (2 types) and applications (3 subareas), in this chapter, we will summarize the current applications of DL in surgery as shown in Table 11-1.[16-59]

DEEP LEARNING FOR PREOPERATIVE PLANNING

Modeling of Data: Image Analysis and Computer-Aided Diagnosis/Prognosis

Medical image analysis, including methods such as image segmentation, registration, classification, and denoising, plays a vital role in preoperative planning. Both physicians and computer-integrated systems rely on the effective and accurate analysis of preoperative images, intraoperative real-time images, and perhaps more importantly, the effective linkage of pre- and intraoperative information to perform the key tasks necessary to safely complete an operation. Identification of lesions and abnormities from preoperative medical images, a typical image classification task in DL applications, can provide diagnostic information to surgeons during surgical planning (eg, the capability of detecting intracranial hemorrhage, calvaria fractures, midline shift, and mass effect from head computed tomography [CT] scans).[19] Image/volume segmentation provides precise anatomic identification of organs and possible lesions within those organs at a pixel- or voxel-level, allowing for surgical planning for both resection and reconstruction.[16]

DL algorithms have been widely used for segmentation in medical imaging, performing direct image-to-image/volume-to-volume learning and inference to learn the image features of a segmentation target. For example, DL has achieved superior performance in tasks such as 3-dimensional (3D) liver segmentation from CT scans and 3D heart and vessel segmentation from magnetic resonance imaging (MRI) scans.[20] Preoperative planning for procedures is usually performed through annotation and analysis on high-quality, 3D axial images such as CT/MRI. During an operation, however, imaging may be limited to low-quality, 2-dimensional (2D) images such as fluoroscopy or ultrasound. In these cases, DL algorithms designed for efficient registration and instantiation can be helpful to enable slice-to-volume registration and volumetric reconstruction from a single 2D image.[17]

Modeling of Action: Policy Inference for Clinical Decision Support

A major challenge in automating elements of surgery lies in the difficulty of modeling, predicting, and managing patient-specific postoperative complications. This is even difficult for clinicians with significant domain expertise. DRL has shown promise in providing complex assessments of surgical prognosis and optimization of management plans through advanced clinical decision support (CDS) systems. Unlike traditional CDS systems where clinical guidelines are implemented to identify potential conflicts or warnings based on predefined rules, DRL analyzes patient data to assess for the development and progression of complications and then assess the effect of decisions for treatments (ie, actions) through a learning-based approach from accumulated records of treatments.[26] By learning a more discriminative representation of treatment data and learning the decision policy for taking corresponding actions based on a patient's status, DRL could discover an optimized treatment plan or even automatically explore new treatment options beyond those available in existing patient records.[21] DRL-based treatment plans that have been published in the literature include those treating sepsis,[22] managing diabetes,[23] treating lung cancer,[24] and recommending medications in intensive care.[25]

DEEP LEARNING FOR NAVIGATION AND TRACKING

Modeling of Data: Image- and Video-Guided Surgical Navigation and Tracking

Automated tracking and localization in minimally invasive surgery focuses on estimating the relative position of instruments (eg, shaft/tip) to the environment, based on electromagnetic, optical, and image/video information.[27] Position estimation and the corresponding contextual information related to instruments and tissues are vital for providing visual and tactile feedback to surgeons. DL solutions have been proposed for instrument segmentation from real-time endoscopic video[30] for cholecystectomy surgeries[34] and from microscopic images for retinal microsurgery.[35] Some examples of these applications have been covered in Chapters 6 and 7.

An interesting application of the work performed in tool segmentation is real-time retargeting (ie, estimating the position of the endoscope to identify whether the endoscopic images are from the same location). This type of work is highly important for applications such as optical biopsy where endomicroscopic images are acquired for diagnosis and to guide treatment.[36] Furthermore, standard laparoscopes are only 2D and thus lack depth information, increasing the difficulty of 3D spatial orientation and navigation. DL has been applied in tasks of depth estimation and camera localization,[31] allowing 3D images to be created from strictly 2D video sources. Depth estimation has also been combined with direct pose estimation by DL, for example, in the application of identifying the location of an ingestible wireless endoscopy capsule during inspection of the gastrointestinal tract.[37]

To better navigate the dynamic and complex intracorporeal environment, correct and robust control of an imaging device (eg, the endoscope) is essential, and a technique in robotic control known as simultaneous localization and mapping (SLAM) has been used to improve performance in automated control of the endoscopic camera.[32] A combination of DL-based analysis of high-fidelity preoperative imaging (eg, segmentation, registration, as discussed earlier) and DL-assisted navigation of the target operative area during minimally invasive surgery can be achieved through estimation of a 3D pose model (eg, modeling position and configuration of the body relative to axial imaging).[33] Training and performance on this type of task can be challenging due to fast movements of the endoscope, which creates noise and artifacts in the acquired images.[32] DL algorithms have thus been developed to enable accurate analysis of such images within a complex motion sequence.[37]

Modeling of Action: Surgical Training by Operative Modeling and Assessment

One important field of research in the application of AI is training care team members (eg, surgeons, assistants, other physicians) to perform procedures. This is especially of interest with the rapid introduction of new technologies (eg, robotic systems) that require more time-consuming and costly training programs.[39] As described in greater depth in Chapters 7 and 8, a major area of investigation for DL in surgical training is the automatic and objective assessment of surgical performance, often from the analysis of motion and video data.[38] Previous studies have shown that automated assessment of surgical skill is feasible and could serve as an effective solution for delivering procedural feedback.[41]

▌ DEEP LEARNING FOR OPERATION CONTROL

Modeling of Data: Surgical Interaction and Operative Procedure

During an operation, surgeons must coordinate the use of surgical devices not just for themselves but for their assistants as well. For example, during laparoscopic surgery, a dedicated assistant is usually required to maneuver the laparoscopic camera, and the assistant needs to synchronize with the surgeon.[43] In efforts to develop more efficient interactions between surgeons and devices, DL-based solutions for recognizing a surgeon's various movements or instructions have been developed. Fujii et al[43] describe a system that models a surgeon's eye movements via a segmentation and classification framework, and then the system can control a robotic arm to hold the endoscope without a human camera assistant. In addition, speech recognition by DL, which has been widely applied in personal devices, has also been used in a voice-controlled robot (eg, the robotic assist scope holder [AESOP])[44] with motion-to-image calibration.[45] Other mechanisms to improve control of devices include a monitor for facial motions[46] and a head-mounted infrared emitter.[47]

Another important and closely related application of DL in surgical interactions is the capability to provide feedback to surgeons by automatically estimating the applied forces of tools and providing a signal to the surgeon.[48] This is particularly important because current robotic systems do not provide haptic feedback of any kind. Force estimation can be based on computer vision methods for modeling surface deformation in acquired images, motion control parameters, proximal-end measurements, or a combination of all of these factors.[49]

Aside from modeling of surgical interactions between the surgeon and devices, modeling of an operative procedure aims to transform a surgeon's movements into structured representations of tasks. This is an essential component for both surgical assessment in training (as discussed earlier and in Chapter 7) and for learning robotic control sequences from human demonstrations (which will be discussed later). In other words, the training of both humans and computers needs to be based on an effective representation of a model surgeon's actions. DL-based modeling of a procedure thus mainly focuses on the recognition of surgical tools and surgical hand gestures (eg, grabbing the needle, passing the needle) from video and/or kinematics data[50-52] or from an accelerometer-based pen-type sensing device[53] and classifying them into discrete tasks (eg, suturing). For example, the region proposal network (RPN), which is a recent advancement of DL for computer vision tasks, has been applied by Sarikaya et al[50] for jointly predicting and localizing tools.

Modeling of Action: Surgical Control Learning and Modeling

An increasing number of surgical procedures have been performed robotically, increasing interest in applying developments in the fields of automation and control theory to surgical robotics. Advanced AI-assisted control methodologies have enabled modeling, learning, and executing control sequences of surgical procedures in a dynamic and complex environment. As an example, preliminary (non-DL) attempts at performing fully automatic surgical procedures, such as suturing in an open surgery environment, have shown improved performance with better consistency and quality and fewer mistakes for knot tying during an intestinal anastomosis in a live porcine model.[5] DL-based methods such as RNN have also been applied for this task, learning the trajectories of surgeon's actions and using internal memory to distinguish between identical inputs that require different actions at different points along a given trajectory.[54] Trajectory planning has also been modeled by an artificial neural network (ANN) architecture that learns from human actions.[55]

Among the novel control techniques developed in recent decades, reinforcement learning (RL) and its DL-based version, DRL, have become the most prominent methods for learning and modeling a control sequence.[13] RL aims at training computational agents to effectively interact with the environment through "actions" in a sequential and iterative way. During the training, agents usually have an observation of their environment (termed *state*) at each iteration with a final specific goal to achieve (termed *value*), which may not be observable until the end. Agents are then trained to learn an action-value function (termed *policy*), measured by the cumulative value of an action within a specific state, where the learning can be based on trial and error (ie, self-supervised) and/or human demonstration.[13] RL has already been successfully applied in surgical AI, such as performing cutting tasks by controlling the STIFF-FLOP flexible robot with learning from human demonstration[56] to sew personalized stent grafts.[57]

DRL further improves the effectiveness of RL by learning the optimized policy directly from raw high-dimensional input, such as images or videos. A few early attempts have been made in applying DRL for surgical procedures, such as robots that were trained by demonstration, showing much faster operative speed and smoother motion trajectory than humans on a 2-handed knot-tie task.[58] For a pattern-cutting task, a DRL-based policy network was trained to optimize both the choice of pinch point and cutting trajectory and was tested on the da Vinci Research Kit (dVRK) simulation with improved performance compared to traditional models.[59]

CONCLUSION

Surgical applications of DL have undergone varied and extensive preliminary investigation, yet the field remains in its infancy. As DL continues to make significant advances in pattern recognition and model generation, it will likely be a technology that will have major impact on the development of CDS systems, surgical devices, and surgical robotics.

REFERENCES

1. Camarillo DB, Krummel TM, Salisbury JK. Robotic technology in surgery: past, present, and future. *Am J Surg.* 2004;188:2-15.
2. Gomes P. Surgical robotics: reviewing the past, analysing the present, imagining the future. *Robot Comput Integr Manufact.* 2011;27:261-266.
3. Vitiello V, Su-Lin L, Cundy TP, Guang-Zhong Y. Emerging robotic platforms for minimally invasive surgery. *IEEE Rev Biomed Eng.* 2013;6:111-126.
4. Yang G, Cambias J, Cleary K, et al. Medical robotics: regulatory, ethical, and legal considerations for increasing levels of autonomy. *Sci Robot.* 2017;2:4.
5. Shademan A, Decker RS, Opfermann JD, Leonard S, Krieger A, Kim PCW. Supervised autonomous robotic soft tissue surgery. *Sci Transl Med.* 2016;8:337ra64.
6. Yang G, Bellingham J, Dupont P, et al. The grand challenges of science robotics. *Sci Robot.* 2018;3:14.
7. Haidegger T. Autonomy for surgical robots: concepts and paradigms. *IEEE Transact Med Robot Bionics.* 2019;1:65-76.
8. Yu K-H, Beam AL, Kohane IS. Artificial intelligence in healthcare. *Nat Biomed Eng.* 2018;2:719-731.

9. LeCun Y, Bengio Y, Hinton G. Deep learning. *Nature*. 2015;521:436-444.

10. Krizhevsky A, Sutskever I, Hinton G. ImageNet classification with deep convolutional neural networks. *Commun ACM*. 2017;60:84-90.

11. Litjens G, Kooi T, Bejnordi BE, et al. A survey on deep learning in medical image analysis. *Med Image Anal*. 2017;42:60-88.

12. Shen D, Wu G, Suk H-I. Deep learning in medical image analysis. *Annu Rev Biomed Eng*. 2017;19:221-248.

13. Silver D, Huang A, Maddison CJ, et al. Mastering the game of Go with deep neural networks and tree search. *Nature*. 2016;529:484-489.

14. Graves A, Mohamed A-R, Hinton G. Speech recognition with deep recurrent neural networks. Accessed October 6, 2020. https://arxiv.org/abs/1303.5778.

15. Esteva A, Robicquet A, Ramsundar B, et al. A guide to deep learning in healthcare. *Nat Med*. 2019;25:24-29.

16. Lessmann N, van Ginneken B, de Jong PA, Išgum I. Iterative fully convolutional neural networks for automatic vertebra segmentation and identification. *Med Image Anal*. 2019;53:142-155.

17. Balakrishnan G, Zhao A, Sabuncu MR, Guttag J, Dalca AV. VoxelMorph: a learning framework for deformable medical image registration. *IEEE Trans Med Imaging*. 2019;38:1788-1800.

18. Ferrante E, Paragios N. Slice-to-volume medical image registration: a survey. *Med Image Anal*. 2017;39:101-123.

19. Chilamkurthy S, Ghosh R, Tanamala S, et al. Deep learning algorithms for detection of critical findings in head CT scans: a retrospective study. *Lancet*. 2018;392:2388-2396.

20. Dou Q, Yu L, Chen H, et al. 3D deeply supervised network for automated segmentation of volumetric medical images. *Med Image Anal*. 2017;41:40-54.

21. Liu S, Feng M. Deep reinforcement learning for clinical decision support: a brief survey. Accessed October 6, 2020. https://arxiv.org/abs/1907.09475.

22. Komorowski M, Celi L, Szolovits P, Ghassemi M. Continuous state-space models for optimal sepsis treatment: a deep reinforcement learning approach. Accessed October 6, 2020. https://arxiv.org/pdf/1705.08422.pdf.

23. Asoh H, Shiro M, Akaho S, Kamishima T. An application of inverse reinforcement learning to medical records of diabetes treatment. Accessed October 6, 2020. http://www.ke.tu-darmstadt.de/events/PBRL-13/papers/02-Asoh.pdf.

24. Tseng HH, Luo Y, Cui S, Chien T, Ten Haken RK, Naqa IE. Deep reinforcement learning for automated radiation adaptation in lung cancer. *Med Phys*. 2017;44:6690-6705.

25. Wang L, Zhang W, He X, Zha H. Supervised reinforcement learning with recurrent neural network for dynamic treatment recommendation. Accessed October 6, 2020. https://arxiv.org/pdf/1807.01473.pdf.

26. Mnih V, Kavukcuoglu K, Silver D, et al. Human-level control through deep reinforcement learning. *Nature*. 2015;518:529-533.

27. Zhao Z, Voros S, Weng Y, Chang F, Li R. Tracking-by-detection of surgical instruments in minimally invasive surgery via the convolutional neural network deep learning-based method. *Comput Assist Surg*. 2017;22:26-35.

28. Wen R, Tay W-L, Nguyen BP, Chng C-B, Chui C-K. Hand gesture guided robot-assisted surgery based on a direct augmented reality interface. *Comput Methods Programs Biomed.* 2014;116:68-80.

29. Rong W, Mei Z, Xiangbing M, Zheng G, Fei-Yue W. 3-D tracking for augmented reality using combined region and dense cues in endoscopic surgery. *IEEE J Biomed Health Inform.* 2018;22:1540-1551.

30. Islam M, Atputharuban DA, Ramesh R, Ren H. Real-time instrument segmentation in robotic surgery using auxiliary supervised deep adversarial learning. *IEEE Robot Automation Letters.* 2019;4:2188-2195.

31. Shen M, Gu Y, Liu N, Yang G-Z. Context-aware depth and pose estimation for bronchoscopic navigation. *IEEE Robot Automation Letters.* 2019;4:732-739.

32. Song J, Wang J, Zhao L, Huang S, Dissanayake G. MIS-SLAM: real-time large-scale dense deformable SLAM system in minimal invasive surgery based on heterogeneous computing. *IEEE Robot Automation Letters.* 2018;3: 4068-4075.

33. Davison AJ, Reid ID, Molton ND, Stasse O. MonoSLAM: real-time single camera SLAM. *IEEE Trans Pattern Anal Mach Intell.* 2007;29:1052-1067.

34. Nwoye C, Mutter D, Marescaux J, Padoy N. Weakly supervised convolutional LSTM approach for tool tracking in laparoscopic videos. *Int J Comput Assist Radiol Surg.* 2019;14:1059-1067.

35. Rieke N, Tan DJ, Amat Di San Filippo C, et al. Real-time localization of articulated surgical instruments in retinal microsurgery. *Med Image Anal.* 2016;34:82-100.

36. Ye M, Giannarou S, Meining A, Yang G-Z. Online tracking and retargeting with applications to optical biopsy in gastrointestinal endoscopic examinations. *Med Image Anal.* 2016;30:144-157.

37. Turan M, Almalioglu Y, Araujo H, Konukoglu E, Sitti M. Deep EndoVO: a recurrent convolutional neural network (RCNN) based visual odometry approach for endoscopic capsule robots. *Neurocomputing.* 2018;275:1861-1870.

38. Ahmidi N, Lingling T, Sefati S, et al. A dataset and benchmarks for segmentation and recognition of gestures in robotic surgery. *IEEE Trans Biomed Eng.* 2017;64:2025-2041.

39. Tan X, Chng C-B, Su Y, Lim K-B, Chui C-K. Robot-assisted training in laparoscopy using deep reinforcement learning. *IEEE Robot Automation Letters.* 2019;4:485-492.

40. Lerner MA, Ayalew M, Peine WJ, Sundaram CP. Does training on a virtual reality robotic simulator improve performance on the da Vinci® surgical system? *J Endourol.* 2010;24:467-472.

41. Ahmidi N, Poddar P, Jones JD, et al. Automated objective surgical skill assessment in the operating room from unstructured tool motion in septoplasty. *Int J Comput Assist Radiol Surg.* 2015;10:981-991.

42. King D, Tee S, Falconer L, Angell C, Holley D, Mills A. Virtual health education: scaling practice to transform student learning: using virtual reality learning environments in healthcare education to bridge the theory/practice gap and improve patient safety. *Nurse Educ Today.* 2018;71:7-9.

43. Fujii K, Gras G, Salerno A, Yang G-Z. Gaze gesture based human robot interaction for laparoscopic surgery. *Med Image Anal.* 2018;44:196-214.

44. Nathan C-AO, Chakradeo VO, Malhotra KO, Agostino HO, Patwardhan RO. The voice-controlled robotic assist scope holder AESOP for the endoscopic approach to the sella. *Skull Base*. 2006;16:123-131.

45. Zinchenko K, Chien-Yu W, Kai-Tai S. A study on speech recognition control for a surgical robot. *IEEE Trans Indust Inform*. 2017;13:607-615.

46. Nishikawa A, Hosoi T, Koara K, et al. FAce MOUSe: a novel human-machine interface for controlling the position of a laparoscope. *IEEE Trans Robot Automation*. 2003;19:825-841.

47. Kommu SS, Rimington P, Anderson C, Rane A. Initial experience with the Endo-Assist camera-holding robot in laparoscopic urological surgery. *J Robot Surg*. 2007;1:133-137.

48. Aviles AI, Alsaleh SM, Hahn JK, Casals A. Towards retrieving force feedback in robotic-assisted surgery: a supervised neuro-recurrent-vision approach. *IEEE Transact Haptics*. 2017;10:431-443.

49. Li X, Cao L, Tiong AMH, Phan PR, Phee SJ. Distal-end force prediction of tendon-sheath mechanisms for flexible endoscopic surgical robots using deep learning. *Mech Mach Theory*. 2019;134:323-337.

50. Sarikaya D, Corso JJ, Guru KA. Detection and localization of robotic tools in robot-assisted surgery videos using deep neural networks for region proposal and detection. *IEEE Trans Med Imaging*. 2017;36:1542-1549.

51. Zappella L, Béjar B, Hager G, Vidal R. Surgical gesture classification from video and kinematic data. *Med Image Anal*. 2013;17:732-745.

52. Oyedotun O, Khashman A. Deep learning in vision-based static hand gesture recognition. *Neural Comput Appl*. 2017;28:3941-3951.

53. Renqiang X, Juncheng C. Accelerometer-based hand gesture recognition by neural network and similarity matching. *IEEE Sensors J*. 2016;16:4537-4545.

54. Mayer H, Gomez F, Wierstra D, Nagy I, Knoll A, Schmidhuber J. A system for robotic heart surgery that learns to tie knots using recurrent neural networks. *Adv Robot*. 2008;22:1521-1537.

55. De Momi E, Kranendonk L, Valenti M, Enayati N, Ferrigno G. A neural network-based approach for trajectory planning in robot–human handover tasks. *Front Robot AI*. Accessed October 6, 2020. https://www.frontiersin.org/articles/10.3389/frobt.2016.00034/full.

56. Calinon S, Bruno D, Malekzadeh MS, Nanayakkara T, Caldwell DG. Human–robot skills transfer interfaces for a flexible surgical robot. *Comput Method Programs Biomed*. 2014;116:81-96.

57. Bidan H, Menglong Y, Yang H, Vandini A, Su-Lin L, Guang-Zhong Y. A multirobot cooperation framework for sewing personalized stent grafts. *IEEE Trans Industrial Inform*. 2018;14:1776-1785.

58. van Den Berg J, Miller S, Duckworth D, et al. Superhuman performance of surgical tasks by robots using iterative learning from human-guided demonstrations. Accessed October 6, 2020. https://ieeexplore.ieee.org/document/5509621.

59. Thananjeyan B, Garg A, Krishnan S, Chen C, Miller L, Goldberg K. Multilateral surgical pattern cutting in 2D orthotropic gauze with deep reinforcement learning policies for tensioning. Accessed October 6, 2020. https://bthananjeyan.github.io/brijen_files/2017-icra-cutting-final.pdf.

ARTIFICIAL INTELLIGENCE IN ROBOTIC SURGERY 12

Daniel Naftalovich, Camille Stewart, Joel Burdick, and Yuman Fong

HIGHLIGHTS

- Artificial intelligence (AI) and robotics can benefit surgery together and individually.
- Not all robotic surgical systems are AI systems. Robots involve hardware and feedback. (Remember: sense-think-act.)
- AI-enhanced robotics has the potential to enable automation in surgery at *varying levels of autonomy*, including assistance (currently in use), supervised/conditional autonomy (in prototype use), and full autonomy (in development).
- Future applications of AI could include virtual assistants and mentors, improved situational awareness, and an interface to a collective surgical consciousness.

▌INTRODUCTION

The field of surgery can gain a great deal from the convergence of artificial intelligence (AI) and robotic technologies. These related but distinct topics—as elaborated in this chapter—stand to benefit from substantial synergy. At this time, the goal of combining robotics with AI for many is to break down surgical tasks into subtasks, which can be recognized through computer vision and machine learning and then be automated using surgical robots. This is to increase procedural efficiency, accuracy, and safety while decreasing surgeon focus on automatable/rote tasks and overall fatigue, which could enable the surgeon to have increased vigilance and focus on the more complex aspects of the procedure. Future possibilities range from virtual robotic assistants that physically move in response to natural language commands or automatic visual interpretation of surgical scenes, virtual mentors that can make remote physical adjustments in the operative field that are available on demand, and autonomous robotic executions of surgical tasks or whole procedures. In this chapter, we provide an introduction to robotics and how robotics interacts with AI. This is followed by a review of the literature on robotics, AI, and the convergence of robotics and AI in the operating room, including additional possibilities for robotics and AI in the future.

▌ INTRODUCTION TO ROBOTICS

Robots Are Cyber-Physical Systems That Sense, Think, and Act

Cyber-physical systems are systems that have both computational (software) and physical (hardware) components.[1] AI (see Chapter 1) refers to a set of techniques within the computational aspects of automated decision making and thus fits in the "cyber" part of cyber-physical systems. Automation systems do exist that are purely algorithmic/computational, without physical components, and such systems are *not* robotic systems.[2] Similarly, automation systems also exist that are purely mechanical/physical, without computation, and such systems are *not* AI systems. Such systems are also *not* robotic, as robots by definition involve some aspect of computation, at least by the definition chosen in this chapter of robots as cyber-physical systems that sense, think, *and* act with feedback control. Multiple definitions exist for robots and for AI and have been debated and discussed for decades. Furthermore, *not all robotic systems are AI systems*, as the computational aspects of a robotic system may not be particularly intelligent. Robotic systems with AI have both physical components for sensing, computation, and actuation, as well as algorithmic intelligence within the computational subsystem, such as effective natural language processing, sophisticated computer vision, or use of artificial neural networks.

Robots are machines that sense, think, and act and have a substantial physical manifestation. Such a thinking machine may be more or less sophisticated in its manner of thought, depending on its particular design and implementation. On the complex end of the spectrum, a machine's manner of thought may be "intelligent" or resembling intelligence, and deemed as AI. On the simple end, such little complexity of thought may be present that the machine may be hardly considered as a robot at all, instead being deemed simply a machine, rather than a substantially thinking machine. In this chapter, such a view is taken, in which *machines of trivial nature of thought are not considered robots.*

Machines "think" via computation, which is the process of calculating and converting information. A key component of a robotic system is software, which serves as the "thinking" algorithm. Physically,

Key Point

Here we refer to automation systems without physical components aside from the physical processor(s) on which they operate. Ultimately, computation is performed by some physical matter, such as vacuum tubes, transistors, biological neurons, or quantum interactions.

software in a robot is implemented within the processor and supporting components, such as computer, memory, and storage. Software often exists also outside of robotic systems, in standalone computers that are not necessarily connected to sensors and actuators. *Computer systems lacking substantial interaction with the physical world are not considered robotic.*

Robots are fundamentally equipped with sensors that observe the physical world and actuators that physically affect the world.[1] *Actuation* is the process of moving or forcing something in the physical world. A typical actuator of robotic systems is an electric motor, which converts electrical energy into rotational motion. Other common actuators include pneumatic actuators and suction mechanisms. *Sensing* is the process of capturing information from some physical phenomenon in the world. Typical sensors of robotic systems include motion detectors, cameras, microphones, ultrasound probes, and detection of other electromagnetic waves. *All robots have some combination of sensors and actuators.*

Not all combinations of sensors and actuators are robots because robots also necessarily involve computation at a substantial level. A trivial connection from a sensor to an actuator is not considered a robot. Furthermore, autonomy of a robot can be thought of in levels.[3] For example, consider an automatic parking gate that has a keypad sensor to detect the user's input of a security code and has an electric motor to open the parking gate. Because the interconnection logic from the keypad sensor to the actuator is a trivially simple algorithm (if the correct code is entered, the gate opens), this system may be considered not particularly robotic, or at least not *autonomous*. This system is an example of an *automatic* gate, but it is not particularly autonomous because it does not involve substantial thinking or decision making.

Feedback occurs when sensors are used to gather information *during* the function of a robot, and actuation is influenced in response to the sensor measurements.[4,5] Intentional use of feedback to achieve a target is known as *closed-loop control.* A typical example of a closed-loop control system is temperature regulation in a home or an oven: a thermostat receives from the user a temperature set point and measures the temperature from a thermometer (the sensor) and turns on the air conditioning or oven flame (the actuator) in order to bring the sensed temperature to the reference target temperature. When feedback is not present in a control system, it is known as open-loop control. An example of open-loop control of temperature is a pot on a stovetop flame: the flame is set initially and has the intention of bringing the temperature of the pot to a high temperature, but no sensor is used to measure the pot's temperature and to adjust the flame size in response. *A key feature of robotic systems is the*

Key Point

The keyboard and mouse, for example, of a typical personal computer are sensors, as they sense the keypresses of a user's fingers or the motion of the user's hand. The computer display and computer speakers are examples of actuators that a personal computer typically uses to physically influence the world based on information that is sent to these components (the display affects photons of light, and the speakers affect air molecules). Other sensors that are often connected to computers include microphones and cameras, and other actuators may include printers. Many different sensors and actuators can be easily connected through USB cables.

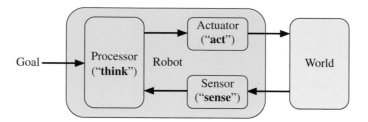

Figure 12-1 • Sense-think-act feedback cycle of robotic systems. Robots physically interact with the world via sensing and actuation. Robots are by definition reprogrammable to new goals from user input.

Key Point

The *Sense-Think-Act* loop is known in the engineering literature as the *control loop* and is often drawn slightly differently to emphasize the comparison between the reference signal (the goal) and the observed sensor measurements.

The difference between the reference and the observed value that is meant to be controlled is known as the *error*.

use of feedback control in a closed-loop fashion. The closed-loop feedback nature of robots can be summarized as the *sense-think-act* loop, shown in Figure 12-1.

AI Is a Subset of Computation

Not all software is AI. AI models are generally structured as input-output models that receive an input signal and produce an output, much like a closed-loop system in which a signal arrives from a sensor and is ultimately sent to an actuator. Additionally, AI models involve *training from data*, not just manual engineering like some closed-loop systems. A common machine learning structure for AI is that of artificial neural networks, and common applications are for natural language processing and computer vision.[6] *AI can enable more complex decision making* than classic feedback control alone and thus lead to greater autonomy in robotic systems, including in surgery.

Figure 12-2 compares AI, closed-loop, and open-loop computation on a spectrum of complexity and autonomy and also emphasizes that

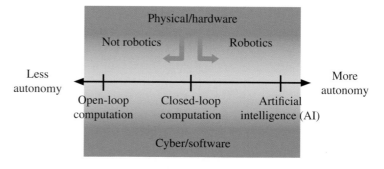

Figure 12-2 • Spectrum of computation and hardware in automation.

robotic systems include nontrivial closed-loop software or AI along with physical hardware.

SURGICAL ROBOTIC TECHNOLOGY WITHOUT AI

A number of robotic systems that can assist in the operative theater exist that do not currently use AI.[7] The first such robot used on a human patient was the Programmable Universal Machine for Assembly (PUMA) 200, which assisted in the performance of a neurosurgical biopsy in 1985.[8] Since that time, a number of surgical robotic systems have been developed,[9] including computerized robotic systems with some level of automation. For example, the PROBOT prostatectomy system took user-defined ultrasound measurements to automate resection of prostatic tissue.[10] The best known and most well-studied surgical robot is the da Vinci robotic system for minimally invasive surgery (Intuitive Surgical, Sunnyvale, CA). This system is a leader-follower setup that includes a surgeon console, patient cart, and vision cart. It is the primary multiarm robotic system for minimally invasive surgery, with US Food and Drug Administration (FDA) approval in the United States obtained in the year 2000. It enables the user to perform surgery with laparoscopic instruments connected to the docked robotic patient cart. The surgeon then works while sitting at the surgeon console (master tool manipulator) remote from the follower robot (patient side manipulator) and patient. The system uses 3 operative arms, enabling the user to function as his or her own assistant with foot pedal control. Specialized laparoscopic instruments used with this particular system have wristed articulation with multiple degrees of freedom, and the dual-lens camera enables 3-dimensional visualization at the surgeon console.

The da Vinci robotic system is most commonly used for intraabdominal and thoracic procedures.[11] Despite a large body of literature comparing robotic laparoscopic to traditional laparoscopic surgery, there are no studies showing superiority of the robotic platform. There are, however, a number of positive elements related to robot-assisted laparoscopic surgery. These include improved ergonomics with diminished surgeon fatigue,[12,13] decreased reliance on hand dominance,[14] shortened learning curve and faster skill retention of trainees,[15] and superior visualization with magnification and a 3-dimensional view.[16-18] As currently available, this robotic system does not use substantial AI in the sense that it does not actively use natural language processing, computer vision, or artificial neural networks. As mentioned in this book's chapter regarding tracking of intraoperative events, these robotic platforms can also serve as data collection platforms.

Beyond the da Vinci robotic system, there are other multiarm robots for minimally invasive surgery that are less well studied and are in various phases of development.[19] The Senhance Robotic System (TransEnterix, Morrisville, NC) is a multiarm robotic platform for minimally invasive surgery, approved by the FDA in 2017, that provides remote haptic feedback and uses eye tracking to center the laparoscopic camera. This platform, unlike the da Vinci, uses typical laparoscopic-type instruments that do not articulate.[20] In addition, there are many other robotic arm systems that are used to assist in the operating room. These are most often used in neurosurgery, orthopedics, and ophthalmology and typically represent medical applications of computer-aided planning/computer-aided milling that also do not use true AI. They do not automate the entire procedure and are constrained to a specific registration within their environment.

Robotic systems used in neurosurgery include Neuromate (Renishaw, New Mills, United Kingdom), SurgiScope (ISIS Robotics, SurgiMedia, Saint-Ismier, France), ROSA (Zimmer Biomet, Warsaw, IN), Renaissance (Mazor Robotics, Caesarea, Israel), and iSYS1 (Medizintechnik GmbH, Kitzbühel, Austria). These robots are used to direct the trajectory of drills or needles by registering previously obtained axial images (computed tomography or magnetic resonance imaging) to robotic software. The robot then aligns with the patient and assists in reaching targets within the brain with submillimeter accuracy for biopsy. This technology can be used for tissue ablation, electrode placement, or catheter placement.[21,22] The effect these robots have on accuracy and postoperative outcomes remains in question due to heterogeneity and poor quality of studies.[23]

Robotic systems used in orthopedics include TSolution-One (formerly Robodoc; THINK Surgical, Freemont, CA) and MAKO Robotic Tactile Guidance System (Stryker, Kalamazoo, MI). These platforms are for image-based robotic milling performed during joint arthroplasty[24] and facilitate an ideal joint mechanical axis. Preoperative imaging is loaded into the system and intraoperatively registered, followed by robotic milling of the existing tissues to fit preselected 3D implant data. Data exist demonstrating that these robots are more accurate and consistent intraoperatively[25,26]; however, robot abandonment and conversion to a traditional procedure occur in 10% to 20% of procedures.[27,28] These types of robotic procedures may also be associated with more operative revisions[28] and do not have long-term data showing differences in functional outcomes.[25,27,28] The NAVIO Precision Freehand Sculpting System (Navio, Blue Belt Technologies, Plymouth, MN) is a similar milling system that does not require a preoperative axial image but does require intraoperative alignment and "painting" anatomic surfaces with an optical probe to register the patient's anatomy. The surgeon intraoperatively demarcates bone that needs to be milled away and then uses a handheld device that is linked with the computer model of the bone. When the burr is moved outside of the cutting zone, the burr retracts and stops milling.[29] Case-control studies suggest improved accuracy with this system compared to conventional techniques.[30]

Given the micrometer-level precision that is required for ophthalmologic surgery, robotic assistance devices have been developed to sense minimal force and also filter out tremor. These robots, including the Steady-Hand Robot (Johns Hopkins University, Baltimore, MD) and Micron (Carnegie Mellon University, Pittsburgh, PA), are still early in their use and are not widely available.[31] The Steady-Hand Robot is a table-mounted robotic system wherein the surgeon and the robot hold a pen-like tool simultaneously.[32] Micron is a handheld instrument that uses optical sensors to detect tool motion and adjusts tip motion accordingly.[33] Forces sensed at the tool tip are conveyed to the operator with auditory signals. Both systems use mathematical filtration algorithms and are able to eliminate high-frequency hand tremors (>2 Hz) by 60% to 80%.[34] Humans have a known physiologic hand tremor with a frequency of 8 to 10 Hz[35] that translates up to 38 μm of motion during retinal surgery.[36] Tremor does not differ significantly between surgeons and is known to increase 7% per hour of operating.[37] High-frequency hand tremor can be eliminated on existing robotic platforms using classic mathematical filters that do not use AI.[38] AI can also be used to improve tremor filtration for leader-follower–operated robotic instruments, as reported by Guo et al,[39] in which an algorithm (support vector machine) discriminates tremor from intentional motion with 92% accuracy. There are also a number of other robotic devices under development for ophthalmologic use that may have autonomous capabilities in the future.[40]

The FreeHand (Freehand 2010, Cardiff, United Kingdom) and its predecessor EndoAssist (Armstrong Healthcare, High Wycombe, United Kingdom) are automated camera holders that were developed to control an endoscopic camera by the surgeon's head movements with activation by a foot pedal.[19,41-43] This is considered robotic because it uses feedback control to move the camera to the reference position that the user provides but, again, does not use AI to do so.

Pupil tracking has been proposed to automate manipulation of a endoscopic camera when gaze is fixed outside of a central area.[44] Work has been done using wearable eye-tracking glasses that connect to a robotic arm with a laser pointer. Translation of eye movement to a location on the laparoscopic monitor has been performed using various sensors, which then triggers a robotic arm to point the laser at the registered location. A recent study showed a median error for the point of fixation of 4 cm, with a 2-second delay between detection of the fixation and activation of the robot.[45] This system uses robotics but does not use computer vision in the AI sense because neural networks or a trained model is not used to move the robotic arm.

■ AI TECHNOLOGY WITHOUT ROBOTICS IN SURGERY

Computer vision as a form of AI can be applied in the operating theater, even without substantial hardware such as an associated robotic system. The challenges of using AI computer vision in the operating room should be acknowledged, however, because simple tasks for the surgeon may be profoundly complex for a computer. An example of this is with thread detection. Thread is difficult for a computer to identify because it is continuous but deformable, self-occludes (at least one segment of thread is visually blocked with every knot thrown, and this is distinct from being tangled), can be occluded by a number of other objects within the surgical field (instruments, tissues), changes visible length after tying or being off screen, and changes actual length by cutting. Visually identifying thread becomes even more difficult with thinner sutures and with more self-occlusions (eg, a surgeon's knot). Additionally, operative cameras typically have imperfect vision due to condensation or an unclean lens. In Hu et al,[46] the authors helped resolve these issues using artificial neural networks (specifically, deep convolutional neural networks) to identify curvilinear structures that have a color gradient from one end of the thread to the other. Their neural network performs better with suture that has a multicolor repeating pattern. Jackson et al[47] used processes similar to those used to identify roads from satellite images (ie, 3-dimensional nonuniform rational B-spline [NURBS] curve modeling). Both use computer processes that identify points along the thread and then use spline algorithms to smooth the lines between the points. Computer vision techniques such as probabilistic road mapping and reinforcement learning have also been created to identify structures that must be avoided during the operation and to plan operative motions around these forbidden zones.[48] Issues with these algorithms, however, are that they assume that target structures are clearly distinguishable from surroundings without changing color (eg, from blood) and do not take into account that the surgical field is often moving.[48]

Computer vision can be used to recognize certain steps in an operation. One method to recognize surgical steps was proposed by

Fard et al,[49] in which motion (kinematic) data were collected from the robotic arms while performing predefined tasks on a phantom model. Mathematical models (specifically, a combination of k-nearest neighbors and dynamic time warping) were then used to classify tasks, enabling matching/recognition with future tasks and resulting in 89% to 100% recognition of suturing, needle passing, and knot tying with only 10% of the task completed.[49] Additional predictive algorithms have been designed to identify significant features within the operative field based on camera dwell time.[50] Volkov et al[51] examined video of laparoscopic sleeve gastrectomy and classified 7 predefined portions of the procedure based on simple cues, including color, position within an 8×8 grid, shape, and texture. Per the authors, these cues functioned better in the surgical environment because many predefined structures and tools have varying shapes and sizes, are often deformable, and are only partially visualized by the camera. Using a coreset algorithm for the k-segment mean problem for video segmentation and summarization algorithm, they reported 93% accuracy reporting the phase of the procedure. These processes could potentially aid in the future by robotic autonomous assistance or with augmented reality visual overlays during surgical procedures.

With the availability of data, an AI system could combine data to form a collective surgical consciousness (see later chapters in this book). The dvLogger is a robotic surgical recording device that collects da Vinci robotic performance metrics including motion tracking, Cartesian coordinates of instruments, and video footage of use. Chen et al[52] reviewed data from 70 vesicourethral anastomoses from prostatectomies and found that posterior bladder neck stitches were consistently performed using a forehand underhand maneuver, whereas the anterior bladder neck sutures were placed with backhand underhand gestures. These findings were used to create a standardized tutorial for trainee education. In the future, this type of analysis could be performed by an AI platform, and this information could be used to assist in robotic automation or guidance of surgeons using robotics in surgery.

Natural language processing also has many potential uses in the operating room. Machines that execute verbal commands could potentially take over some tasks. Although obtainable with current technologies, machines enabled with this technology are not currently used in the operating room. Examples such as telling a light to turn on and off would only use AI by natural language processing because they would not require substantial robotic hardware. More complex processes, such as telling a light to move, would use both AI and a robotic hardware component, as described in the next section.

▌AI AND ROBOTIC TECHNOLOGY IN SURGERY

As stated at the beginning of this chapter, some goals of combining robotic surgery with AI are to increase procedural efficiency, accuracy, and safety and to decrease surgeon focus on automatable/rote tasks and overall fatigue. The hope is that this will enable the surgeon to have increased vigilance and focus on the complex and less automatable aspects of the procedure. We are currently at the infancy of robotics with AI in the operating room. Potential for this goes beyond automation or autonomy and may one day include virtual AI surgical assistants using additional robotic arms, AI mentoring with instrument position adjustment, and integration with the collective surgical consciousness. Following is a description of the work done thus far, bringing us close to these goals.

Autonomous knot tying combines computer vision to view the suture and interpret it and additional software to manipulate the suture to tie a knot using the robot. It requires tracking of effective suture length to keep constant tension on the suture because insufficient tension results in loose knots or open wounds and too much tension results in torn tissue. This can be simplified by an interrupted suture pattern, such that tightening can be accomplished by pulling 2 ends of suture in opposite directions parallel to the wound with uniform rate and tension. Running suture adds complexity because suture lengths are not the same on both sides, and as such, the rate and tension on each end are also not the same.[53] These problems have been described at length in the literature.[46,47,53-55] Knoll et al[54] and Osa et al[56] both used a concept of learning by demonstration, where the computer analyzes a library of knot-tying movements and then breaks down each trajectory into a sequence of temporally nonoverlapping steps. Osa et al[56] were able to execute knot tying even when moving the target for suturing and when changing the stiffness of the surface by rapid updating of the needle robotic arm trajectory. Many reports on this subject do not report the time to execute a task; in Lu et al,[55] creating one loop of suture took an average of 408 seconds (6.8 minutes).

Automated suturing similarly requires computer vision, artificial neural networks, and a robotic actuator. Because a needle grasped in a needle driver is not truly fully constrained (rotation and translation along the needle require both haptic and visual feedback to be maintained[57]), needle tracking by computer vision is not a trivial static problem. Sen et al[57] designed a suture needle angular positioner with 2 points of contact for a robot that was effective in reducing needle motion, thereby decreasing the accuracy requirements for needle tracking with computer vision. The needle tracking that was devised in this report required a painted needle to distinguish it from the background but was able to function with partial occlusion (while the needle is being passed through tissues or behind the robot arms) and was able to estimate the needle trajectory. It was noted, however, that the system designed in this study required a larger camera and a larger needle than typically would be used in endoscopic surgery. Tests of the robot performing 4 running suture throws were attempted with a 50% success rate; failure was most often due to incorrect needle regrasp and pull. The Smart Tissue Autonomous Robot (STAR) was similarly developed to perform surgeon-assisted robotic suturing. This is done with computer vision aided by marking tissue with 10 µL of near-infrared fluorescent (indocyanine green [ICG]) solution along the cut edges of the target tissue. Force sensors provide the appropriate amount of suture tension, and software is used to generate an optimized suture plan. Research on this system has shown that distance between sutures was more consistent with STAR compared with trained surgeons alone and had higher leak pressure.[58] It should be noted that autonomous suturing in this system does require a human assistant and that the average time for an end-to-end porcine bowel anastomosis with the STAR was 50 ± 15 minutes, including 5 ± 2 minutes to mark the tissues, as compared to 8 minutes for an open anastomosis sewn manually. STAR was also used to develop algorithms that divide tissue with electrocautery along a straight line marked by ICG. It was more precise than human operators for cutting along the line and did so with less char.[59] These authors also used the STAR system to autonomously create intersecting straight cuts in a geometric shape based on ICG markings to denote a perimeter. Both of these systems do not technically use computer vision with a neural network, but do approach autonomous function by integrating a collection of mathematical and experimental techniques with a robotic actuator.

▌CONCLUSION

In conclusion, there are numerous potential advantages that robotics and AI can offer within the field of surgery. Currently, applications are typically separate from each other and are not used in the majority of operations performed today. A substantial amount of work is ongoing. As engineers and physicians continue to collaborate, robotic and AI systems will mature and improve, and we anticipate they will play an increasing role in the operative suite in the future.

▌REFERENCES

1. Siciliano B, Khatib O. *Springer Handbook of Robotics*. ed 3. Springer; 2017.
2. Lamb F. *Industrial Automation: Hands-On*. McGraw-Hill Education; 2013.
3. Guang-Zhong Y, Cambias J, Cleary K, et al. Medical robotics: regulatory, ethical, and legal considerations for increasing levels of autonomy. *Sci Robot*. 2017;2:eaam8638.
4. Aström KJ, Murray RM. *Feedback Systems: An Introduction for Scientists and Engineers*. Princeton University Press; 2008.
5. Leigh KJ. *Control Theory: A Guided Tour*. ed 3. The Institution of Engineering and Technology; 2012.
6. Müller AC, Guido S. *Introduction to Machine Learning with Python: A Guide for Data Scientists*. O'Reilly Media; 2016.
7. Desai JP, Patel RV. *The Encyclopedia of Medical Robotics*. World Scientific Publishing Co.; 2018.
8. Kwoh YS, Hou J, Jonckheere EA, Hayati S. A robot with improved absolute positioning accuracy for CT guided stereotactic brain surgery. *IEEE Trans Biomed Eng*. 1988;35(2):153-160.
9. Leal Ghezzi T, Campos Corleta O. 30 years of robotic surgery. *World J Surg*. 2016;40(10):2550-2557.
10. Harris SJ, Arambula-Cosio F, Hibberd RD, et al. The Probot— an active robot for prostate resection. *Proc Instn Mech Eng H*. 1997;211(4):317-325.
11. Stewart CL, Ituarte PHG, Melstrom KA, et al. Robotic surgery trends in general surgical oncology from the National Inpatient Sample. *Surg Endosc*. 2019;33(8):2591-2601.
12. Tarr ME, Brancato SJ, Cunkelman JA, Polcari A, Nutter B, Kenton K. Comparison of postural ergonomics between laparoscopic and robotic sacrocolpopexy: a pilot study. *J Minim Invasive Gynecol*. 2015;22(2):234-238.
13. Szeto GP, Poon JT, Law WL. A comparison of surgeon's postural muscle activity during robotic-assisted and laparoscopic rectal surgery. *J Robot Surg*. 2013;7(3):305-308.
14. Mucksavage P, Kerbl DC, Lee JY. The da Vinci® Surgical System overcomes innate hand dominance. *J Endourol*. 2011;25(8):1385-1388.
15. Moore LJ, Wilson MR, Waine E, Masters RS, McGrath JS, Vine SJ. Robotic technology results in faster and more robust surgical skill acquisition than traditional laparoscopy. *J Robot Surg*. 2015;9(1):67-73.
16. Wilhelm D, Reiser S, Kohn N, et al. Comparative evaluation of HD 2D/3D laparoscopic monitors and benchmarking to a theoretically ideal 3D pseudodisplay: even well-experienced laparoscopists perform better with 3D. *Surg Endosc*. 2014;28(8):2387-2397.
17. Lusch A, Bucur PL, Menhadji AD, et al. Evaluation of the impact of three-dimensional vision on laparoscopic performance. *J Endourol*. 2014;28(2):261-266.
18. Herron DM, Marohn M, The SAGES-MIRA Robotic Surgery Consensus Group. A consensus document on robotic surgery. Society of American Gastrointestinal and Endoscopic Surgeons (SAGES) and Minimally Invasive Robotic Association

(MIRA) Robotic Task Force. Accessed August 7, 2018. https://www.sages.org/publications/guidelines/consensus-document-robotic-surgery/.

19. Peters BS, Armijo PR, Krause C, Choudhury SA, Oleynikov D. Review of emerging surgical robotic technology. *Surg Endosc*. 2018;32(4):1636-1655.

20. deBeche-Adams T, Eubanks WS, de la Fuente SG. Early experience with the Senhance®-laparoscopic/robotic platform in the US. *J Robot Surg*. 2019;13(2):357-359.

21. Fomenko A, Serletis D. Robotic stereotaxy in cranial neurosurgery: a qualitative systematic review. *Neurosurgery*. 2018;83(4):642-650.

22. Kajita Y, Nakatsubo D, Kataoka H, Nagai T, Nakura T, Wakabayashi T. Installation of a neuromate robot for stereotactic surgery: efforts to conform to Japanese specifications and an approach for clinical use—Technical notes. *Neurol Med Chir (Tokyo)*. 2015;55(12):907-914.

23. Vakharia VN, Sparks R, O'Keeffe AG, et al. Accuracy of intracranial electrode placement for stereoencephalography: a systematic review and meta-analysis. *Epilepsia*. 2017;58(6):921-932.

24. Shenoy R, Nathwani D. Evidence for robots. *SICOT J*. 2017;3:38.

25. Cobb J, Henckel J, Gomes P, et al. Hands-on robotic unicompartmental knee replacement: a prospective, randomised controlled study of the Acrobot system. *J Bone Joint Surg Br*. 2006;88(2):188-197.

26. Bell SW, Anthony I, Jones B, MacLean A, Rowe P, Blyth M. Improved accuracy of component positioning with robotic-assisted unicompartmental knee arthroplasty: data from a prospective, randomized controlled study. *J Bone Joint Surg Am*. 2016;98(8):627-635.

27. Liow MHL, Chin PL, Pang HN, Tay DK, Yeo SJ. THINK surgical TSolution-One® (Robodoc) total knee arthroplasty. *SICOT J*. 2017;3:63.

28. Honl M, Dierk O, Gauck C, et al. Comparison of robotic-assisted and manual implantation of a primary total hip replacement. A prospective study. *J Bone Joint Surg Am*. 2003 Aug;85-A(8):1470-8.

29. Lonner JH, Smith JR, Picard F, Hamlin B, Rowe PJ, Riches PE. High degree of accuracy of a novel image-free handheld robot for unicondylar knee arthroplasty in a cadaveric study. *Clin Orthop Relat Res*. 2015;473(1):206-212.

30. Batailler C, White N, Ranaldi FM, Neyret P, Servien E, Lustig S. Improved implant position and lower revision rate with robotic-assisted unicompartmental knee arthroplasty. *Knee Surg Sports Traumatol Arthrosc*. 2019;27(4):1232-1240.

31. Roizenblatt M, Edwards TL, Gehlbach PL. Robot-assisted vitreoretinal surgery: current perspectives. *Robot Surg*. 2018;5:1-11.

32. Taylor R, Jensen P, Whitcomb L, et al. A steady-hand robotic system for microsurgical augmentation. *Int J Rob Res*. 1999;18(12):1201-1210.

33. Riviere C, Ang WT, Khosla P. Toward active tremor canceling in handheld microsurgical instruments. *IEEE Trans Rob Autom*. 2003;19(5):793-800.

34. Gonenc B, Handa J, Gehlbach P, Taylor RH, Iordachita I. A comparative study for robot assisted vitreoretinal surgery: micron vs. the steady-hand robot. *IEEE Int Conf Robot Autom*. 2013:4832-4837.

35. Stiles R. Mechanical and neural feedback factors in postural hand tremor of normal subjects. *J Neurophysiol*. 1980;44(1):40-59.

36. Singh SPN, Riviere CN. Physiological tremor amplitude during retinal microsurgery. Proceedings of the IEEE 28th Annual Northeast Bioengineering Conference (IEEE Cat. No.02CH37342), Philadelphia, PA, 2002, pp 171-172.

37. Slack PS, Coulson CJ, Ma X, Pracy P, Parmar S, Webster K. The effect of operating time on surgeon's hand tremor. *Eur Arch Otorhinolaryngol*. 2009;266(1):137-141.

38. Oppenheim A, Willsky A, Hamid S. *Signals and Systems*. ed 2. Pearson; 1996.

39. Guo S, Shen R, Xiao N, Bao X. A novel suppression algorithm of isometric tremor for the vascular interventional surgical robot. 2018 13th World Congress on Intelligent Control and Automation (WCICA), Changsha, China, 2018, pp 135-140.

40. Mango CW, Tsirbas A, Hubschman JP. Robotic eye surgery. In: Spandau U, Scharioth G, eds. *Cutting Edge of Ophthalmic Surgery*. Springer; 2017.

41. Aiono S, Gilbert JM, Soin B, Finlay PA, Gordan A. Controlled trial of the introduction of a robotic camera assistant (EndoAssist) for laparoscopic cholecystectomy. *Surg Endosc*. 2002;16(9):1267-1270.

42. Gilbert JM. The EndoAssist robotic camera holder as an aid to the introduction of laparoscopic colorectal surgery. *Ann R Coll Surg Engl*. 2009;91(5):389-393.

43. Stolzenburg JU, Franz T, Kallidonis P, et al. Comparison of the FreeHand® robotic camera holder with human assistants during endoscopic extraperitoneal radical prostatectomy. *BJU Int*. 2011;107(6):970-974.

44. Ali SM, Reisner LA, King B, et al. Eye gaze tracking for endoscopic camera positioning: an application of a hardware/software interface developed to automate Aesop. *Stud Health Technol Inform*. 2008;132:4-7.

45. Kogkas AA, Darzi A, Mylonas GP. Gaze-contingent perceptually enabled interactions in the operating theatre. *Int J Comput Assist Radiol Surg*. 2017;12(7): 1131-1140.

46. Hu Y, Gu Y, Yang J, Yang GZ. Multi-stage suture detection for robot assisted anastomosis based on deep learning. 2018 IEEE International Conference on Robotics and Automation (ICRA), Brisbane, Queensland, Australia, 2018, pp 1-8.

47. Jackson RC, Yuan R, Chow DL, Newman W, Çavuşoğlu MC. Real-time visual tracking of dynamic surgical suture threads. *IEEE Trans Autom Sci Eng*. 2018;15(3):1078-1090.

48. Baek D, Hwang M, Kim H, Kwon D. Path planning for automation of surgery robot based on probabilistic roadmap and reinforcement learning. 2018 15th International Conference on Ubiquitous Robots (UR), Honolulu, HI, 2018, pp 342-347.

49. Fard MJ, Pandya AK, Chinnam RB, Klein MD, Ellis RD. Distance-based time series classification approach for task recognition with application in surgical robot autonomy. *Int J Med Robot*. 2017;13:3.

50. Ji JJ, Krishnan S, Patel V, Fer D, Goldberg K. Learning 2D surgical camera motion from demonstrations. 2018 IEEE 14th International Conference on Automation Science and Engineering (CASE), Munich, Germany, 2018, pp 35-42.

51. Volkov M, Hashimoto DA, Rosman G, Meireles OR, Rus D. Machine learning and coresets for automated real-time video segmentation of laparoscopic and robot-assisted surgery. 2017 IEEE International Conference on Robotics and Automation (ICRA), Singapore, 2017, pp 754-759.

52. Chen J, Oh PJ, Cheng N, et al. Use of automated performance metrics to measure surgeon performance during robotic vesicourethral anastomosis and methodical development of a training tutorial. *J Urol*. 2018;200(4):895-902.

53. Kang H, Wen JT. Autonomous suturing using minimally invasive surgical robots. 2000 IEEE International Conference on Control Applications, Anchorage, AK, 2000, pp 742-747.

54. Knoll A, Mayer H, Staub C, Bauernschmitt R. Selective automation and skill transfer in medical robotics: a demonstration on surgical knot-tying. *Int J Med Robot*. 2012;8(4):384-397.

55. Lu B, Chu HK, Huang KC, Cheng L. Vision-based surgical suture looping through trajectory planning for wound suturing. IEEE Transactions on Automation Science and Engineering, vol. 16, no. 2, April 2019, pp 542-556,

56. Osa T, Sugita N, Mitsuishi M. Online trajectory planning and force control for automation of surgical tasks. IEEE Transactions on Automation Science and Engineering, vol. 15, no. 2, April 2018, pp 675-691.

57. Sen S, Garg A, Gealy DV, McKinley S, Jen Y, Goldberg K. Automating multi-throw multilateral surgical suturing with a mechanical needle guide and sequential convex optimization. 2016 IEEE International Conference on Robotics and Automation (ICRA), Stockholm, 2016, pp 4178-4185.

58. Shademan A, Decker RS, Opfermann JD, Leonard S, Krieger A, Kim PC. Supervised autonomous robotic soft tissue surgery. *Sci Transl Med*. 2016;8(337):337ra64.

59. Opfermann JD, Leonard S, Decker RS, et al. Semi-autonomous electrosurgery for tumor resection using a multi-degree of freedom electrosurgical tool and visual servoing. *Rep U S*. 2017;2017:3653-3659.

NATURAL LANGUAGE PROCESSING AND ARTIFICIAL INTELLIGENCE FOR CLINICAL DOCUMENTATION

13

David Y. Ting

HIGHLIGHTS

- Currently, most of the data in electronic health records reside in free-text documentation—often unstructured—that is useless for artificial intelligence (AI) training without preprocessing.

- Natural language processing (NLP) plays the dual function in health care AI of unlocking meaning from free-text and other unstructured documentation while also advancing and improving the creation of clinical documentation in the first place.

- Regarding the capture of data, NLP-based applications (eg, computerized voice recognition, clinical documentation improvement, ambient voice assistants, and ambient virtual scribes) have proven their ability to decrease the burden of clinicians in producing clinical documentation.

- Regarding the curation of data on the back end, NLP provides the mechanism that transforms clinical data from an amorphous and unhelpful state to a form that makes deep insight and explainable AI possible. These NLP use cases include data mining research, computer-assisted coding, automated registry reporting, clinical trial matching, prior authorization, clinical decision support, risk adjustment and hierarchical condition category (HCC) coding, computational phenotyping and biomarker discovery, and population surveillance.

❙ INTRODUCTION

Natural language processing (NLP) is a subfield of artificial intelligence (AI) and machine learning (ML) that concentrates on the capture, interpretation, and manipulation of human-generated spoken or written data (see Chapter 5). Most surgeons are already well exposed to the pervasiveness of NLP in their nonclinical daily lives, whether it is using Google Maps to request driving directions, using autocorrect while composing text messages, selecting automatic email responses suggested by Microsoft Outlook365, using Apple's Siri to set a calendar appointment, or asking Amazon's Echo to play songs from a favorite recording artist. In each of these scenarios, the pathway is essentially the same: first, the human's spoken voice or keystrokes are captured electronically. Then those signals are processed, using a combination of probabilistic and deep-learning models to predict an initial output of recognizable words and phrases. Then these data drive further machine predictions (eg, "this is a request for information" or "this is a command"), which ultimately drive an action (eg, "display directions to 55 Fruit Street in Boston" or "play the next song in the Bon Jovi library").

In health care, NLP is increasingly the critical front end that captures and curates information necessary to power training, insights, predictions, and executable output from AI. Regarding the capture of data, NLP-based applications, such as computerized voice recognition, voice assistants, and virtual scribes, have already proven their ability to decrease the burden of clinicians in producing clinical documentation. Many surgeons today, inundated by myriad reporting, billing, and documentation requirements, are either burning out under the administrative burden of typing and dictating[1] or have bypassed the documentation process almost entirely by implementing boilerplate templates (that make every case and every patient appear to be a clone of the next) or by hiring expensive nurse practitioners or other staff merely to delegate the job of documentation. However, by decreasing time and effort required to document clinical activities, findings, diagnoses, assessments, and plans, NLP offers busy clinicians the opportunity to focus on improving the content of what they document, as well as devoting attention to clinical care itself.

With respect to the curation of data on the back end, NLP provides the mechanism that transforms clinical data from an amorphous and unhelpful state to a form that makes deep insight and explainable AI possible. To wit, tens of billions of dollars have been invested to implement electronic health records (EHRs) nationwide (largely in response to the 2009 Health Information Technology for Economic and Clinical Health Act and its "EHR Meaningful Use" requirements), and surgeons and health care leaders have been sold the promise that such an investment should have yielded petabytes of data to feed hungry neural networks and deep-learning systems.[2] However, unfortunately, the current reality is that most of the data in EHRs still reside in free-text documentation (eg, progress notes, operative notes, radiology reports, pathology results). In most cases, that unstructured documentation is useless for AI training, let alone predictive analytics, without an initial step of processing, parsing, curating, and annotating the natural language so that ML can be effective.

Thus, NLP plays the dual function in health care AI of unlocking and unleashing meaning from free-text and other unstructured documentation, while playing an equally important role in advancing and improving the creation of clinical documentation in the first place. Because of the particularly important role of NLP and AI in producing and consuming clinical documentation, this chapter will be devoted to exploring these aspects. In addition, the challenges of current-state NLP and the promise of future documentation solutions will be highlighted.

PLACING NLP AND CLINICAL DOCUMENTATION USE CASES INTO CONTEXT

A 2018 Chilmark Research Market Scan report entitled, "Natural Language Processing: Unlocking the Potential of a Digital Healthcare Era," identified 12 use cases of NLP in health care and categorized them in regard to their levels of maturity in the marketplace, ranging from well-established mainstay use cases with proven return on investment (eg, speech recognition and computer-assisted coding), emerging NLP health care use cases that are primed for immediate impact (eg, clinical trial matching and prior authorization), or next-generation NLP health care use cases that will be increasingly important as health care moves more toward value-based purchasing (eg, ambient virtual scribes and population surveillance).[3] An additional use case not highlighted by the Chilmark Research report is the rising use of ambient voice assistants, the clinical cousins to Amazon Echo, Google Home, and Microsoft Cortana. A review of these 13 use cases reveals 2 sides of the interplay between NLP and clinical documentation: in some use cases, NLP makes it easier, more efficient, and less burdensome to produce useful clinical documentation. In other cases, NLP makes it possible to consume existing documentation for AI purposes: to extract meaning and insights from unstructured text in order to advance patient care quality, to improve cost-effective clinical practice, to fulfill regulatory or research requirements, or to do all of these.

Table 13-1 summarizes and contextualizes the 13 NLP health care use cases, with commentary on how NLP either impacts the production

Table 13-1   PLACING NLP HEALTH CARE USE CASES IN CONTEXT

Classification	NLP Use Case in Health Care	Description	Interplay With Clinical Documentation
Established NLP health care use cases with proven return on investment	Speech recognition	Signal processing transforms recorded voice waveforms into recognizable text that can be transferred directly into the medical record or indirectly into transcription services or command processors	**Data production:** By reducing typing, decreases the clinicians' burden of documentation production while also enabling the capture of richer, more nuanced documentation than can be achieved through use of templates, drop-down lists, or macros in the EHR
	Clinical documentation improvement	Real-time or near-real-time analysis of documentation prompts the clinician to add or refine documentation	**Data production:** Improves the content of clinical documentation, allowing it to better support coding and compliance requirements, as well as provide additional clinical insights, such as acuity, sidedness, timing, and so on
	Data mining research	Provide tools that parse, index, and search through large unstructured text-based data sets	**Data consumption:** These sophisticated query tools can accomplish within seconds results that would previously requires days of manual "chart biopsy" by trained human reviewers or surgeons seeking clinical insights
	Computer-assisted coding	Provide analytics to predict with high accuracy and recall the ICD-10 codes, billing levels, and Current Procedural Terminology (CPT) codes for a case, based on the available documentation	**Data consumption:** Removes the busy surgeon from the administrative burden of completing billing and coding tasks; instead, the surgeon can focus on providing documentation that supports the billing codes while being clinically useful
	Automated registry reporting	Query vast numbers of patient charts, apply surgical society definitions to extract relevant facts and then automatically populate appropriate patient registries (eg, American Joint Replacement Registry [AJRR], National Surgical Quality Improvement Program [NSQIP] registry)	**Data consumption:** Reduces the cost and administrative burden of manually searching through documentation in patient charts and then transferring existing facts into registries

Emerging NLP health care use cases that promise immediate impact	Clinical trial matching	Search through structured and unstructured documentation to identify patients with specific conditions, histories, demographics, and so on, and then match those patients to research protocols that could appropriately recruit those patients	**Data consumption:** Reveal clinical insights from documentation (eg, appropriate phenotypic matches) to accelerate the research trial process
	Prior authorization	Once third-party payer requirements to justify a specific clinical order are known, query the available structured and unstructured documentation to find clinical justification and autonomously report back to the payer	**Data consumption:** Relieves one of the top-ranked causes of administrative burden by surgeons and nonprocedural clinicians alike
	Clinical decision support (CDS)	In real-time, extract clinical facts from unstructured documentation that can be compared against vetted clinical algorithms, and then provide clinical guidance (eg, drug-disease interactions, history of anticoagulation, cardiac risk)	**Data consumption:** Versions of CDS can also give guidance on appropriate procedures and other order type, improving not only patient safety but also cost-effectiveness
	Risk adjustment and hierarchical condition categories (HCCs)	Query the patient documentation for evidence of clinical acuity and HCC codes, which are then used for scoring risk-adjusted patient panels and justifying increased payments under value-based contracts	**Data consumption:** Automates what would otherwise require intensive human chart reviews to extract evidence from chart documentation
Next-generation and future NLP health care use cases	Ambient virtual scribe	Conventional speech recognition is augmented by signal processing techniques that allow for recognition of multiple speakers in the room; AI then predicts the clinical context of the conversation and produces a synthesized narration of the patient-clinician interaction	**Data production:** Reduces the burden of clinical documentation even further by removing the clinician from the need to produce a first draft of the documentation; has advantages over human scribes by being real time and always available and, through machine learning, is constantly self-improving

(continued)

Table 13-1 PLACING NLP HEALTH CARE USE CASES IN CONTEXT (CONTINUED)

Classification	NLP Use Case in Health Care	Description	Interplay With Clinical Documentation
	Ambient voice assistants	Using the same technology behind ambient virtual scribes, transform spoken voice signals into executable commands	**Data production:** In addition to instantiating orders, reading out results, scheduling tasks, and control of robotics or other equipment, virtual assistants can invoke documentation macros and tee up documentation tasks (eg, consent forms, patient questionnaires)
	Computational phenotyping and biomarker discovery	Search patient records, including radiology reports, to identify patients with specific clinical phenotypes and diseases, and then map against lab results, genomes, and other biomarkers to discover novel associations	**Data consumption:** A discovery tool that uses NLP to analyze text in clinical documentation in the way earlier image-based AI used machine learning methods to provide pattern-based recognition of lung nodules, breast cancer, and strokes by examining pixels in radiology images
	Population surveillance	Use automation to read through clinical notes, radiology reports, and pathology reports to monitor rates of screening and detection	**Data consumption:** Replaces a costly human-based manual process that can only monitor a small sample of cases per year with an automated process that can provide true rates by examining nearly all cases with great efficiency and predictive accuracy

AI, artificial intelligence; EHR, electronic health record; ICD-10, International Classification of Diseases, Tenth Revision; NLP, natural language processing.

of clinical documentation or enables the consumption of existing clinical documentation for further AI processing or direct clinical operations.

From the 13 NLP health care use cases described in Table 13-1, 4 can be described as being positioned on the input side of the AI data flow: speech recognition, clinical documentation improvement, ambient virtual scribes, and ambient voice assistants. The remainder can be considered to lie on the output side: data mining research, computer-assisted coding, automated registry reporting, clinical trial matching, prior authorization, clinical decision support, risk adjustment and hierarchical condition category (HCC) coding, computational phenotyping and biomarker discovery, and population surveillance. On both the input and output sides of the data flow, there are opportunities for the entrepreneurial surgeon to leverage NLP and AI to advance clinical documentation along the following 4 domains:

- Working with data scientists to advance the academic development of NLP methodologies, including the probabilistic (statistically driven) and deep-learning approaches described in Chapter 5.
- Engaging third-party vendors (examples of which will be mentioned later in this chapter) to implement one or several NLP health care use cases in a surgical division or practice, with an eye toward improving practice productivity, patient care quality, and reimbursement and/or reducing documentation burden.
- Advocating with institutional leadership to integrate one or several NLP health care use cases to address clinician administrative burden, reducing staff burnout and returning surgeons and their patients to face-to-face interactions, as opposed to the face-to-computer monitor interactions all too common today.
- Developing best-of-class NLP-driven clinical documentation solutions that can interoperate with current EHRs and clinical data repositories, can be integrated with clinical workflows, and can compete in the commercial marketplace. For the foreseeable future, the health care NLP market appears to be poised for continual growth. Allied Market Research has predicted that the cognitive computing market will be worth $13.7 billion across multiple industries by 2020, representing a 33.1% compound annual growth rate over current levels. In 2014, NLP composed 40% of that market's total revenue, and it is projected to continue to be a major opportunity within the field through the rest of the decade, with an estimated $6.5 billion in spending on text analytics by the year 2020.[4] Another research firm, Markets and Markets, projects NLP overall will be a $16.07 billion market by 2021, with health care representing a key vertical.[5]

With such an array of use cases and growth potential for NLP in health care documentation, it is worth examining more deeply some of the archetypal use cases of NLP to understand how they came about historically, how they work, how the AI has advanced over time, and where the technology is going in the future, including derivative use cases.

SPEECH RECOGNITION

History and Early Technology Behind Speech Recognition

Any exploration of NLP's strong impact on the production of clinical documentation should begin with understanding the history and evolution of speech recognition (SR), variously known as computerized voice recognition, automatic SR, and speech to text. In short, what began as an exercise in signal processing 5 decades ago has given rise in health care to computerized note transcription, voice commands, voice assistants, and ultimately virtual scribes. All these current and near-future technologies trace their ancestry to the Automatic Digit Recognizer, or Audry, created by Bell Labs in 1952.[6]

What Audry could do—recognize one person speaking the digits 0 through 9—seemed inauspicious even in that day. However, the overall architecture of Audry was not so far afield of how SR and its spin-offs work today (Figure 13-1). To wit, automatic SR begins with the capture of the human voice through a microphone, which converts sound waves to an analog electrical signal. An analog-to-digital converter digitizes that signal and sends the digital waveform to a signal processor, which applies mathematical transforms to reduce and quantize the data so they can be consumed by the next stages: recognition search, language modeling, and speech modeling.

The recognition search step compares spoken utterance to the language model (What are you allowed to say?) and the speech model (What should those words and the distinct units of sound in those words look like?) by scoring each potential match against what amounts to a lookup table containing a list of hypotheses.

The language model limits the scope of the recognition search by applying deterministic constraints (Is this utterance acceptable or not acceptable?) or probabilistic constraints (What is the probability this interpretation of the utterance is more appropriate than an alternative?). As examples, most existing command recognition systems use deterministic grammars, which limit the recognition algorithm to matching a limited set of unambiguous instructions: Does the utterance match a known

Traditional Speech Recognition

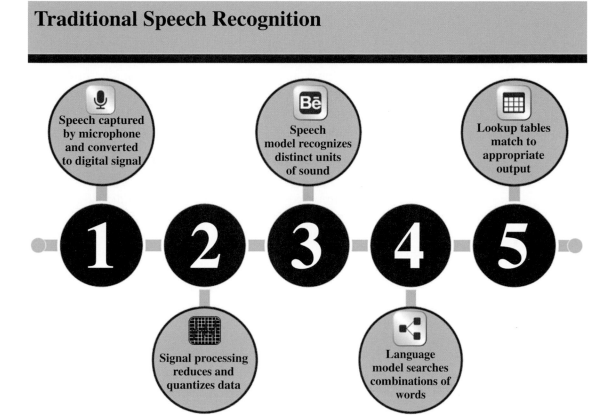

Figure 13-1 • Traditional speech recognition process.

list of commands, such as "open new document," "scroll right," or "close window"? In contrast, most dictation systems use probabilistic language models to predict whether utterances fit with frequently used patterns of speech.

The speech model asks what symbols make up reasonable words and phonemes (distinct units of sound in the language), for instance, p, b, d, and t in the English words pad, pat, bad, and bat. Given a segment of utterance, the speech model informs how well that segment matches the expectation of the word or phonemes the segment is meant to represent. A robust speech model should account for durational, acoustic, and other phonetic variability between people; for instance, it must account for various dialects and accents within the same language. Because there could be several million parameters, the speech model should be trainable and be able to adjust automatically.

Early forms of SR could only recognize about 10 words. In 1962, IBM created an SR tool, called Shoebox, that could recognize 16 words (10 digits plus mathematical functions). With that tool, a user could say, "One plus one," and the system would output "two." In the 1970s, the Department of Defense and US government made major investments toward accelerating development of similar brute-force systems. These still relied on parsing speech into phonetic units but mapped them with a node system. One of the largest examples of such a system, Carnegie Mellon's Harpy, had 15,000 nodes. Thus, at that point, SR systems could recognize 1000 words with different pronunciations of the same words.

However, even a decade later, the best SR systems had expanded only to 20,000 words. Compared to the 60,000-word vocabulary of an average high school graduate, this achievement was underwhelming. There were 2 reasons for the relatively slow growth of the capability of SR. First, the best speech models used between the 1980s through the 2000s were built upon a complex mathematical system of probability, called hidden Markov models (HMM).[7] Briefly, these models work by taking raw audio waveforms, parsing them into small pieces, and then trying to identify which phoneme was spoken with each piece of speech. Each word is thus represented by a chain, with each node in the chain the phonetic units making up the word. The nodes are connected by links, or phonemes. Numbers are assigned to these phenomes according to the probability that certain phonemes naturally fit when chained together (Figure 13-2). In this way, SR driven by HMMs accounted for differences in accents and cadences. For example, both "potato" and "po-tah-to" were recognized. Unfortunately, one irritating requirement of these systems was that users were forced to dictate using discrete speech; in other words, rather than saying a natural sentence such as, "This is a 34-year-old woman with appendicitis," the user was forced to pause between each word: "This … is … a … 34- … year- … old … woman … with … appendicitis." And by the 1990s, it was clear that this brute-force methodology of HMM would present a limitation even with increases in computer processing speed.

The second barrier to advancement in SR was indeed the limited computing power of the day. But the early 1980s to 1990s saw the advent of faster microprocessors and cheaper memory chips, and raw computing capacity increased to allow a more continuous SR experience. Under the pioneering leadership of founder Ray Kurzweil, Kurzweil Technology produced the first example of large-vocabulary SR software in this era. By the mid-1990s, as 16-bit desktop computers became widespread, continuous SR became commercially available; but the cost of such systems was prohibitive outside of large institutional customers. As an example, Dragon Voice Recognition debuted in 1994 at an eyewatering $9000 per

Probabilistic Speech Recognition

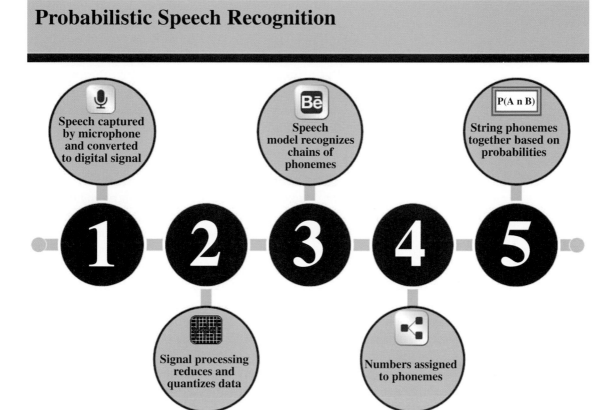

1 — Speech captured by microphone and converted to digital signal

2 — Signal processing reduces and quantizes data

3 — Speech model recognizes chains of phonemes

4 — Numbers assigned to phonemes

5 — String phonemes together based on probabilities

Figure 13-2 • Probabilistic speech recognition process.

user. Fast-forwarding to today, even blazingly fast, 64-bit, single–central processing unit (CPU) desktop computers are being supplanted by cloud computing, where processing is distributed over the internet across hundreds, if not thousands, of fast CPUs. This form of massively parallel processing enables Apple's Siri and Microsoft's Cortana to process millions of words and phrases simultaneously. The availability of cloud computing has also opened the possibility of deploying SR systems to thin client devices and mobile devices, because the SR systems are no longer tethered to expensive, high-capacity local CPUs.

The Role of Neural Networks and Cloud Computing in SR

Through the early 2000s, an essential aspect of SR that remained in infancy was speech *understanding*. Early software could predict which phonemes generally fit together, but the systems could not predict words in context. Even today, computers have difficulty understanding what a sentence *means*. Two turn-of-the-century developments disrupted that truism: cloud computing and artificial neural networks. With processors working in parallel in a virtual cloud, SR became enabled to listen to more than just one word at a time; rather, it could look for other words for context and use probabilities to determine what the user is trying to say. More significantly, neural networks and the associated deep ML extended beyond the brute-force combination of cloud processing and the HMM with a new algorithmic paradigm.

Geoffrey Hinton, a cognitive psychologist, computer scientist, and arguably the godfather of deep learning, developed a concept where computer programs learn dynamically and evolve based on changing inputs to the system. The inspiration behind the concept, called neural networks, was based on the human brain. Namely, the brain has 100 billion neurons, 7000 synapses between neurons, and 20,000 to 70,000 inputs per second between these synapses. The strength of these neurons "computing" together in parallel results in what is perceived as the "knowledge" of the brain. Neural networks simulate this activity in a computer and are designed to work roughly in the same way as the brain, where each node in the artificial neural network is like a synapse between neurons.

With traditional HMM-based SR, systems were engineered by human designers to parse sound waves, perform Fourier analysis, and look for features and patterns. In contrast, neural networks learn their own features, then hunt for features within features, and so on. This process is called deep learning and has led to enormous improvements in the speed and accuracy of SR. Most saliently, SR systems can leverage this deep-learning model for language understanding tasks. By way of methodology, current-generation SR systems represent words as lists of numbers. For example, the word "Paris" might be represented by a list of several hundred numbers. A deep-learning system could take the numbers for "Paris," then subtract "France," add Italy, then look at the numbers that remain. The closest answer might include the list of numbers that represents Rome. By analogy, this process begins to give the AI an "understanding" that Paris and Rome are associate subsets of France and Italy. And further deep learning would associate them with the notion of "cities."

This way, SR systems powered by neural networks and deep learning can amass millions of examples of similar analogical reasoning. Examples would include the following:

Paris – France + Italy = Rome
Baseball – Ball + Racket = Tennis
Summer – Sun + Snow = Winter

In other words, the combination of cloud computing (massive processing capability), inexpensive and expandable cloud storage systems (massive memory capacity), and neural networks (deep learning) now affords SR systems the ability to capture, store, add to, and refine massive databases of analogies. The end effect begins to approach machine understanding of language. And this evolution has led to a current generation of continuous SR tools that are able to interpret and execute complex commands and synonyms of commands (ie, voice assistants), as well as synthesize clinical documentation from natural interactions between humans in an exam room (ie, virtual scribes).

Evolution in the Use of SR

Limited by extremely narrow vocabularies, second-generation SR systems of the 1970s were relegated to simple command interpretation tasks: "Dial 5-5-5-7-8-3-2." Over the next 2 decades, as third-generation SR matured with the advent of HMM algorithms, increased microprocessor speed, and increased computer memory, early adopters, including surgeons interested in replacing costly human-powered documentation transcription services, began to experiment with expensive commercial systems. But their documentation was limited to courtroom-style flat transcription of only what the surgeon said into the microphone: "The … patient … was … prepped … for … the … OR."

In the early 2000s, advances in hardware, including beam-forming noise-canceling microphones, even faster microcomputers, and more robust SR algorithms allowed for more affordable software solutions, such as Dragon Medical and IBM Via Voice. Performance levels started to allow nearly continuous SR (ie, no need to pause between words) because the systems were recognizing entire phrases at a time and recognizing and predicting appropriate word combinations: "The patient was prepped for the OR." To optimize accuracy and recall, while keeping data files small enough in size to be saved on a desktop computer's hard drive, these systems generally restricted the user to fixed vocabulary sets (eg, "Family Practice Vocabulary" vs "General Surgery Vocabulary"). Furthermore, these systems still had difficulty adjusting to user variation in accents, dialects, and speaking rate; thus, users were generally required to spend hours reading predetermined samples of text in order to "train" the SR by creating a profile of each user's speech patterns.

During that decade, while speech accuracy was often claimed by vendors to be as good as 95% to 97%, adoption of SR systems remained relatively low. And among clinicians, usage stayed in the purview of early adopters and technology enthusiasts. Simply, the hassle of training the

SR, learning the quirks of "talking to the machine," and editing the 3% to 5% of seemingly random errors was too high an adoption barrier. However, behind the scenes, although surgeons were slow to adopt SR, transcription services quietly made the transition from fully manual medical transcription to back-end SR (BESR).[8]

With traditional transcription, vendors charged per line, per page, or per minute to listen to voice recordings (usually microcassette tapes) of surgeons and then manually typed the text into unstructured "free-text" files that were then printed to paper or uploaded to an EHR. However, long-sighted vendors, recognizing the potential of technology, inserted SR between the tape recordings and the human transcriptionists, allowing the machine intelligence to produce a first draft upon which the transcriptionist would proofread, edit, and finalize. Unknown to clinicians who relied on these expensive transcription services, most major transcription vendors eventually switched to using BESR, resulting in decreased documentation turnaround time, decreased cost, and increased profits for the vendors.

The fourth generation of SR software arrived in the early 2010s, when vendors, including Nuance and M*Modal, began migrating their speech processing to the cloud. Removing the processing and user voice data files from local computers on users' desks and aggregating the data and computing onto Health Insurance Portability and Accountability Act (HIPAA)-compliant private clouds allowed for a number of important innovations: (1) massive amounts of data, now aggregated in a single datastore, could feed neural networks and deep learning, resulting in continuous ML and AI improvement; (2) no need for user voice training, as the system could learn and adjust to accents on its own; (3) less downtime from corrupted profiles or data files; (4) significantly improved SR accuracy and recall, now approaching 99%; (5) noticeably faster response time; (6) ability to deploy the SR on very thin clients, including Android and iOS mobile phones and tablets; and (7) much easier enterprise deployment and management by large organizations, including entire hospitals and health delivery systems.

Simultaneous to software improvements, advances in the quality of noise-canceling microphones built into mobile phones and tablets soon made it possible for Nuance (Power Mic Mobile) and M*Modal (Fluency Direct Mobile) to replace the need for tethered dedicated dictation microphones with mobile apps. Now the busy surgeon could step out of an operating room, pull out a mobile phone, and quickly dictate an operative note directly into the EHR. Behind the scenes, the mobile app captures the voice waveform, encrypts the data, and transmits the data over the internet to the SR vendor's secure cloud server. At no point are the voice data actually stored on the user's device or on the customer's own servers (which are used only to manage customer accounts and handle data transmission through its own network). At the vendor, the data are processed through its neural network, which interprets the appropriate output, either documentation or commands (eg, navigation commands, editing commands, EHR macros, and so on). That output is then routed back to the customer's server, which sends the output to the user's end point, which is typically the local EHR session. The experience for the user is that he or she speaks into a wireless microphone, and words, orders, mouse movements, and menu clicks happen directly in the EHR, right at the station where the user is working, instantaneously.

Presently, with the combination of fourth-generation SR AI, cloud processing, and mobile end points, most of the major barriers to adoption of SR in surgery have been addressed. The accuracy and recall of SR are on par with human transcriptionists, and indeed, human transcription services actually leverage SR in their own workflows. The response time of SR is nearly instantaneous. The availability of SR is ubiquitous, for as long as the surgeon is standing in front of the EHR (or holding a mobile version of it in his or her hand) and has a mobile device, that surgeon can navigate or dictate immediately. Finally, the turnaround time for placing documentation into the EHR is nonexistent, which exceeds what is possible with traditional dictation services or even human scribes in the exam room.[9]

These advancements have finally inspired a level of clinician adoption that makes SR for clinical documentation mainstream. In one typical case, at Massachusetts General Hospital (MGH) in Boston, Massachusetts, voice recognition had been offered and supported at the institutional level since before 2010. But even in 2014, when the organization underwent a major EHR transition and 42% of clinicians expressed experiencing burnout largely driven by use of the ambulatory EHR, the adoption of a potentially burden-relieving tool like SR was only 150 physicians out of a clinical faculty of 2500. At that point, MGH and Partners HealthCare (the corporate enterprise of which MGH and the Brigham and Women's Hospital were founding members) implemented a third-generation SR system, Nuance's Dragon Medical, and 2 years later, they upgraded to the fourth-generation Dragon Medical One. Today, encouraged by the improved SR performance and ease of implementation, over 1200 users have been trained on SR at MGH, and across Partners HealthCare's 6000 faculty physicians, the active user base approaches 3100 with 9200 hours of dictation captured per month. These results are comparable to those of a 2018 national survey of physicians, which estimated that 62% of doctors currently use SR in their EHRs, 4% are currently implementing SR, and 11% plan to adopt SR over the coming 2 years.[10]

Results of SR in Health Care

Formal studies of clinician productivity and documentation quality have shown favorable outcomes from the implementation of SR in the clinical domain. However, the caveat in interpreting these findings is that, given rapid acceleration of SR ML in recent years, most studies to date have examined older generation SR software; thus, the performance of the most recent fourth-generation SR should be expected to exceed that published in current reports. A 2014 systematic review by Maree Johnson and colleagues[11] examined the effects of SR on report turnaround time (RTT) and found that RTT of clinical notes was significantly reduced, particularly in the emergency department, endocrinology, radiology (where the reduction was 81%), and surgical pathology (with 22%-36% reduction). A study by Zick and Olsen[12] reported a $334,000 annual cost reduction because of reduced turnaround time seen after SR was implemented in the emergency department.

In regard to quality of reports, a survey of 7 studies (all published before 2014) found that human transcription slightly exceeded the accuracy of computer SR, with the highest average accuracy rate of 99.6% for human transcription and 98.5% for SR.[11] However, generally, studies have shown lower accuracy rates of SR, including a study performed in 2016 at the Brigham and Women's Hospital and Colorado Health System that showed an error rate for SR of 7.4%, translating to an accuracy of 92.6%.[13]

Lesson for Implementation of SR in Health Care

Although the increasing adoption and advantages of SR in clinical documentation are favorable overall, it is important to interpret the range of user experience as well as the true performance of SR in light of the complex interactions among implementation factors. First, the range of clinicians is diverse, ranging from residents who grew up as "digital natives" to surgeons nearing retirement age who would rather not be bothered with new workflows. Second, the untrained style of each user differs, where one surgeon may prefer to think and dictate in short snippets, halting every few seconds, while another may speak rapidly, mumbling in run-on sentences. Third, the environment may differ, where some surgeons may dictate in a quiet office, while others document in a noisy intensive care unit against the backdrop of alarms and ongoing conversations. Finally, the available technology may differ, including the provision (or lack) of noise-canceling recording equipment, the processing power and memory capacity of workstations, the availability of cloud infrastructure, the vocabularies chosen (eg, a vocabulary specific to general surgery versus a general-purpose administrative vocabulary set), the ability of the SR to accommodate regional and foreign accents, and the AI (SR engine) implemented by the vendor.

Considering these variables, the following best practices for implementation of SR for clinical documentation can be gleaned:

- Although users tend to eschew training of any length, the best results and experience come from investing in user training. Even limited training, including online videos lasting 15 to 20 minutes or training delivered in a hands-on classroom setting over an hour or two, makes the difference between acceptable SR accuracy with a good user experience versus user frustration. The training content should include how to properly set up, handle, and control the recording device (either wireless or tethered); how to speak clearly and with proper cadence; how to select the appropriate vocabularies; how to correct errors in a way that trains the AI (rather than leads the SR to continually repeat the same mistakes); and how to navigate and edit using voice commands. Users should be taught to speak in longer phrases, because current AI models perform better when given more context with which to predict correct word choices. More advanced training could incorporate how to create and use voice commands to execute complex orders, drop in text macros (eg, a normal physical exam or recent lab results), or route consult letters and reports to multiple recipients.
- For third-generation SR systems that require individual user voice training, it is incumbent that users take the time—even if it is an hour or more—to train the voice model. As good news, with latest-generation cloud-based SR, this training step is decreased and often entirely unnecessary because the accuracy of such systems is generally excellent "out of the box."
- An investment in proper hardware is critical. For instance, departments should consider provisioning noise-canceling microphones or purchasing licenses for smartphone wireless microphones, especially for surgeons and other clinicians working in noisy clinical settings.
- The SR software must be well-integrated with the EHR. The simple act of needing to log in separately to the EHR and the SR system could mean the difference between a busy surgeon choosing to take advantage of SR or defaulting to manual typing. Thus, good implementation means creating a seamless way for users to access SR directly in the EHR, with single sign-on. The user profile

(eg, vocabulary edits, voice model, configuration preferences) must travel automatically and instantaneously with the user as he or she moves from one workstation to the next.

DERIVATIVES OF SPEECH RECOGNITION

Voice Assistants

In the 2000s, the internet proliferated, and companies like Google had captured enough information to use neural networks on a commercial scale. In 2008, Google introduced voice search, and in 2011, Apple bundled its voice assistant Siri, with iOS version 5. Thus, the 2010s became the decade of the ambient voice assistants. Today, in the consumer space, Apple's Siri, Microsoft's Cortana, Amazon's Alexa, Google Voice Assistant, and (in China) Baidu's Voice Assistant are widely adopted, with 46% of Americans using voice assistants for fact search and purchases and an estimated 55% of US households predicted to have a voice-powered smart speaker installed by 2022. Lesser-known voice assistants, such as Hound from SoundHound, Bixby from Samsung, Alice from AIVC, and Dragon Mobile Assistant by Nuance, have also received favorable reviews and point toward a proliferation of specialized voice assistants in the consumer market.[14] Each of these can be considered "ambient" voice assistants, in that they can be authorized by the user to constantly listen to the environment for an invocation word (eg, "Alexa" or "Hey Google"), at which point the AI considers subsequent voice input to be a command to be executed.

In health care, the ability to use voice to control cursor movements, scroll through menus, and execute lists of commands has been packaged with SR systems from the beginning. However, the usability of these voice command systems has heretofore been limited by the fact that to access these features, users had to be at a workstation where the SR was installed, had to log into the system, and had to press a button on a noise-canceling microphone to activate the voice command. What has changed since the introduction of consumer smart speakers is the concept of *ambient* voice assistants in the exam room. Here, a device in the exam room (or a mobile app on the surgeon's smartphone) is constantly listening for an invocation word. Upon recognizing the invocation, the AI can reach into the EHR and other clinical data repositories to provide clinically relevant services, such as "Show me the patient's last 5 CBCs," "Schedule a return appointment for 3 weeks," or "Order my preoperative test panel."

Contemporary virtual assistants, such as Nuance's Dragon Medical Virtual Assistant and M*Modal's virtual assistant, are built upon the vendors' core SR platforms. The assistants are bolstered by health care–grade authentication and encryption—a critical feature lacking in consumer-level assistants like Siri or Echo—and benefit from the same cloud-based learning models that help the SR AI continually improve. Typically, these virtual assistants are accessed via the EHR or EHR mobile app. The next step in health care virtual assistants is to bundle the software with an exam room appliance (similar to Amazon's Echo or Google's Home devices) that provides biometric voice identification and obviates the need for a separate user-carried microphone or mobile device.

Ambient Virtual Scribes

The final mile in terms of front-end SR that relieves the burden of creating and consuming clinical documentation is the concept of the ambient virtual scribe. Systems like Nuance's Ambient Clinical Intelligence merge the core SR technology of Dragon Medical One with a hardware device containing a microphone and video array that can separate the voice streams of 2 speakers in an exam room, typically the clinician and the patient. Having differentiated the input data from each speaker, the software can provide a real-time transcript of the conversation in the room; and further, AI is applied to translate and summarize key information into clinical terminology. For example, if the surgeon says to the patient, "I see you are here to follow up your gallbladder removal," the output placed into the documentation might read instead, "The patient is here to follow up status-post cholecystectomy."

Naturally, the hardware and software are combined with the ambient virtual assistant, as described previously, so that the surgeon can request test results and order labs by saying the invocation phrase: "Hey, Dragon." In addition, as the virtual scribe creates documentation, the system can apply NLP to extract medical facts, including predicting billing codes, and suggest HCCs, which the clinician can approve and finalize prior to finalizing the note. And having predicted what additional codes could be counted if the surgeon simply documented a few additional features (eg, acuity, sidedness, specificity), the virtual scribe could prompt the surgeon to clarify those facts prior to closing the documentation. In effect, such a system would represent the confluence of computer-assisted coding and clinical and documentation improvement, as being offered by the market leaders, M*Model and Nuance, as well as start-ups like Codametrix, with its Automated Coding Tool.

The potential for ambient virtual scribes to impact the efficiency, cost-effectiveness, and burden relief associated with clinical documentation is enormous. In many surgical specialties, the burnout-inducing burden of documentation, coding, and data review has prompted the hiring of armies of nurse practitioners, physician assistants, in-room scribes, and transcriptionists. Over time, the transfer of clinical documentation to AI, where notes and coding are created in real time directly from the surgeon-to-patient interaction, will dramatically reduce the dependence on costly human intermediaries. And as an additional benefit, nurse practitioners, physician assistants, and (in academic settings) residents and fellows can be tasked to more meaningful clinical work. However, most experts predict the availability of ambient virtual scribes beyond early, controlled demonstrations will not be before 2024 to 2027.

NLP AND THE CONSUMPTION OF CLINICAL DOCUMENTATION

Whereas SR and its derivatives, including ambient voice assistants, virtual scribes, and real-time clinical documentation improvement, represent applications of NLP that aid the creation of clinical documentation, manifold use cases exist to apply NLP toward the consumption of clinical documentation. As mentioned previously, AI can read through clinical documentation—even as it is being produced by a virtual scribe—and predict procedural, classification, and billing codes. For example, Health Fidelity's MedLEE NLP engine incorporates a comprehensive ontology and rules engine tuned to specific health care risk adjustment and hierarchical condition categories; in 2016, the UPMC Health Plan used the solution to achieve a $62 million increase in annual revenue.[15] However, beyond the billing and coding function, NLP can assist researchers, quality officers, population health managers, health information managers, and front-line clinicians.

NLP has been applied toward sifting through patients' self-narratives on screening questionnaires to predict diagnoses for specific diseases, such as posttraumatic stress disorder. In other cases, NLP could examine the speech patterns of schizophrenic patients and identify with 100% accuracy which were likely to experience an onset of psychosis.[4] It has also been used to read through the unstructured narrative text in a patient's medical record to provide clinical decision support at the point of need (eg, predict postsurgical complications). NLP can reduce a major administrative burden by leveraging information from physician notes to alleviate delays and administrative errors associated with prior authorizations. In addition, in streamlining medical policy assessment, NLP can compile and compare clinical guidance from public sources to define the most appropriate care guidelines for care delivery.

Clinithink is an example of a specific NLP platform that shows promise for automated registry reporting as well as clinical trial recruitment and computational phenotyping and biomarker discovery. In a study conducted with Mount Sinai's Icahn School of Medicine, the company's NLP engine searched unstructured patient charts, looking for opportunities to match patients with potential clinical trials. Clinithink generated 10 times more patient matches in one-quarter of the time previously required. In collaboration with San Diego's Rady Children's Hospital, the platform broke records for the fastest screening of newborn infants for rare diseases, completing a full genomic and phenomic analysis in 19.5 hours.[15]

Another NLP vendor, Linguamatics, provides text mining for life sciences, population health management, and precision medicine. Eighteen of the 20 largest pharmaceutical companies, along with payers and providers, report saving as much as 85% of the time spent conducting cohort discovery by using the company's platform.[15]

In regard to population, registry, and quality reporting examples, at the University of California Los Angeles, researchers combined NLP analysis of unstructured radiology reports with International Classification of Diseases, Ninth Revision (ICD-9) codes and lab data to identify patients with cirrhosis with extremely high levels of sensitivity and specificity. And researchers from the University of Alabama (UAB) found that NLP identification of reportable cancer cases was 22.6% more accurate than manual review of medical records. The UAB system quickly differentiated cancer patients whose conditions should be reported to the Cancer Registry Control Panel from those who were not appropriate for inclusion in the registry.[4]

CHALLENGES WARRANTING FUTURE DEVELOPMENT

With NLP in health care having moved from being a promising AI subfield to a mature business tool, the need to address and resolve several standing issues is increasingly salient. The foremost challenge is the interdependent issues of the availability of data, the infrastructure to access them, and the evolving privacy policies governing the access and use of those data. Clinical care organizations are awash with unstructured text data and are producing terabytes of new data on a daily basis. And the current generation of NLP tools designed to self-improve through deep learning neural networks are finally at a maturity that organizations and individual clinicians stand to reap enormous insights and efficiencies. However, obtaining permission to share those data with solution vendors, consolidating those data from hundreds of disparate systems into curated data lakes for ML, and integrating the output with EHRs, reporting systems, and real-world clinical workflows have become the limiting factors.

A second challenge involves the lack of alignment within clinical organizations around how to prioritize the implementation and development of NLP. Anand Shroff, founder and chief development officer of Health Fidelity, says, "Unless there is agreement on which use cases deliver the most value to the organization, it is difficult to find long-term funding for the use of NLP in the enterprise."[15] He adds that the most common initiatives focus on quality of care, documentation improvement, risk stratification, and adjustment cohort selection for clinical trials and outcomes research.

The third challenge is meaningfully integrating NLP into the clinical workflow. Currently, NLP is already embedded in EHRs, where it is most commonly used to enhance clinical search. For example, if the surgeon types "liver" into the clinical search box, the answer should return not only the term "liver" but also clinically related terms, such as "hepatic," "hepatocellular," and "LFTs." Yet, unstructured clinical notes and narrative text still present a major problem for computer scientists because clinical notes are often written or dictated in cryptic, abbreviated, and often ambiguous shorthand, which is eminently understandable by clinicians in the field but befuddling to even the smartest NLP algorithms. Consider the following as an example: "44 y.o. w/ diab, htn, POD #2 s/p appy no f/n/v/d. +BS +BM. Ready for dc this PM." Although the data scientist may be tempted to make life easier for NLP by demanding that surgeons change the way they speak and write in the EHR, the challenge here is to avoid disrupting the clinicians' thought process and workflow; otherwise, the clinicians would experience more burden using NLP than not.

On the contralateral side of capturing valid results out of documentation, developers must face the equal challenge of displaying clinical decision support data within the workflow. Surgeons already complain about the "banner blindness" imposed by inconsequential or overly abundant decision support alerts. And without intentionality in how and when to display results, the wealth of potential insights and facts extracted by NLP threatens to further disrupt the surgeon's ability to focus on what is clinically relevant.

Finally, although many data science pundits predict that, because of AI, health care will move increasingly away from structured data and toward consuming insight-rich unstructured information, the current reality is that structured data will always remain critical in some way. Many organizations are attempting to leverage NLP to fill in the gaps of structured data on the back end, but this endeavor too presents a major challenge. Lack of standardization of data elements, poor data governance policies, and wide variation in the data structures of EHRs and complementary applications have left a gaping hole to be filled.

CONCLUSION

NLP and AI for clinical documentation offer a growing set of technologies that promise to bridge the gap between the seemingly limitless amount of unstructured data generated daily in health care and the limits of what humans can meaningfully manage. In an environment where 35% to 65% of US physicians are burned out and where the administrative burden of using the EHR is often cited as a major driver for that burnout, NLP and its branches—SR, voice assistants, ambient virtual scribes, clinical documentation improvement, computer-aided coding, and so on—offer hope to struggling surgeons and other clinicians that relief is possible. And for researchers, finance officers, revenue cycle managers, population health coordinators, quality and safety leaders, health information managers, third-party payers, regulators, and other consumers of clinical documentation, NLP opens new opportunities for efficiency and insight.

All these benefits are predicated on the continual development of health care– and specialty-specific algorithms, further improvements in computer processing and data storage systems, better access to data (while reconciling with and evolving data privacy, sharing, and governance standards), and greater attention paid to engineering clinically sensitive workflows and data displays for those who create the documentation as well as those who consume it.

REFERENCES

1. del Carmen MG, Herman J, Rao S, et al. Trends and factors associated with physician burnout at a multispecialty academic faculty practice organization. *JAMA Netw Open.* 2019;2(3):e190554-e190554.
2. Emani S, Ting DY, Healey M, Lipsitz SR, Karson A, Bates DW. Physician beliefs about the meaningful use of the electronic health record: a follow-up study. *Appl Clin Inform.* 2017;8:1044-1053.
3. Natural language processing: enabling the potential of a digital healthcare era. Chilmark Research Market Scan Report, July 2018. Accessed October 6, 2020. https://www.chilmarkresearch.com/chilmark_report/nlp-market-scan-report/.
4. Bresnick J. What is the role of natural language processing in healthcare? HealthITAnalytics, September 29, 2019. Accessed October 6, 2020. https://healthitanalytics.com/features/what-is-the-role-of-natural-language-processing-in-healthcare.
5. Natural language processing market by type (rule-based, statistical, and hybrid), technologies (recognition, IVR, OCR, speech recognition, text processing, pattern & image recognition), by deployment type, vertical & by region: global forecast to 2021. Markets and Markets Research Pvt Ltd, July 2016. Accessed October 6, 2020.

https://www.globenewswire.com/news-release/2015/06/25/747403/0/en/
Natural-Language-Processing-Market-by-Type-Rule-Based-Statistical-
and-Hybrid-Technologies-Recognition-IVR-OCR-Pattern-Image-Recognition-
Worldwide-Forecast-to-2020.html.

6.   Sadewo B. Speech recognition: life before Siri, and what's to come. Android Authority, October 27, 2013. Accessed October 6, 2020. https://www.androidauthority
.com/speech-recognition-life-before-siri-and-whats-to-come-67994/.

7.   Huang X, Jack M, Ariki Y. *Hidden Markov Models for Speech Recognition.*
Edinburgh University Press; 1990.

8.   Calabrese K, Doggett S, Jones J, et al. *Speech Recognition Best Practices: Relevance and Application of BESR Implementation Best Practices in Healthcare
Documentation.* Association for Healthcare Documentation Integrity; 2016.

9.   Myers E. Speech recognition accuracy: past, present, future. Temi.com,
October 25, 2017. Accessed October 6, 2020. https://www.temi.com/blog/
speech-recognition-accuracy-history/.

10. Landi H. Survey: 62 percent of docs use speech recognition, but cite concerns
about accuracy. Healthcare Innovation, September 26, 2018. Accessed October
6, 2020. https://www.hcinnovationgroup.com/clinical-it/news/13030744/survey-
62-percent-of-docs-use-speech-recognition-but-cite-concerns-about-accuracy.

11. Johnson M, Lapkin S, Long V, et al. A systematic review of speech recognition
technology in health care. *BMC Med Inform Decis Mak.* 2014;14:94.

12. Zick RG, Olsen J. Voice recognition software versus a traditional transcription
service for physician charting in the ED. *Am J Emerg Med.* 2001;19(4):295-298.

13. Zhou L, Blackley SV, Kowalski L, et al. Analysis of Errors in dictated clinical
documents assisted by speech recognition software and professional transcriptionists. *JAMA Netw Open.* 2018;1(3):e180530.

14. Ryan K. Who's smartest: Alexa, Siri, and or Google Now?" Inc.com, June 3,
2016. Accessed October 6, 2020. https://www.inc.com/kevin-j-ryan/internet-
trends-7-most-accurate-word-recognition-platforms.html.

15. Chavis S. Hidden treasure: the value of unstructured documentation. *For the
Record.* 2018;30(9):10. Accessed October 6, 2020. https://www.fortherecordmag
.com/archives/1018p10.shtml.

ETHICS OF ARTIFICIAL INTELLIGENCE IN SURGERY

14

Frank Rudzicz and Raeid Saqur

HIGHLIGHTS

- The 4 key principles of biomedical ethics from a surgical context are autonomy, nonmaleficence, beneficence, and justice.
- Implications of fairness and the taxonomy of algorithmic bias in artificial intelligence (AI) system design are important factors in the ethics of AI.
- The ethical paradigm shifts as the degree of autonomy in AI agents evolves.
- Ethics in AI is dynamic, and continuous revisions are needed as AI evolves.

▌INTRODUCTION

Surgery manifests in an intense form of practical ethics. The practice of surgery often forces unique ad hoc decisions based on contextual intricacies in the moment, which are not typically captured in broad, top-down, or committee-approved guidelines. Surgical ethics are principled, of course, but also pragmatic. They are also replete with moral contradictions and uncertainties; the introduction of novel technology into this environment can potentially increase those challenges.

A discussion about ethics is often a discussion about choice. Wall et al[1] defined an ethical problem as "when an agent must choose between mutually exclusive options, both of which either have equal elements of right and wrong, or are perceived as equally obligatory. The essential element that distinguishes an ethical problem from a tragic situation is the element of choice." Moreover, choosing between options often involves identifying factors by which those options are *not* exactly equal, and the method one uses to weigh these factors can draw upon a set of ethical frameworks that, themselves, can be somewhat incongruous.

At their core, artificial intelligence (AI) systems—and machine learning (ML) more specifically—are also designed to make choices, often by categorizing some input among a set of nominal categories. In the past, the choices these systems made could only be evaluated by their correctness—their accuracy in applying the same categorical labels that a human would to previously unseen inputs, like whether or not an image contains a tumor. As these systems are increasingly used in less quixotic (or more critical) scenarios, we are asking of them to make choices for which even humans struggle to find correctness.[2,3] Indeed, when software is more accurate than the most correct humans,[4,5] but it is validated by labels *provided by* humans, the very nature of the process—and its application into practice—is called into question. Indeed, we may no longer consider that the human and the machine are in contrast to one another, or even that one simply uses the other; rather, we may consider that surgeons and their tools are in a sense a single, hybrid, active entity. We shape our tools, and thereafter, our tools shape us, as Marshall McLuhan described.

The expectations of surgery and ML are similar in some ways. Both surgeons and ML algorithms are meant to solve complex problems quickly with a dispassionate technical skill, and neither have traditionally been defined by their bedside manner.[6] However, surgeons are regularly faced with profound ethical and moral dilemmas, often on a daily basis, as a fundamental matter of their profession, whereas establishing practical ethical frameworks in AI has only just recently begun to take shape.

In this chapter, we approximate root cause analyses,[7] in which the factors that cause ethical dilemmas are predictable and therefore learnable through observation. Wall et al[1] identified broad categories of these factors in which differences (in understanding and otherwise) may lead to conflict in the surgical domain in general. These are summarized in the part of this chapter. Subsequently, we also explore the ethical dilemmas arising from the intertwining of AI and surgery.

▌ETHICAL ASPECTS OF SURGERY

As issues of choice permeate ethics, it is no surprise that one has a choice of moral frameworks to apply in surgery. For instance, we may apply the *prima facie* duty theory.[8] This is a standard widely used in biomedical ethics to provide first principles, or ground rules, for making ethical decisions in health care. These principles are (1) respect for patient autonomy, (2) nonmaleficence, (3) beneficence, and (4) justice. However, these principles are not sufficient and can themselves create conflict and ethical dilemma. It is useful to understand these key principles to realize the inherent tension among them and how they can give rise to ethical dilemmas in real-world scenarios.

Autonomy dictates that each medical care provider should respect patients' choices with regard to their medical care. This principle is often put into action through informed consent, although it also means that a physician should be willing to consider alternate treatment methods if a patient rejects the original plan deemed best by the physician. However, the degree to which this principle can be upheld is often hard to clearly discern. Wall et al[1] pointed out that autonomy is continuously present in classical medical ethics, but in surgery, it is clearly not, because while the patient is under anesthesia, shared decisions cannot be made.

Nonmaleficence in bioethics is often juxtaposed with the Hippocratic oath "to do no harm." This requires that doctors not provide treatments or perform interventions that are needlessly harmful to patients. Surgery is somewhat unique in that to achieve some treatment goal, one has to temporarily do some harm, but that harm is typically necessary, with minimized effects.

Beneficence is the duty of physicians to maximize benefits and minimize harm to patients. In surgery, beneficence is a subjective measure in that the risks taken should be commensurate with the benefits received, ascertained in the context of the patients' goals and values.

Justice stipulates that equals be treated equally and nonequals (appropriately) unequally.[9] In health care, justice is often described in terms of the "fairness" of the distribution of resources, including medical goods and services, or benefits and burdens of medical research. True fairness may be forever unobtainable, especially when constraints like resource scarcity force decisions that otherwise would not be necessary. Indeed, the very definition of *fairness* may be unbound. Is a utilitarian view of fairness preferable to one focused on each individual? Are systemic or institutional constraints more pressing than an individual's? Consider the case of admitting a critically ill patient to an at-capacity intensive care unit (ICU). If available resources cannot be redistributed to accommodate the new patient, then prioritizing patients suddenly becomes necessary, and the weighting of criteria in that prioritization may be an unsolved problem.

Those 4 key principles are not absolute, either in combination or even individually. For instance, a patient's aptitude or cognitive faculties can modulate his or her autonomy. Consider the case of a patient with advanced dementia or other cognitive impairment. To what extent can an understanding of the fundamental risks be truly shared between doctor and patient? To what extent is informed consent *truly and completely* informed when the administration of the process cannot assess for the level of information even in cognitively healthy individuals? To what extent does autonomy *depend* on situational awareness?

Alternatively, Little[10] identified 5 moral pillars (or categories) more specific to the surgical experience that touch on the ethical, relational, existential, and experiential aspects, drawing on his own practice and various pieces of literature.[11,12] These are as follows:

> **Rescue:** Surgery involves a severe power relationship in which patients choose to surrender themselves to the surgical team,[13] but it is a surrender with the expectation of rescue. Little[10] suggested that this first pillar of surgical ethics must be acknowledged and negotiated between patient and surgeon and can serve as the basis for a shared understanding between them. If the rescuer is a human, the patient may have certain expectations as to the surgeon's emotional involvement and their subsequent urgency in the rescue relationship. If the rescuer is increasingly augmented by automation, where no emotional urgency of rescue may be expected, this pillar may begin to crumble.
>
> **Proximity:** Surgery is at the extreme of the medical gaze, in which the surgeon has a physical proximity to the patient and their inner workings that even the patient themselves cannot typically observe. Proximity to the patient is not only physical, however, but emotional and personal, and often the surgeon will install limits on this type of proximity as a means of self-preservation to avoid the penalties of closeness or the pains of failure.[10] Unemotional aspects of automation clearly do not require layers of emotional protection, but they introduce other facets to consider. For example, if a purely data-driven analysis of a patient or case reveals patterns that are too intricate or complex for the typical doctor-patient relationship to capture, to what extent can they be acted upon? If they are acted upon, how can they be rationalized or explained? This is discussed later in this chapter.
>
> **Ordeal:** The ordeal of surgery requires that a patient concede autonomy, face risk and possibly mortality, suffer physical pain and discomfort, and disrupt the flow of their lives. When the benefits of rescue override the trauma of the ordeal, those aspects are usually tolerated. Sometimes, the depth of the ordeal is not fully grasped prior to a surgery, and negative outcomes predictable to the surgeon but not the patient may raise conflict after the fact. Cassel[14] suggested that relieving suffering and curing disease are in fact twin obligations and that a

technically adequate procedure may not be a sufficient intervention if the nature of the suffering is not also considered.

Aftermath: Physical and psychological scars persist after surgery, and surgical ethics must accommodate both objective and subjective aspects of these experiences. Little[10] does not make it explicit, but the scope of the aftermath may depend on intraoperative factors, and adverse events that may be common nevertheless can directly magnify the aftermath, including risks of readmission, death, lifelong injury, or other postoperative complications. For these reasons, it will be crucial to minimize the scope and profundity of the aftermath by using data-driven analytics, including AI, in the prediction and prevention of adverse events.[15,16]

Presence: Because patients surrender themselves to the surgical team, they will typically expect or desire a certain degree of access to that team (at least, to the extent that the access is initiated by them). Personal attributes of charisma, confidence, and empathy may not be as important as the stamina, cognitive abilities, and mere time that a surgeon can present to their patients. Being available gives a sense of comfort and protection. From this perspective, it does not matter if an AI remains less personable than a surgeon; it may be *more* relevant that the information processed by automated processes is continuously available and interpretable to a patient.

Rather than broad principles, Wall[17] outlined a set of questions with definite possible responses, clustered by category, that can be used to identify the root cause or causes of an ethical dilemma, as re-created in Table 14-1. These questions can be adapted to the scenario, as flexibility is often necessary in clinical contexts, but the point is to have some objective set of fundamental variables from which a computation of ethics is to be made.

In contrast to the more traditional *prima facie* duty theory or the moral pillars of Little,[10] each of which broadly outlines qualitative principles, Little's framework of identifying atomic facts of a case may be more suited to a quantitative *computation* of ethics.[10] That is, given that we have a set of objective facts, then one ought to be able to compute an objective ethical outcome given an objective transfer function with sufficient parameters. In other words, if one has a set of variables $X = \{x_1, x_2, \ldots, x_N\}$ that answer, for example, the questions in Table 14-1, we may seek a mathematical function $f(\cdot)$ that takes X as its input and outputs some numerical score $S = f(X)$ of the *utility* for one decision over all others. Whether ethics can ever be truly *calculated* in the medical context should be open to debate, but it is worth noting that this sort of cost-benefit calculation is

Table 14-1	QUESTIONS TO ASK PRIOR TO THE DECISION-MAKING PROCESS, ACCORDING TO WALL[17]
Stakeholders	Who are the primary stakeholders? Are there additional medical providers who should be involved? Does the patient have additional people who should be involved?
Facts	What is the diagnosis? What are the options for intervention? What are the expected outcomes for each intervention (including no intervention)? What does each of the stakeholders understand about the medical facts? Are there additional facts relevant to the case?
Goals and values	What are the goals of each of the primary stakeholders? Are there any conflicts among the various goals? What are the values of the primary stakeholders? Are there any conflicts among the identified values?
Norms	What are the relevant ethical norms? What are the relevant legal norms? What are the relevant institutional norms? What are the relevant professional norms? Are there conflicts among the identified norms?

precisely what artificial agents perform when deciding on what action to take in AI's subfield of reinforcement learning.[18]

ETHICAL ASPECTS OF USING AI IN SURGERY

In the preceding section, we presented multifarious frameworks for surgical ethics, discussed the *prima facie* duties of human surgeons as full ethical agents animated by certain key principles,[8] and outlined questions to ask when analyzing ethical problems.

ML in practice includes all of the risks typical of software generally—malware and hackers, software bugs and lack of dependability, and disparities and inequities inherent in the society in which the software is used. In surgery, applications of AI are largely confined to the agents performing specific and defined tasks initiated and controlled entirely by human surgeons or clinicians, although recent advances such as the Smart Tissue Autonomous Robot (STAR) have begun to perform *in vivo* and *ex vivo* surgical tasks more effectively than humans, albeit in quite specific and controlled conditions.[19] AI may also be used as a clinical decision support system prior to surgery or other acute care.[20] In such circumstances, the ethical paradigm may be fully enveloped using de-ontological (ie, defined duty) ethics. In this framework, an AI system is an *implicit ethical agent*, and the burden of responsibility of machine behavior falls on the human designers and developers of the machine agent or AI system. Thus, we focus on ethical issues faced by human designers in developing AI systems in the current context.

Privacy of (Mostly Patient) Data

The decision-making capability of an AI system emanates from an underlying mapping between relevant inputs and an output decision. Regardless of the specific learning mechanism, training a production-grade AI system for surgical applications usually requires a nontrivial amount of sensitive patient data. The *privacy* of such patient data is therefore an automatic-choice topic in many discussions concerning ethics of AI in surgery, because it can be argued that personal medical data are the most sensitive kind of user data available. Hence, the safeguarding of users' medical data is of the utmost importance and a primary concern when applying AI in surgery. In this way, the data-hungry algorithms of modern ML are traditionally described as being at odds with modern ethical approaches to patient data, but this need not be the case[21] because there are various emerging tools, including *federated learning*, that can keep an individual's data decentralized and while still approximating the performance of a system with access to a more complete data set.[22] An alternative approach to keeping patient data private is *differential privacy* in which the outputs of a statistical system are provably uninformative as to whether an individual's data are included.[23] This is accomplished, essentially, by judiciously adding noise in a way that does not fundamentally hinder the accuracy of the system but makes an adversarial attack nearly impossible, even with auxiliary information.[24] Other algorithmic protections to patient privacy are constantly being developed.

Keeping pace with the development of AI systems, there has been a recent surge in regulatory measures addressing data privacy. A prominent example is the European General Data Protection Regulation (GDPR), which stipulates stringent data privacy measures not only for direct patient care, but also for research.[25] The American Health Insurance Portability and Accountability Act (HIPAA) provides similar stipulations. These measures are somewhat limited by their jurisdictional interpretations. Juxtaposing GDPR with HIPAA, we see that although these regulations may have similar overarching intents, their scopes are different. HIPAA focuses on health care data from patient records but does not cover alternate sources of health data generated outside of covered entities, such as life insurance companies or applications on smart devices (eg, fitness bands, smart watches).[26] These frameworks also offer incomplete models of ethics. For example, the duty of patient autonomy and their right to informed consent alludes to "a right to explanation" of all decisions made by automated or AI systems.[27] The right to explanation was widely expected to be legally mandated by GDPR once enforced[28]; however, in reality, GDPR only mandates a *right to be informed*—that is, patients could receive meaningful information (Articles 13-15), however limited, about the logic involved, as well as the significance and envisaged consequences of automated decision support systems. In this area, GDPR appears to lack precise language to explicitly state well-defined rights and safeguards against AI-based automated decision making, which, therefore, may limit its ineffectiveness. However, given the complexity and state of explainability in modern AI models, it is currently infeasible to stipulate and enforce the full scope of a "right to explainability" for AI systems, which we discuss in more detail in later in this chapter. Indeed, given the novelty of ML generally, there remains significant confusion over which laws and regulations might apply.[29]

Although the focus of the discussion on privacy has typically been on patient data, there are also, naturally, concerns about the privacy of the surgeon and their teams. As AI is increasingly being used by tools that assess or analyze aspects of the surgery itself,[16] concerns may be raised around increased legal risk or even changes to behavior (and therefore performance) given that one knows he or she is being recorded. Jurisprudence reveals a few principles in Western law applicable to recording surgical procedures, touching on the same issues of privacy as for the patient, with the addition of the importance of professional secrecy.[30]

Fairness and Algorithmic Bias in AI

The issue of fairness in using AI systems primarily concerns the inadvertent *algorithmic biases* and *statistical biases* inherent in the design and functioning of an AI system. Due to the magnitude and severity of the consequences that these biases may engender, including in social, legal, and medical domains, the topic of *fairness* ranks as one of the top recurring themes in machine medical ethics and AI ethics in general. Biased AI systems can have various deleterious effects in multiple domains, and the types of algorithmic biases can impact the surgical cases presented in the other chapters of this book.

Decision support systems powered by AI—designed with controls for fairness—may be used to augment human judgment and reduce both conscious and unconscious biases.[31] In contrast, unintended statistical biases caused by differences in sampling (or insufficient controls, such as data regularization) may reflect and amplify existing cultural prejudices and inequalities.[32] This is reflected in a litany of research confirming racial[32-35] and gender bias[36] emanating from insufficiently examined autonomous decision support systems. For example, comprehensive studies by Kehl and Kessler[37] and Flores et al[38] showed systemic racial bias in algorithms used to predict recidivism, with implications for the US criminal justice system. In natural language computing, models of language derived from general texts using neural networks have learned a host of gender biases with which we may not be comfortable (eg, that a man is to a woman as a programmer is to a homemaker, or as a surgeon is to a nurse).[36] Although progress can be made in minimizing biases against identifiable groups, because ML is meant to uncover complex nonlinear relationships in the data, it is quite possible that groups (or procedures, or treatments, etc) that are less well identified in the societal zeitgeist will be isolated by these pattern-finding algorithms and nevertheless not be detected by the system's users.[39]

Gianfrancesco et al[40] and Vayena et al[41] focused their discussions predominantly on *training data bias*, which concerns the quality and representativeness of data used to train ML and AI systems. A taxonomy of biases in ML may be dichotomized into those originating from either (1) technical or computational sources or (2) inappropriate use or deployment of algorithms and autonomous systems. Statistical bias in training data falls under the first category. Adhering to the iconic aphorism "garbage in, garbage out," bias in the input will result in a biased model. For example, existing medical data sets have had much higher ratios of white adult males (ie, an overrepresentation bias) than exist in the actual population.[42] A lack of diversity in sampling manifests in biased data and, without special controls in place, therefore results in biased models that may not behave as expected for underrepresented groups.[43] Similarly, electronic medical record (EMR) data can suffer from missing samples and incorrect labels,[40] with unintended downstream effects. The suboptimal performance for underrepresented social groups creates an ethical bottleneck.

Other sources of technical or computational bias include algorithmic *focus* and *processing* bias. The *focus bias* emanates from the differential usage of information in training AI systems. For example, developers may deliberately include or exclude certain features (ie, types of inputs) when training a model, thereby causing it to deviate from the statistical standard if those attributes have a strong main effect on the outcome or interaction effects with other variables. *Algorithmic processing bias* occurs when the algorithm itself is biased, as in the use of statistically biased estimators, which may result in a significant reduction of model variance on small sample sizes (ie, the bias-variance trade-off[44]). Thus, developers may embrace algorithmic processing as a bias source in order to mitigate or compensate for other types of biases.[45]

The potential effects of biases emanating from technical and computational sources of AI in surgery could have direct effects on patient safety and system integrity. For example, training data bias could dramatically impact a preoperative risk stratification prior to surgery. Underrepresentation of demographic clusters may also cause inaccurate risk assessments, and thus, AI-driven decisions, such as which patient is treated first or offered resources in the ICU after surgery, will be flawed.

Transfer of context bias and *interpretation bias* are 2 remaining sources of algorithmic bias that constitute inappropriate use or deployment of algorithms and AI systems.[45] The transfer of context bias is introduced when an algorithm or trained model is used outside the context of its training. An unwarranted application or extension of an AI system outside of its intended contexts will not necessarily perform according to appropriate statistical, moral, or legal standards. For example, an ML model trained only with simulated surgical data being deployed to analyze real-life patient surgeries would not be appropriate. Transfer of context bias may also arise when translating a model from a research hospital directly to a rural clinic. Once again, the ML community has identified the challenge and has begun to tackle this challenge, as in off-policy learning,[46] but as these challenges become more subtle, so too do their solutions; hence, it is crucial that all stakeholders are kept up to date about the state of the art.

Consider the case of automated intraoperative video analyses during surgery. Contextual bias *may* occur if one ignores what may appear to be trivial caveats (eg, whether the operating surgeon is right- or left-handed) or if one presumes that the same level of resources is available across operating rooms and hospitals. Methods to mitigate against this include ensuring variance in the data set, being sensitive to overfitting on training data, and having humans-in-the-loop to examine new data as they are deployed, for starters.

Finally, *interpretation bias* concerns the misinterpretation of an algorithm's output by either a human user or by the broader system within which the algorithm functions. Developers are rarely able to fully specify all possible scenarios in which their algorithms or models are to be used. For example, biased judgments about causal structure or strength can be easily misused in biased ways by AI systems if not carefully accounted for.

Transparency and Explainable AI

The best-performing modern AI models predominantly use deep neural networks, which can be abstracted and thought of as black box, noninterpretable function approximators. Thus, even though such models can be used to achieve high prediction accuracies, one cannot *a priori* coherently explain or attribute the influence of particular features of input on the resulting predictions in a causative manner, nor necessarily describe the model itself in human-graspable terms—at least, not by default.

Consider a simplified binary classifier that takes in patient data x and outputs whether the patient has cancer or not, y (ie, $y = +1$ for cancer, $y = -1$ otherwise). The input data here could be a patient's biographical information, cell culture images, and so on. To train the model, input-label pairs $(x,y) \in X \times \{\pm 1\}$ are sampled from a data distribution D; the goal is to learn a classifier $C : X \to \{\pm 1\}$ that predicts a label y^0, corresponding to a particular new input x^0. We can define a *feature* to be a function mapping from the input space X to the real numbers, with the set of all features being $F = \{f : X \to R\}$. In this case, the patient's weight, height, age, body mass index, and so on could be considered features, represented by normalized real numbers. For an arbitrary black box deep neural network, the precise influence that function F has in the mapping of X to a binary prediction $y \in R$ will be lost in the layers upon layers of artificial neurons, or at the very best, the mapping will be so complex as to be uninterpretable. Thus, even if an ML system is able to predict cancer with very high accuracy, one could not infer or attribute which features $f \in F$ caused this prediction, and hence, one may find it difficult to take interventional action, if the causes of the diagnosis, especially the modifiable ones, are unknown.

If a system's output cannot be interpreted, it invalidates its use in a broad swath of domains when formulating *health care policies*. In a surgery setting, if more diagnostic and therapeutic interventions become based on AI, the autonomy of patients in decisional processes may also be undermined. Already, an increasing reliance on automated decision-making tools has reduced the opportunity for meaningful dialogue between the health care provider and patient.[47] However, the current ethical debate of whether (or how) the details of an AI system should be disclosed to patients is still in its infancy. A bigger ongoing concern is whether such black box algorithms, whose self-learned rules may be too complex to reconstruct and explain, should be used in medicine.[48] Although some have called for a duty to transparency to dispel the opacity of such systems,[28] others have justified limited requirements—for example, the *right to be informed*, instead of the *right to explanation*, suffices to adequately protect the morally relevant interests of patients when AI algorithms are used to provide them with care.[49]

If ML is in its infancy, then the subfield tasked with making its inner workings explainable is so embryonic that even its terminology has yet to recognizably form.[50] However, several fundamental properties of explainability have started to emerge. Among these, Lipton[51] argued that ML should be *simultaneous* (its behavior should be graspable holistically), *decomposable* (its components or inputs should also be understandable), and *algorithmically transparent* (the shape of the solution, and the method to get there, should be somewhat intuitive). Moreover, explanations can be textual, visualized, local to a data point under consideration, or in terms of other examples (prototypical or critical).

The benefits of adding explainability and transparency to the decision-making process are illustrated by a case study in anesthesiology,[52] where a clinical decision support system was used to predict hypoxemia in patients in real time during surgeries. The system was trained on EMR data combined with minute-by-minute vitals data over 50,000 surgeries and helped to increase the rate of anticipating hypoxemia from 15% to 30% during surgeries. However, the system not only made predictions, but also provided real-time interpretable risks in terms of an automatically selected subset of contributing factors. This allowed for easier early intervention because the results could be associated with modifiable factors. Additionally, this system can help improve the clinical understanding of hypoxemia risk during anesthesia care by providing general insights in the exact changes in risk induced by patient characteristics or surgical procedure.[53]

RESPONDING TO CHALLENGES, DUTIES OF HUMAN DESIGNERS, AND INSTITUTIONAL INTERVENTIONS

Monitoring the integration of AI in surgery will involve every health care worker it affects. In particular, the surgeon-in-chief, in consultation with a committee of stakeholders, can embody the institutional memory and authority to ensure that progress is managed effectively and safely.[54] In the current context, the responsibility of a machine's behavior apparently falls on its human designers and developers. Stahl and Coeckelbergh[55] argued that an effective way for handling contingencies is to minimize the gap between AI researchers and the different stakeholders (or the subsequent users) of the systems they create. They propose the responsible research and innovation framework including ethical considerations built in to research (ie, at a nascent stage of technical development). Clearly, part of this will involve a more effective dialogue between developers and stakeholders, including around potential ethical contingencies.

AI and ML are often referred to as the source of risks when discussing their use in health care, but the contrapositive is rarely discussed: What are the ethical risks of *not* integrating these into practice, especially in situations where their effects can only be positive? What are the risks of maintaining the status quo, which has been so replete with cognitive error?

Innovation in surgery is a process rather than an event and is commonly the result of creative attempts to solve individual problems.[56] The process will help filter good ideas from bad ones through multiple layers of scrutiny. However, too many filters may be prohibitively dense and keep the best novel ideas from impacting care in the short term. In traditional thyroidectomy, the risks of permanent hypoparathyroidism and recurrent laryngeal nerve injury are only 1% to 2%. If a method guided by AI can reduce those risks by a half, it may take thousands of procedures with the new method to observe any statistically significant change, which an individual surgeon may never observe, at least not in a short time frame. However, a repository of AI-based analytics, aggregating these thousands of cases from hundreds of sites, would be able to discern and communicate those significant patterns. This is the promise of scale that AI delivers.

However, scale itself can provide a subtle but concrete mode of failure that is unique to AI. Amodei et al[57] describe several problems in AI safety that often evade discussion, including the following:

- Avoiding negative side effects involves placing bounds on the negative consequences, or on impact generally, of an AI system in the pursuit of its goals. Because AI systems will typically be used in environments not identical to those in which they were trained, it is important for such systems to identify those bounds themselves, automatically.
- Avoiding reward hacking means setting goals that do not have "short cuts" or hidden paths to optimization that might be unexpected. For example, a system in the same vein as that of Lundberg et al,[52] designed to not only predict but also *avoid* adverse events, may incur a penalty for every such detected event and, if not carefully controlled, may learn to ignore such detections to avoid cost.
- Scalable oversight includes questions of how an AI system can explicitly evaluate its performance, especially in the long tail of the many potential atypical or rare cases, when the size of the data grows beyond human intervention.
- Robustness to distributional shift ensures that a system behaves robustly, or can generalize its behavior, to new data that are

fundamentally different than the data on which it was trained. For example, a system trained in a large, modern, and expensively outfitted integrated operating room should be able to maintain a level of performance even in smaller, more modestly outfitted environments.

These aspects can manifest in subtle ways, often eluding human scrutiny (which further emphasizes the need for explainable systems). In the literature, case studies are often described by contrasting extreme but recognizable aspects. Although this can help to familiarize one's self with the types of frameworks traditionally used in ethics (see earlier discussion), real-life ethical dilemmas are often not so extreme and occur at the boundaries of more subtly differing aspects. Due to the domain-specific subtleties and complexities of AI systems, it is imperative to have domain- and industry-specific guiding frameworks for applications of AI. The continued technologic advancement in AI will sow rapid increases in the breadths and depths of their duties. Extrapolating from the progress curve, we can predict that machines will become more *autonomous*. We observe a concomitantly accelerating emergence of frameworks for algorithmic fairness and impact assessment by governments and institutional authorities, including the Government of Canada's Algorithmic Impact Assessment[58] and the Harm Assessment Risk Tool framework in the United Kingom.[59] Although these (and similar) frameworks have common overarching intentions, due to the unprecedented pace of innovation, it will remain difficult to produce complete frameworks that can provide total guidance for dispelling ethical challenges and thereby ensuring ethical AI systems. Some recent frameworks have attempted to occupy the niche between health care and AI, including a notable framework by Luxton,[60] who reiterates that theoretical approaches and expert knowledge must be current (which is an ever-increasing challenge itself) and evidence supported. Among his considerations for ethical codes, guidelines, and uses of AI systems in health care are:

- Disclosing the services of an AI system, and their limits, to patients.
- Ensuring education of an AI system's users around capabilities, scope, and limitations, and for these to be communicable during informed consent.
- Requiring human supervision and monitoring for adverse outcomes and risks (although this of course presumes that human monitoring and intervention would not in themselves cause error and risk).

- Following applicable privacy laws and best practices.
- Ensuring that the AI system follows established clinical best practices.
- Ensuring that the AI is used within a continuity of care sensitive to the emotional nature of patient interactions.
- Providing a mechanism for patient feedback and queries.
- Identifying specifications for use, including limits on autonomy.
- Testing safety and ethical decision making in diverse situations.
- Including data logs and audit trails.
- Considering cultural sensitivity and diversity in designing AI systems.

Luxton[60] also nevertheless emphasizes that "formal ethical principles can never be substituted for an active, deliberative, and creative approach." In this way, AI development will need to be guided by an ad hoc interpretation of principles in the same way that surgeons are merely guided by the principles we discussed before, such as the *prima facie* theory or Little's moral pillars.[10]

The rise in autonomy necessitates an increased focus on the ethical horizon that we need to scrutinize. The discussion may soon transcend from deontological (defined duties) ethics to teleological (consequentialist) ethics. In surgery, some questions that may arise regarding AI may include the following[61]: What limits do we place on AI autonomy? Can a surgical robot refuse to perform a surgery? How do we attribute the responsibilities of machine behavior in this scenario? That is, who is responsible if the machine performs poorly? Does a robot surgeon support or compete with physicians and their assistants? We intentionally refrain from elaborating and exploring these questions; a prescriptive plan for future AI systems would be, in some sense, like making life choices by gazing into a crystal ball. However, it will be important to remember (1) that the nature of ethical challenges of AI in surgery will remain dynamic for some time, due to the evolving and constantly shifting technologic capabilities, and (2) that increasing AI autonomy will drastically expand the ethical paradigm and the challenges that come with it.

Ethical considerations of applying AI in health care generally often involve adhering to data protection and privacy requirements; fairness (broadly construed) across data sourcing, development, and deployment; and the maintenance of certain standards for transparency.[41] Like ethical decision making in current practice, ML will not be effective if it is merely designed carefully by committee; it requires exposure to the real world.

▌REFERENCES

1. Wall A, Angelos P, Brown D, Kodner IJ, Keune JD. Ethics in surgery. *Curr Prob Surg*. 2013;50(1):99-134.

2. Schwartz CE, Ayandeh A, Finkelstein JA. When patients and surgeons disagree about surgical outcome: investigating patient factors and chart note communication. *Health Qual Life Outcomes*. 2015;13(1):1-8.

3. Jordan DA, McKeown KR, Concepcion KJ, Feiner SK, Hatzivassiloglou V. Generation and evaluation of intraoperative inferences for automated health care briefings on patient status after bypass surgery. *J Am Med Inform Assoc*. 2001;8(3):267-280.

4. Esteva A, Kuprel B, Novoa RA, et al. Dermatologist-level classification of skin cancer with deep neural networks. *Nature*. 2017;542(7639):115.

5. Devlin J, Chang MW, Lee K, Toutanova K. BERT: pre-training of deep bidirectional transformers for language understanding. Accessed October 6, 2020. https://www.aclweb.org/anthology/N19-1423/.

6. Angelos P. Surgical ethics and the future of surgical practice. *Surgery*. 2018;163(1):1-5.

7. DuBois JM. *Ethics in Mental Health Research: Principles, Guidance, and Cases*. Oxford University Press; 2008.

8. Emanuel EJ. The beginning of the end of principlism: principles of biomedical ethics by Tom L. Beauchamp and James F. Childress. *Hastings Center Rep*. 1995;25(4):37.

9. Jonsen AR, Siegler M, Winslade WJ. *Clinical Ethics: A Practical Approach to Ethical Decisions in Clinical Medicine*. McGraw-Hill Medical; 1982.

10. Little M. Invited commentary: is there a distinctively surgical ethics? *Surgery*. 2001;129(6):668-671.

11. McCullough LB, Jones JW, Brody BA, eds. *Surgical Ethics*. Oxford University Press; 1998.

12. Frank AW. *At the Will of the Body*. Houghton Mifflin Co.; 1991.

13. Brody H. *The Healer's Power*. Stanford University Press; 1993.

14. Cassel EJ. The nature of suffering and the goals of medicine. *N Engl J Med*. 1982;306(11):639-645.

15. Jung JJ, Jüni P, Lebovic G, Grantcharov T. First-year analysis of the operating room black box study. *Ann Surg*. 2020;271(1):122-127.

16. Goldenberg MG, Jung J, Grantcharov TP. Using data to enhance performance and improve quality and safety in surgery. *JAMA Surg*. 2017;152(10):972.

17. Wall A. *Ethics for International Medicine: A Practical Guide for Aid Workers in Developing Countries*. Dartmouth College Press; 2012.

18. Abel D, MacGlashan J, Littman ML. Reinforcement learning as a framework for ethical decision making. *AAAI Workshop Tech Rep*. 2016;WS-16-01:54-61.

19. Panesar S, Cagle Y, Chander D, Morey J, Fernandez-Miranda J, Kliot M. Artificial intelligence and the future of surgical robotics. *Ann Surg*. 2019;270(2):223-226.

20. Lynn LA. Artificial intelligence systems for complex decision-making in acute care medicine: a review. *Patient Saf Surg*. 2019;13(1):1-8.

21. Rohringer T, Budhkar A, Rudzicz F. Privacy versus artificial intelligence in medicine. *Univ Toronto Med J*. 2019;96:1.

22. Bonawitz K, Eichner H, Grieskamp W, et al. Towards federated learning at scale: system design. Accessed October 6, 2020. https://arxiv.org/pdf/1902.01046.pdf.

23. Wu X, Li F, Kumar A, Chaudhuri K, Jha S, Naughton JF. Bolt-on differential privacy for scalable stochastic gradient descent-based analytics. Accessed October 6, 2020. https://adalabucsd.github.io/papers/2017_Bismarck-BoltOnDP_SIGMOD.pdf.

24. Dwork C. Differential privacy: a survey of results. In: Agrawal M, Du D, Duan Z, Li A, eds. *Theory and Applications of Models of Computation. TAMC 2008. Lecture Notes in Computer Science*. Springer; 2008:1-19.

25. McCall B. What does the GDPR mean for the medical community? *Lancet*. 2018;391(10127):1249-1250.

26. Cohen IG, Mello MM. HIPAA and protecting health information in the 21st century. *JAMA*. 2018;320(3):231-232.

27. Goodman B, Flaxman S. EU regulations on algorithmic decision-making and a right to explanation. Accessed October 6, 2020. https://arxiv.org/abs/1606.08813.

28. Wachter S, Mittelstadt B, Floridi L. Why a right to explanation of automated decision making does not exist in the general data protection regulation. *Int Data Privacy Law*. 2017;7(2):76-99.

29. Cortez N. *The Evolving Law and Ethics of Digital Health*. Springer International Publishing; 2018.

30. Henken KR, Jansen FW, Klein J, et al. Implications of the law on video recording in clinical practice. *Surg Endosc*. 2012;26(10):2909-2916.

31. Anderson M, Anderson SL. Machine ethics: creating an ethical intelligent agent. *AI Magazine*. 2007;28(4):15-18.

32. Sweeney L. Discrimination in online ad delivery. October 6, 2020. https://arxiv.org/ftp/arxiv/papers/1301/1301.6822.pdf.

33. Barr A. Google Photos mistakenly tags black people as "gorillas," showing limits of algorithms. *The New York Times*, 2015. Accessed October 6, 2020. https://bits.blogs.nytimes.com/2015/07/01/google-photos-mistakenly-labels-black-people-gorillas/.

34. Bass D, Huet E. Researchers combat gender and racial bias in artificial intelligence. *Bloomberg*. Accessed October 6, 2020. https://www.bloomberg.com/news/articles/2017-12-04/researchers-combat-gender-and-racial-bias-in-artificial-intelligence.

35. Garcia M. Racist in the machine: the disturbing implications of algorithmic bias. *World Policy J*. 2016;33(4):111-117.

36. Bolukbasi T, Chang KW, Zou JY, Saligrama V, Kalai AT. Man is to computer programmer as woman is to homemaker? Debiasing word embeddings. Accessed October 6, 2020. https://arxiv.org/abs/1607.06520.

37. Kehl DL, Kessler SA. Algorithms in the criminal justice system: assessing the use of risk assessments in sentencing. Accessed October 6, 2020. https://dash.harvard.edu/bitstream/handle/1/33746041/2017-07_responsivecommunities_2.pdf.

38. Flores AW, Bechtel K, Lowenkamp CT. False positives, false negatives, and false analyses: a rejoinder to machine bias: there's software used across the country to predict future criminals, and it's biased against blacks. *Fed Probation*. 2016;80:38.

39. Char DS, Shah NH, Magnus D. Implementing machine learning in health care: addressing ethical challenges. *N Engl J Med*. 2018;378(11):979-981.

40. Gianfrancesco MA, Tamang S, Yazdany J, Schmajuk G. Potential biases in machine learning algorithms using electronic health record data. *JAMA Intern Med*. 2018;178(11):1544-1547.

41. Vayena E, Blasimme A, Cohen IG. Machine learning in medicine: addressing ethical challenges. *PLoS Med*. 2018;15(11):e1002689.

42. Landry LG, Ali N, Williams DR, Rehm HL, Bonham VL. Lack of diversity in genomic databases is a barrier to translating precision medicine research into practice. *Health Aff*. 2018;37(5):780-785.

43. Adamson AS, Smith A. Machine learning and health care disparities in dermatology. *JAMA Dermatol*. 2018;154(11):1247-1248.

44. Geman S, Bienenstock E, Doursat R. Neural networks and the bias/variance dilemma. *Neural Comput*. 1992;4(1):1-58.

45. Danks D, London AJ. Algorithmic bias in autonomous systems. Accessed October 6, 2020. https://www.cmu.edu/dietrich/philosophy/docs/london/IJCAI17-AlgorithmicBias-Distrib.pdf.

46. Rakelly K, Zhou A, Quillen D, Finn C, Levine S. Efficient off-policy meta-reinforcement learning via probabilistic context variables. Accessed October 6, 2020. https://arxiv.org/abs/1903.08254.

47. Vayenaid E, Blasimmeid A, Cohen IG. Machine learning in medicine: addressing ethical challenges. *PLoS Med*. 2018;15(11):e1002689.

48. Price W, Nicholson II. Black-box medicine. *Harv J Law Technol*. 2014;28:419.

49. Selbst AD, Powles J. Meaningful information and the right to explanation. *Int Data Privacy Law*. 2017;7(4):233-242.

50. Adadi A, Berrada M. Peeking inside the black-box: a survey on explainable artificial intelligence (XAI). *IEEE Access*. 2018;6:52138-52160.

51. Lipton ZC. The mythos of model interpretability. Accessed October 6, 2020. https://arxiv.org/abs/1606.03490.

52. Lundberg SM, Nair B, Vavilala MS, et al. Explainable machine-learning predictions for the prevention of hypoxaemia during surgery. *Nat Biomed Engineer*. 2018;2(10):749.

53. Gordon L, Grantcharov T, Rudzicz F. Explainable artificial intelligence for safe intraoperative decision support. *JAMA Surg*. 2019;154(11):1064-1065.

54. Das S, McKneally M. The surgeon-in-chief should oversee innovative surgical practice. *Am J Bioethics*. 2019;19(6):34-36.

55. Stahl BC, Coeckelbergh M. Ethics of healthcare robotics: towards responsible research and innovation. *Robot Auton Syst*. 2016;86:152-161.

56. Angelos P. Surgical ethics and the challenge of surgical innovation. *Am J Surg*. 2014;208(6):881-885.

57. Amodei D, Olah C, Steinhardt J, Christiano P, Schulman J, Mané D. Concrete problems in AI safety. Technical report, 2016. Accessed October 6, 2020. https://arxiv.org/pdf/1606.06565.pdf.

58. Reisman D, Schultz J, Crawford K, Whittaker M. Algorithmic impact assessments: a practical framework for public agency accountability. Technical report, 2018. Accessed October 6, 2020. https://ainowinstitute.org/aiareport2018.pdf.

59. Oswald M, Grace J, Urwin S, Barnes GC. Algorithmic risk assessment policing models: lessons from the Durham HART model and experimental proportionality. *Inform Commun Technol Law*. 2018;27(2):223-250.

60. Luxton DD. Recommendations for the ethical use and design of artificial intelligent care providers. *Artif Intell Med*. 2014;62(1):1-10.

61. Bendel O. Surgical, therapeutic, nursing and sex robots in machine and information ethics. In: van Rysewyk S, Pontier M, eds. *Machine Medical Ethics. Intelligent Systems, Control and Automation: Science and Engineering*, vol 74. Springer; 2015.

POLICY IMPLICATIONS OF ARTIFICIAL INTELLIGENCE IN SURGERY

15

Benjamin H. Jacobson, Megan B. Diamond, and Winta T. Mehtsun

HIGHLIGHTS

- Current regulation for surgery and surgical procedures is sparse and decentralized.
- Incorporation of artificial intelligence (AI) into surgery presents unique and challenging problems that necessitate novel regulation.
- Regulation for surgical AI must focus on ensuring safety, efficacy, equity, and privacy.
- Beyond regulation, policy must adapt to clarify patient rights, malpractice liability, and adequate surgical training and competency maintenance.

▎ INTRODUCTION

In robotics, risk calculation, electronic health record analysis, and other elements of surgery, artificial intelligence (AI) is rapidly expanding into surgical care. Its technical utility in increasing precision, improving dexterity, and reducing tremor is being explored across multiple procedures but most notably in microsurgery and image-guided orthopedic surgery (see Chapter 12).[1,2] There is also potential for AI to augment surgeon performance beyond the operating room and across the care continuum. When it comes to ensuring good patient outcomes, nuanced decisions outside of the operating room (eg, who to operate on, the timing of an intervention, and expedient recognition of complications postoperatively) are equally as important as the decisions made inside the operating room. AI tools are currently in development to allow for data-driven optimization of patient selection and the use of predictive analytics to determine which patients are at higher risk of complications.[3,4] As AI technology evolves and integration into surgical care becomes a reality, it is imperative that policies are in place to ensure safety, efficacy, and equity for patients; to delineate accountability; and to mitigate the consequences of AI integration for health care providers.

Despite the abundance of surgical operations and the significant consequences that they can have for patients, no centralized state or federal agency approves new surgical procedures or directly regulates surgical procedures that are used today.[5] The current surgical regulatory framework is decentralized and occurs indirectly through the regulation of surgeons, hospitals, and devices or drugs that are used during and after operations. This regulation is enforced by bodies including the American Board of Surgery, The Joint Commission, and the US Food and Drug Administration (FDA), respectively. In this context, AI presents new and unique challenges that will undoubtedly require regulation. Without a centralized surgical regulatory infrastructure, these novel policy needs will require diverse policy innovations. This chapter intends to outline these challenges and the policy approaches that might address them.

Before moving into an exploration of health policy, surgery, and the ways in which new AI technologies interact with the current policy framework, it will be helpful to outline a few of the key features of AI technologies that make them challenging from a regulatory perspective. These aspects of AI will appear repeatedly throughout this chapter, and the following section is intended to provide a brief overview of relevant concerns associated with each of these AI attributes. Although there are many unique and complex aspects of AI, the focus here will be on those most relevant to surgery and health policy, namely the requirement for large amounts of data, the ability to evolve and change, and the black box that prohibits understanding of internal mechanisms.

▌ KEY AI CHALLENGES

AI Requires Large Quantities of High-Quality Medical Data

Most AI algorithms are, at their core, complex methods of identifying patterns in data. Generally, this pattern recognition is accomplished through iterative training and improvement as the algorithm observes more and more data (see Chapter 3). Ultimately, the quality and effectiveness of the algorithm are dependent on the quantity and quality of the data on which the algorithm is trained. The more training data an algorithm can access, the more training it can undergo and, therefore, the more it can optimize its performance. When those data are something such as images of handwritten numbers or historical rainfall records, the need for large amounts of high-quality data is not particularly concerning from a privacy or ownership perspective. With medical data, however, there is immediate and reasonable apprehension about distribution and use of data at any quantity, much less in the quantities required for AI research and implementation.

AI Can Evolve

Not only is AI capable of evolving and changing, but this is often viewed as one of its greatest strengths. In contrast to stagnant medical products such as devices or drugs, which never improve upon the version that is tested and marketed, many AI algorithms can continually improve as they are implemented by learning from the data on which they are acting. The ability to improve iteratively and to learn more every time they are used greatly increases the ceiling of capability for these algorithms and partially solves the need for large data sets by allowing some of the training to happen during implementation. Although this capacity for evolution is a benefit to development and performance, it presents a significant challenge when it comes to regulatory approval.[6] Further, this continuous transformation opens the door for many other concerns about AI, including inequity and lack of efficacy, to eventually manifest themselves within an algorithm, even if said algorithm was initially trained and tested with great care to avoid such pitfalls.

Some Medical AI Involves Black Box Algorithms With Unknown Inner Workings

In computer science and AI research, a black box is a system in which inputs and outputs can be observed but there is no capacity to understand how outputs are derived from inputs. This inability to "peer under the hood" presents challenges to understanding an algorithm's validity or interpreting unexpected findings. In AI specifically, opaque algorithms can learn patterns and make predictions based on input data but do not explain how their conclusions were drawn or how the input data were used.[7] Much of AI does not operate in the black box space, although there are certain algorithmic classes for which this opacity is inherent. Black box concerns are not new. Despite AI currently experiencing a surge in popularity, there were papers calling attention to the black box problem as early as the 1970s, although the nature of these concerns have shifted in a surgical context.[8] Specifically, the opacity of some AI algorithms increases the difficulty of obtaining proper informed consent, creates complex situations of liability, and heightens the challenges of ensuring safety and equity.

Although the idea of an uninterpretable algorithm sounds concerning, the truth is that we use these black boxes every day. Imagine using voice commands to ask Google Maps for directions. Most people do this regularly without thinking twice about how the chosen directions were selected or even about how one's voice was converted into a comprehended request for directions. Of course, surgery carries much greater stakes than driving directions or smartphone voice assistants, and although we may not be able to peer into the black box, it must be taken seriously. Although the opaqueness of algorithms may not be in and of itself concerning, it leads to many potentially problematic situations. As such, there must be sufficient regulation to guarantee safety, efficacy, and equity.

▍INTEGRATING AI CHALLENGES AND HEALTH POLICY

To effectively explore the ways in which AI interfaces with the current health policy framework, it is necessary to outline that framework and establish the primary goals of government policy in relation to health care and medical innovation. The policy framework presented here will focus on 2 major policy categories relevant to surgeons. The first of these policy subdivisions is regulation, which encompasses ensuring the safety and efficacy of surgical innovations, ensuring fairness and equity in surgical care, and ensuring the privacy and confidentiality of health care information. The second key policy category is legal purview, which includes protecting patient rights and creating legal standards for malpractice and medical errors. Each of these policy roles will be explored through a brief discussion of the current policy framework before moving into a discussion of the ways in which new AI technologies challenge this framework and an exploration of how policy should evolve in pursuit of a sound regulatory landscape governing AI in surgery.

Ensuring Safety and Efficacy

Understanding the current regulatory framework in medical innovation must begin with a discussion of the FDA, which plays a critical regulatory role in approval of medical innovations. Although the FDA was initially granted regulatory control over only pharmaceuticals, it gained purview over medical devices as well with the Medical Devices Amendment to the Federal Food, Drug, and Cosmetic Act.[9] The FDA's regulatory scope was further expanded with the recognition of Software as a Medical Device (SaMD), extending the FDA's control to the newest class of medical innovations.[10] Recent clarifications to that regulatory scope exclude some health care software including electronic medical records

(EMRs) and some clinical decision support (CDS) software from the definition of device and, therefore, from FDA regulation.[11] These algorithms are excluded because they either do not directly impact patient care, as in the case of EMRs, or because they simply offer advice and information to doctors who must still interpret and make their own decisions, as is the case with many CDS tools.[11] As will be discussed later, many AI technologies do not fit into these exemption requirements and are, therefore, still under the control of the FDA.

Medical devices must receive premarket approval from the FDA, and this approval can proceed through either of 2 avenues, outlined in sections 510(k) and 360(e) of the Medical Device Amendment.[9] The 510(k) approval pathway constitutes demonstrating that a device is a "substantial equivalent" to a device that was marketed prior to 1976, whereas the 360(e) Premarket Approval (PMA) pathway involves a complete and extensive review of the engineering process and of safety data for a novel device. The 360(e) PMA pathway is a more burdensome pathway, taken in only 2% of approvals, but carries the benefit of no manufacturer liability for defects upon approval.[12] Although there was minimal software marketed for health care prior to 1976 and thus no reference products on which to build a 510(k) submission, the FDA has since issued new guidelines allowing for inclusion of software in 510(k) approvals.[13] Although it is not necessary to delve into the details of these approval pathways, it is valuable to note that all devices either must be proven similar to a previous device or must have their design process and workings rigorously examined (Figure 15-1).

To receive approval for a medical device or SaMD, manufacturers must provide the FDA with sufficient evidence that a device is safe and effective, often in the form of a controlled trial. Such a trial generally features blinding, unbiased or random group assignment, and effective and unbiased data collection and analysis.[14] There is an expectation that data on safety and efficacy will continue to be collected and reviewed after approval and marketing of a device, allowing recognition and remediation of issues not identified during the premarket approval process. This postmarket surveillance has been aided by the development of electronic health records, which offer aggregated health outcomes data at the hospital level and simplify the process of collecting and reviewing outcomes data.

Although the current FDA approvals process ensures the safety and efficacy of devices and drugs, the opaque and evolving nature of AI algorithms makes them incompatible with the process as it currently stands. The black box nature of algorithms presents a challenge to the existing policy framework by creating a need to ensure safety and efficacy without

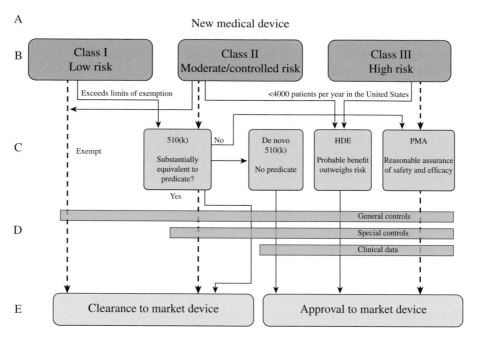

Figure 15-1 • FDA approval can proceed through a range of pathways contingent on the risk, novelty, and value of the product. HDE, humanitarian device exemption; PMA, premarket approval. (Hoffmann, M.J. FDA Regulatory Process. https://www.fda.gov/media/90419/download.)

mechanistic understanding. Although the 21st Century Cures Act excludes some CDS algorithms from FDA oversight, it extends this exclusion only to algorithms "enabling such health care professional to independently review the basis for such recommendations that such software presents so that it is not the intent that such health care professional rely primarily on any of such recommendations to make a clinical diagnosis or treatment decision regarding an individual patient."[15] Although the term *black box* is not explicitly used in this law, the act establishes a clear delineation between interpretable and uninterpretable algorithms and empowers the FDA to regulate fully those algorithms whose inner workings cannot be understood, addressing them under the established device regulation guidelines. Even within these guidelines, the FDA approves devices either through a thorough engineering review or through demonstration of similarity to a previous device [PMA or 510(k), respectively]. Without mechanistic insight, neither of these pathways is viable. As such, regulation and approval of black box AI cannot pass through the traditional SaMD framework and will require a new approach to oversight.

Beyond opaqueness of algorithms, many new AI innovations continue to evolve after implementation, providing benefits including improved functioning in a specific hospital population despite initial training on a general data set or improved specificity to better fit the needs of a specific surgeon or other health care provider.[6] The FDA approvals process and clinical trials are founded on the idea of a static product, with the concept that whatever drug or device is used in patients should be the same one whose safety and efficacy have been rigorously established.[12] The FDA outlines stringent reporting guidelines for any modification to a device after premarket approval that might affect its safety or effectiveness, and no modification can be implemented until the FDA has signed off.[16] This is clearly incompatible with a continuously evolving algorithm because every use and iterative change might alter the safety and effectiveness of the overall AI tool. Not only would it be incredibly burdensome to report a change every time an AI tool was used, but it would also be impossible to predict how usage and evolution would change the algorithm, due to the black box nature of many AI tools, making such preapproval of modifications truly unfeasible.

The issue of evolving algorithms has been specifically addressed by the FDA, with a report outlining ideas for ensuring the continued and perpetual safety of these AI technologies.[17] The FDA framework categorizes AI-based SaMD innovations as either informing clinical management (as in non–black box CDS), driving clinical management (as in black box CDS), or treating and diagnosing (as in autonomous robotic surgery), with greater regulatory attention focused on the latter categories.[6] For those algorithms deemed high risk and also presenting challenges to regulation as outlined earlier, the FDA proposes implementing a Total Product Life Cycle (TPLC) approach to regulation.[6] This approach consists of 4 major steps: validation of the quality and reputation of the manufacturer to ensure trust in careful development and testing, review of safety and efficacy through testing on additional data other than that used for training, establishment of an agreed-upon protocol for changes given the potential needs and evolutionary characteristics of the specific algorithm, and extensive real-world monitoring of performance to ensure safety and efficacy are continuously demonstrated.[6] Manufacturer reviews would help alleviate black box concerns by ensuring that companies are collecting the best possible safety data and are proceeding in a responsible manner that minimizes the risk of undetectable problems that might threaten safety or efficacy. Real-world monitoring helps address the issue of evolution by continuously examining the algorithm as it evolves and providing ample opportunity to flag potential issues and terminate the use of algorithms that have grown problematic.

Ensuring Fairness and Equity

Many of the equity-focused initiatives seen in today's policy landscape are focused not on preventing new disparities and unfairness, but on implementing targeted interventions to reduce and/or eliminate current and long-standing disparities in health care. For example, the Health and Human Services Action Plan to Reduce Racial and Ethnic Health Disparities outlines an extensive plan to strengthen infrastructure and understanding in pursuit of increased equity in health care,[18] whereas the Centers for Disease Control and Prevention has sponsored and highlighted many health interventions focused on specific health behaviors in targeted populations.[19] In a surgery-specific context, the National Institutes of Health recently launched a research focus on disparities in surgical outcomes, providing funding to support research aimed at increasing equity in surgery.[20]

Although many initiatives are focused on being more inclusive, there are also some regulations in place to ensure that existing disparities are not exacerbated. Within the FDA, the Office of Minority Health and Health Equity (OMHHE) aims to "increase the amount of clinical trial data available on racial and ethnic minorities; improve the data quality to determine how minorities react to medical products; and increase transparency and access to available data."[21] Recognizing that drugs and devices may work differently in different populations, the OMHHE works to ensure that new medical innovations are tested on diverse populations and generalizable to the public. The OMHHE seeks to combat recent findings that many clinical trials, especially those focused on oncology and cardiovascular products, enroll at most 2% to 4% African Americans, considerably lower than their representation in the overall US population.[22] This imbalance in testing creates a potential risk that clinical products may be approved and marketed despite posing serious and undiscovered risks to certain minority populations.

Although AI may help uncover the causes of some existing disparities and thus help to reduce existing inequalities, the preventative role of policy in avoiding the introduction of new inequity is most relevant in the context of AI in surgery. To combat introduction of inequity into medicine through the use of AI innovations, it is critical to ensure the quality of data used for training and testing. The issue of data quality is not merely one of standardization or missing data points. Rather, data quality can be mapped to bias and specifically broken down into 2 forms of bias: (1) data that perpetuate existing biases and (2) data not representative of the patients on which the resulting algorithm is used.[23] Attention to these quality issues is critical to preventing AI from contributing to inequity in medicine.

There is a common misconception that AI cannot demonstrate bias because it has no cognitive capacity to do so. People view computers and AI algorithms as strictly logical and objective, observing patterns in data with no emotion or external context. However, when those data are generated by humans, they may well contain biases, and AI algorithms can see those biases as patterns in the data and perpetuate them.[24,25] Essentially, biased data give biased results. For example, in the 1990s, it was shown that African Americans with peripheral vascular disease were less likely to receive revascularization procedures and were instead more likely to receive amputation.[26] If an AI algorithm were trained to recommend procedures based on these data, it would preferentially suggest amputation for African American patients and revascularization for other patients, clearly perpetuating an inequitable and unacceptable medical bias.

Beyond perpetuating human biases, examination of some AI models trained on medical data has shown that the accuracy of predictions varies based on gender and ethnicity.[27] The applications of this observation are multifold. First, it is imperative that the data on which an algorithm is trained are representative of the patients on whom the algorithm will be applied. Along with this, testing and approval of algorithms must be done on diverse patients. This is in line with the work of the FDA OMHHE. One can imagine that an algorithm trained entirely on the medical records of white males would not perform particularly well on an African American woman, nor would an algorithm trained on data from patients at a cutting-edge urban hospital work well on patients from a small, rural hospital. One potential approach to such concerns would be to train an algorithm on a narrow segmentation of patients and only recommend its use on patients fitting that categorization. Yet this strategy raises a second concern, which is that of inequity in design and application. A utilitarian may argue that those patients addressed by the narrow algorithm are helped while nobody is actively harmed; therefore, such an approach is valuable and acceptable. In contrast, others may feel that any inequity should be avoided. Precedent from the FDA suggests acceptance of the former view. In 2005, a heart failure drug, BiDil (hydralazine and isosorbide dinitrate), was approved for use only in black populations after the discovery in clinical trials that it was effective solely in that population.[28] One could argue that the FDA may not feel as comfortable making such an approval for an AI tool that widens a disparity rather than shrinks it. Regardless, it is apparent that health policy must undertake the challenge of answering these difficult questions about bias and the demographic composition of medical data for AI development.

While general concerns involving equity and AI in surgery have now been outlined, it should be noted that opaque algorithms heighten such concerns. Without a clear and explainable demonstration of the patterns discovered by an AI algorithm, it is challenging to establish whether these patterns map to racial or sociodemographic characteristics, nor can it be shown that decisions made by AI did not draw heavily on these demographics in lieu of available medical information.[29] While ensuring fairness and equity with medical AI is always important, it must be approached with particular care when using black box algorithms to ensure that outputs are not biased.

Although EMRs have made it easier to compile and analyze medical data at the hospital level, that data infrastructure remains greatly fragmented on the national level.[30] This limits the quantity of data that can be aggregated by isolating silos of medical information in incompatible islands and imposing a significant burden on anyone undertaking the challenge of assembling a large data set for AI development. Such lack of data aggregation could also prove challenging in postmarket surveillance as part of the TPLC approach, as described earlier in the "Ensuring Safety and Efficacy" section. In addition, beyond the challenge to aggregated quantity, this fractured infrastructure makes difficult the customization of algorithms to different hospitals.[30] Recognizing that safe, effective, and equitable integration of AI into medicine requires accurate representation of target populations in training data sets, algorithms may require adjustment and retraining in specific hospitals and populations. A system in which data live in different formats in each hospital makes adjusting algorithms to specific patient populations highly burdensome, if not outright impossible. Given the numerous challenges data fragmentation presents to AI regulation in surgery, it is an issue that must be addressed if AI is to become ubiquitous in surgery and other medical applications.

Although there are multiple ways to approach overcoming the fragmented data infrastructure currently faced by developers and regulators, there are 2 major paths forward. The first would be to create incentives for good data management and sharing and to build upon systems that have been identified as successful.[30] The second and more extreme approach would be to build an aggregated data portal and to mandate that health care organizations store their clinical data within such a portal (see Chapter 18).[30] Such an aggregated system would make it easier for companies to access high-quality and equitable data and for the FDA to review the data and validate those data as acceptable for algorithm training. Regardless of how such data integration and transparency is achieved, it is clear that new policy ensuring quality of medical data will be critical to ensuring the equity of new AI algorithms and to making certain that they do not perpetuate or initiate biases or disparities in surgical care.

Ensuring Privacy and Confidentiality

An understanding of the importance of privacy and confidentiality in medicine dates back as far as the Hippocratic Oath, which mandates, "What I may see or hear in the course of the treatment or even outside of the treatment in regard to the life of men, which on no account must be spread abroad, I will keep to myself, holding such things shameful to be spoken about."[31] This mandate of confidentiality was explicitly codified in American law with the passage of the Health Insurance Portability and Accountability Act (HIPAA) regulations[32] and was further extended to electronic health records with the Health Information Technology for Economic and Clinical Health (HITECH) amendment.[33] HIPAA regulations apply to all health plans, health providers, and business associates, but notably do not apply to other private companies. These regulations prevent the release, sharing, or sale of any identifiable medical data. It should be noted that deidentified data is not covered under HIPAA and may be shared or sold, so long as those deidentified data do not contain information with which someone could reasonably reidentify individuals within the data set.[34]

These HIPAA regulations provide the first point of potential concern in making health care data available to companies or researchers for AI development. It is clear from HIPAA guidelines that it would be impermissible for hospitals to make identifiable data available, whether publicly or only to a specific external organization. Current rules offer no prohibitions on deidentified data, however, so there is a legal pathway by which organizations can obtain the requisite data to develop AI tools. It should not be forgotten, however, that HIPAA only permits deidentified data if it cannot be reasonably reidentified. Specifically, the Privacy Rule within HIPAA states that "health information that does not identify an individual and with respect to which there is no reasonable basis to believe that the information can be used to identify an individual is not individually identifiable health information."[32] Although this concept of reasonable basis for reidentification may traditionally have been interpreted as referring to phone numbers, addresses, and other information that could easily be linked back to an identity, the rise of AI has forced a reconsideration of what should be considered a reasonable basis for reidentification. Recent research has proven the feasibility of reidentifying individuals within a large data set stripped of protected information using machine learning techniques.[35] In addition, private companies with access to deidentified data could reidentify patients by linking deidentified medical data to other data they possess, such as search terms or locations, and would be within their rights to do so.[36] The capacity for reidentifying medical data raises significant privacy concerns and suggests the current HIPAA privacy guidelines may need reconsideration or clarification to create more stringent standards for deidentification.

If medical data are sufficiently deidentified, HIPAA guidelines do not regulate their distribution and even permit their sale. Beyond privacy, the potential for sale of health care data raises 2 further policy concerns. For one, there is the potential that hospitals may sell their medical data to the highest bidder or in other ways restrict its distribution in the interest of profit.[37] This restrictive sharing is not merely speculation. Memorial Sloan Kettering signed a deal in 2018 to share their tissue slides exclusively with a new AI start-up, igniting significant controversy.[38] Such exclusivity could stifle AI innovation by limiting the availability of the data necessary for algorithm training and development. Additionally, deidentified data are often shared without patient consent. This action is generally considered acceptable given the potential to advance health care research and the minimal potential harm to patients, so long as proper confidentiality and deidentification are maintained.[39] However, once those data are used not just for research but for profit as well, it is not hard to imagine patients demanding a share of the proceeds or objecting outright to the sale of their data.[39] Despite judicial challenges, the Supreme Court of the United States has upheld the right of health care organizations to sell medical data as long as they are not in violation of HIPAA regulations.[40] Although this might prevent an outright ban on sale of medical data, a mandated centralized data portal, as described in the earlier "Ensuring Fairness and Equity" section, could combat this concern by devaluing the data generated by any particular health care organization and ensuring that all developers can access the data necessary to innovate.

Protecting Patient Rights

Although the confidentiality of health care information is an essential patient right, patient rights are also safeguarded through the process of informed consent. Informed consent is particularly relevant in the surgical field given the need for patient approval for all procedures. Although there is not a unified policy definition of informed consent, the American Medical Association suggests that proper informed consent requires fully educating a patient of sound mind on the intended intervention and its potential risks and benefits and then obtaining that patient's permission to proceed.[41] Essentially, patients have a right to know what is being done to them and to make their own appraisal of the risk-benefit trade-off. Although the definition of proper informed consent itself may not be outlined in current health policy, there are certainly laws protecting individual rights and patient rights specifically, and the application of these laws makes informed consent inseparable from health policy. Failure to obtain proper informed consent undermines a patient's autonomy, which in a policy context can strengthen a malpractice lawsuit or, in the case of surgery, lead to a criminal battery charge for undesired physical contact with a patient.[42]

Black box algorithms present a significant barrier to informed consent. Even if a clinician is fully trained and informed about a black box algorithm that will be used as part of their surgical process, that physician is incapable of describing to a patient exactly how that algorithm works and how its conclusions are drawn or what risks may lurk in its opaque structure. Although physicians could share everything they know and still obtain consent from a patient, it is not apparent that this consent would be truly informed. This raises both ethical and legal issues, as patients have a right to know what they are agreeing to and failure to adequately inform a patient could leave a doctor using black box AI tools open to increased liability in the event of a medical or AI error.[43]

Some may feel that concerns about informed consent and AI are unfounded because patients already consent frequently to procedures for which they do not have a full and extensive understanding of the underlying biology. There is a clear difference, however, between lack of mechanistic understanding by a patient and the use of a black box algorithm, as will be illustrated using the example introduced earlier concerning activating Google Maps using voice controls. There is an interesting distinction in this example between a true black box, like the voice recognition algorithm that uses a neural network,[44] and a client-facing black box, like the map algorithm, which likely uses a comprehensible pathfinding algorithm,[45] albeit an algorithm hidden to the client in the interest of maintaining a competitive edge.[46] In medicine, patients are often willing to accept client-facing black boxes, taking drugs or undergoing procedures without demanding a full explanation of the underlying biology and pathway of influence governing the intervention. Patients are comfortable with such a lack of information because they trust that their doctors are aware of the detailed information and would raise any relevant risks or worries. A true black box unknown even to physicians, however, raises greater concerns, and these are the novel consent scenarios that could be created through the incorporation of AI into surgical practice.

To address concerns about consent with opaque AI, policy will need to implement deliberate safeguards to protect patient autonomy and informed decision making. First, even if patients cannot fully understand the underlying structure of an algorithm, they can be presented with the best available safety data to aid in making their own cost-benefit analysis.

The FDA has indicated its intent to collect such data to aid in postmarket surveillance, and such data could be provided not only to FDA regulators but also to physicians with the intention of passing it on to patients to help guide the decision-making process.[6] Furthermore, surveys have shown that many patients are concerned by the use of AI in their care and are especially unwilling to undergo hypothetical surgery under the hand of an autonomous robot.[43] If these AI tools are demonstrated to be safer and more effective, clinicians can indicate this to patients and make their recommendations but must be careful to acknowledge and understand the fears of patients and to not overly pressure them into an AI guided procedure to which they do not wish to consent.[43] In addition, policy should mandate a requisite level of understanding that physicians must have about AI and about the black box problem in order to properly convey these issues to patients and obtain informed consent, whether through training by companies developing AI tools or through incorporation into the medical school curriculum.[47,48]

Malpractice and Medical Errors

When patients or their families feel they have been harmed by insufficient or improper medical care, they can file a malpractice lawsuit. Health policy governs the liabilities and burdens of proof involved in such a case. Although there are many kinds of malpractice, this discussion will be limited to malpractice resulting from a medical device error, as that is the closest analogy to malpractice arising from an error in AI software.

In medical device malpractice cases, there are 3 stakeholders with potential liability: the surgeon, the hospital, and the device manufacturer.[12] Although the hospital is responsible for proper installation and maintenance of a medical device or software tool, most other liability lies with the physician or manufacturer.[12] As described earlier in discussing safety and efficacy, PMA approval can absolve device manufacturers of all liability should a defect in their product cause harm. The much more popular 510(k) approval pathway does not offer this benefit to manufacturers. In these situations, a manufacturer is liable for harms if it can be demonstrated that they should have known their product had a default or that they erred in manufacturing the particular device that caused harm.[12]

Even if a device is properly designed, there are always potential risks to the use of a device or software tool in surgery. If patients are not informed of these risks, it could constitute malpractice, but manufacturers can avoid such liability through the learned intermediary doctrine, which states that it is sufficient for manufacturers to notify physicians of these risks, and physicians are then liable if they do not pass on that information to patients.[49] To fully transfer liability and avoid claims related to device misuse, manufacturers must also fully educate doctors on how devices work and how to use them properly.[12] As a final note, some software tools, including CDS systems, do not place any liability on the manufacturer because these tools are considered to be merely providing information to a clinician who must then evaluate that information and interpret it. In so doing, a physician accepts full responsibility for the outcomes of their decision.[50]

As has been discussed repeatedly, it can be impossible to understand the thought process of a black box algorithm and, therefore, impossible to verify that such an algorithm will never make a mistake. To this point, courts have viewed software as simply a supporting tool to a physician and shifted responsibility for interpreting and acting on the output of such software to the physician.[51] Although this legal precedent offers a general guidance for CDS software, it is unclear whether such precedent will extend to black box algorithms, as they cannot provide doctors with sufficient explanation to permit causal analysis and allow effective clinician oversight and interpretation.

Imagine a situation in which a surgeon receives a recommendation from an AI tool that seems clearly wrong and goes against all of his or her medical training. Should the surgeon follow this recommendation? If he or she does follow this recommendation and serious consequences arise for the patient, is the surgeon liable for those consequences as a result of not overruling the AI? Alternatively, if the AI system has been proven in studies to improve the quality of care, would the surgeon be liable if he or she overrules the system and thus removes what has been demonstrated to be the standard of care?[52] The surgeon in this scenario finds him- or herself in a clear catch-22, in which law offers no clear guidance on how to proceed and every choice seems fraught with the potential for a lawsuit. To ensure surgeons are comfortable in adopting AI tools and incorporating them into surgical practice, a clear legal roadmap will need to offer guidelines on how to proceed in such scenarios.

CDS is not the only role AI might play in surgery, and other uses pose their own concerns for tort and liability. Should AI algorithms begin performing robotic surgery, it is unclear how liability for errors will be assigned. Although precedent establishes that the robot itself cannot be held liable, it is apparent that the manufacturing company, the overseeing surgeon, or the hospital responsible for maintenance could theoretically be liable, and new regulation will need to clarify how these situations should be legally approached.[53]

Surgical Training and Competency

Even if responsible software developers working within a well-developed policy framework create AI tools that are fair, safe, and ethical, injecting these new technologies into surgery without care for the implications could prove dangerous and irresponsible. Health policy, therefore, must not only govern AI, but must also govern AI implementation and the ways in which surgery might change to accommodate it. Specifically, 2 major threats are deskilling of surgeons and errors due to overreliance on AI.

The surgical training process is extensive and includes years of practice and learning before certification.[54] After this certification, however, there is little regulation imposed to ensure that surgeons continue to practice at a peak skill level. Continuing education and decennial exams guarantee some continued learning and engagement with new best practices, but there is no procedure-based exam to ensure maintenance of surgical skills.[54] With the emerging potential for autonomous robotic surgeons, there is the potential for these surgical skills to become less frequently used by human surgeons. Concerningly, this reduction in practice could lead to deskilling and a decline in the capability of surgeons to perform challenging surgeries.[55] With the risks of power outages, broken machinery, or lack of consent by patients for AI-driven surgery, there will always be a need for capable human surgeons, and thus policy must ensure that skills are maintained even as they are less frequently applied. In addition, there is a concern that doctors may grow to overly rely on their AI tools, replacing a healthy dose of skepticism with blind trust and failing to spot and correct errors.[52]

In considering how best to approach maintenance of skills and focus, it is helpful to consider airline pilots and the analogous rise of autopilot tools. Pilots no longer need many of the skills they historically used every time they flew. Yet, in the event of an error, these pilots must be able to perform those skills at an incredibly high level, with stakes of life or death. Research into airline pilots has shown that their physical skills decline over time after completing training because they are generally relying on autopilot to take on many of the flight duties.[56] Even beyond these physical declines, it has been found that pilots suffer declines of focus and mental skills and that wandering minds lead to fewer mistakes being caught.[57] In plane flight, pilot skill maintenance is achieved mostly through the use of flight simulators, which allow pilots to practice their skills without implementing them in real flights where autopilot is the preferred technique. A similar model could be implemented in surgery, where surgical simulators have been shown to improve the performance of surgeons.[58-60] As with many of the regulatory needs outlined in this chapter, a sparse regulatory approach has proved sufficient to this point in maintaining surgical skills. However, the changes ushered in by AI adoption are significant and will require novel regulation to ensure safety and efficacy are maintained moving forward.

CONCLUSION

AI has the potential to transform the delivery of surgical care. Yet, as with any new medical innovation, it is important to examine both the promising and untoward consequences of AI for all stakeholders. This chapter has highlighted the unique aspects of AI that need to be considered for health policy design, including maintaining large amounts of data, deconstructing the black box, and the need for an iterative review process. In addition, key tenets of a health policy framework have been identified, including ensuring safety, efficacy, and equity for patients; maintaining the privacy and confidentiality of patient data; protecting patient rights; ensuring accountability for errors; and ensuring the maintenance of surgical skills. The current sparsity of regulation for surgical procedures may present challenges to more detailed and centralized regulation governing expansion of AI into surgery. Although new regulation may be met with hesitation by some, the integration of AI into the delivery of surgical care may come at a faster pace than we anticipate, and it is paramount to establish sound regulation that will evolve at the pace of technology.

Given the many complexities and cross-cutting problems presented by AI integration, a centralized, multidisciplinary task force composed of surgeons, data scientists, and nongovernmental and governmental members may be optimal in overseeing the expansion of AI in surgery. Regardless of whether novel regulation is achieved through a unified body or through dispersed regulatory action, however, there are clear steps that must be undertaken to ensure a responsible implementation of AI in surgery. Minimum safety and efficacy standards must be established, and these must evolve beyond current FDA criteria because AI is not static and its constructs are not easily delineated. Guidelines regarding data management, protection of patient autonomy, and accountability in the event of errors must also be clearly established. Private-public partnerships can be leveraged for the creation of timely and iterative processes needed to maintain and monitor AI technology and ensure the continuing education of surgical providers. Although it is not yet clear what path forward will be taken in establishing regulation for AI in surgery, it is clear that the unique aspects of AI present serious obstacles to current surgical regulations. Implementing clear and consistent oversight through new regulation is imperative to ensuring that AI can achieve its promise of improving surgical outcomes and efficiency while avoiding the risks of widening disparities or causing harm.

▌ REFERENCES

1. Rappel JK, Lahiri A, Chee Leong T. A digital stereo microscope platform for microsurgery training. In: Cheng SM, Day MY, eds. *Technologies and Applications of Artificial Intelligence*. TAAI 2014. Lecture Notes in Computer Science, vol 8916. Springer; 2014.

2. Zheng G. *Intelligent Orthopaedics: Artificial Intelligence and Smart Image-Guided Technology for Orthopaedics*. Springer Berlin Heidelberg; 2018.

3. Yoo TK, Ryu IH, Lee G, et al. Adopting machine learning to automatically identify candidate patients for corneal refractive surgery. *NPJ Digit Med.* 2019;2(1):59.

4. Bertsimas D, Dunn J, Velmahos GC, Kaafarani HMA. Surgical risk is not linear: derivation and validation of a novel, user-friendly, and machine-learning-based Predictive OpTimal Trees in Emergency Surgery Risk (POTTER) Calculator. *Ann Surg.* 2018;268(4):574-583.

5. Darrow JJ. Explaining the absence of surgical procedure regulation. *Cornell J Law Public Policy.* 2017;27(1):189-206.

6. US Food and Drug Administration. Proposed regulatory framework for modifications to artificial intelligence/machine learning (AI/ML)-based software as a medical device (SaMD): discussion paper and request for feedback. 2019. Accessed October 7, 2020. https://www.regulations.gov/document?D=FDA-2019-N-1185-0001.

7. Castelvecchi D. Can we open the black box of AI? *Nature.* 2016;538(7623):20-23.

8. Rapoport A. A probabilistic approach to networks. *Social Netw.* 1979;2(1):1-18.

9. The Medical Device Amendments of 1976 ("MDA"), Pub. L. No. 94-295, 90 Stat. 539 (1976),

10. International Medical Device Regulators Forum SaMD Working Group. Software as a medical device (SaMD): key definitions. December 9, 2013. Accessed October 7, 2020. http://www.imdrf.org/docs/imdrf/final/technical/imdrf-tech-131209-samd-key-definitions-140901.pdf.

11. US Food and Drug Administration. Report on non-device software functions: impact to health and best practices. December, 2018. Accessed October 7, 2020. https://www.fda.gov/media/119187/download.

12. McLean T. The complexity of litigation associated with robotic surgery and cybersurgery. *Int J Med Robot.* 2007;3:23-29.

13. US Department of Health and Human Services, Center for Devices and Radiological Health, Center for Biologics Evaluation and Research. Guidance for the content of premarket submissions for software contained in medical devices. May 11, 2005. Accessed October 7, 2020. https://www.fda.gov/media/73065/download.

14. US Food and Drug Administration. PMA clinical studies. Published 2019. Accessed September 13, 2019. https://www.fda.gov/medical-devices/premarket-approval-pma/pma-clinical-studies.

15. 21st Century Cures Act, Pub. L. No. 114-255, 130 Stat. 1033 (2016).

16. US Food and Drug Administration. PMA supplements and amendments. Published 2019. Accessed September 20, 2019. https://www.fda.gov/medical-devices/premarket-approval-pma/pma-supplements-and-amendments.

17. US Food and Drug Administration. Statement from FDA Commissioner Scott Gottlieb, M.D. on steps toward a new, tailored review framework for artificial intelligence-based medical devices. April 2, 2019. Accessed October 7, 2020. https://www.fda.gov/news-events/press-announcements/statement-fda-commissioner-scott-gottlieb-md-steps-toward-new-tailored-review-framework-artificial.

18. US Department of Health and Human Services. HHS action plan to reduce racial and ethnic health disparities. April, 2011. Accessed October 7, 2020. https://www.minorityhealth.hhs.gov/npa/files/Plans/HHS/HHS_Plan_complete.pdf.

19. US Centers for Disease Control and Prevention. Strategies for reducing health disparities: selected CDC-sponsored interventions, United States, 2014. April 18, 2014. Accessed October 7, 2020. https://www.cdc.gov/mmwr/pdf/other/su6301.pdf.

20. National Institutes of Health. NIH launches research program to reduce health disparities in surgical outcomes. April 18, 2016. Accessed October 7, 2020. https://www.nih.gov/news-events/news-releases/nih-launches-research-program-reduce-health-disparities-surgical-outcomes.

21. US Food and Drug Administration. Office of Minority Health and Health Equity. Published 2018. Accessed September 9, 2019. https://www.fda.gov/about-fda/office-commissioner/office-minority-health-and-health-equity.

22. US Food and Drug Administration. Drug trials snapshots summary report (2015 and 2016). Accessed October 7, 2020. https://www.fda.gov/drugs/drug-approvals-and-databases/drug-trials-snapshots-summary-report-2015-and-2016.

23. Vayena E, Blasimme A, Cohen IG. Machine learning in medicine: addressing ethical challenges. *PLoS Med.* 2018;15(11):e1002689-e1002689.

24. Rajkomar A, Hardt M, Howell MD, Corrado G, Chin MH. Ensuring fairness in machine learning to advance health equity. *Ann Intern Med.* 2018;169(12):866-872.

25. Gianfrancesco MA, Tamang S, Yazdany J, Schmajuk G. Potential biases in machine learning algorithms using electronic health record data. *JAMA Intern Med.* 2018;178(11):1544-1547.

26. Guadagnoli E, Ayanian JZ, Gibbons G, McNeil BJ, LoGerfo FW. The influence of race on the use of surgical procedures for treatment of peripheral vascular disease of the lower extremities. *Arch Surg.* 1995;130(4):381-386.

27. Chen IY, Szolovits P, Ghassemi M. Can AI help reduce disparities in general medical and mental health care? *AMA J Ethics.* 2019;21(2):E167-E179.

28. Associated Press. FDA approves first race-specific medication. June 23, 2005. Accessed October 7, 2020. http://www.nbcnews.com/id/8336206/ns/health-heart_health/t/fda-approves-first-race-specific-medication/#.X35QyWhKjIU.

29. Khullar D. A.I. could worsen health disparities. *The New York Times.* January 31, 2019. Accessed October 7, 2020. https://www.nytimes.com/2019/01/31/opinion/ai-bias-healthcare.html.

30. Panch T, Mattie H, Celi LA. The "inconvenient truth" about AI in healthcare. *NPJ Digit Med.* 2019;2(1):77.

31. Rothstein MA. The Hippocratic bargain and health information technology. *J Law Med Ethics.* 2010;38(1):7-13.

32. Health Insurance Portability and Accountability Act (HIPAA), 110 Stat. 1936 (1996).

33. Health Information Technology for Economic and Clinical Health (HITECH) Act, 123 Stat. 226 (2009).

34. US Department of Health and Human Services. Summary of the HIPAA privacy rule. Published 2013. Accessed September 3, 2019. https://www.hhs.gov/hipaa/for-professionals/privacy/laws-regulations/index.html.

35. Na L, Yang C, Lo C-C, Zhao F, Fukuoka Y, Aswani A. Feasibility of reidentifying individuals in large national physical activity data sets from which protected health information has been removed with use of machine learning. *JAMA Network Open.* 2018;1(8):e186040-e186040.

36. Cohen IG, Mello MM. Big data, big tech, and protecting patient privacy. *JAMA.* 2019;322(12):1141-1142.

37. Hollis KF. To share or not to share: ethical acquisition and use of medical data. *AMIA Jt Summits Transl Sci Proc.* 2016;2016:420-427.

38. Ornstein C, Thomas K. Sloan Kettering's cozy deal with start-up ignites a new uproar. *The New York Times,* September 20, 2018. Accessed October 7, 2020. https://www.nytimes.com/2018/09/20/health/memorial-sloan-kettering-cancer-paige-ai.html.

39. Rothstein MA. Is deidentification sufficient to protect health privacy in research? *Am J Bioeth.* 2010;10(9):3-11.

40. *William H. Sorrell, Attorney General of Vermont Et Al., Petitioners v. IMS Health Inc. Et Al.* (Supreme Court of the United States, 2011).

41. American Medical Association. Informed consent: code of medical ethics opinion 2.1.1. Published 2019. Accessed September 4, 2019. https://www.ama-assn.org/delivering-care/ethics/informed-consent.

42. Raab EL. The parameters of informed consent. *Trans Am Ophthalmol Soc.* 2004;102:225-232.

43. Schiff D, Borenstein J. How should clinicians communicate with patients about the roles of artificially intelligent team members? *AMA J Ethics.* 2019;21(2): E138-E145.

44. Chan W, Jaitly N, Le Q, Vinyals O. Listen, attend and spell: a neural network for large vocabulary conversational speech recognition. Paper presented at 2016 IEEE International Conference on Acoustics, Speech and Signal Processing, March 20-25, 2016. Accessed October 7, 2020. https://arxiv.org/abs/1508.01211.

45. Yin C, Wang H. Developed Dijkstra shortest path search algorithm and simulation. Paper presented at 2010 International Conference on Computer Design and

Applications, June 25-27, 2010. Accessed October 7, 2020. https://ieeexplore.ieee
.org/document/5541129.

46. Burrell J. How the machine "thinks": understanding opacity in machine learning algorithms. *Big Data Soc.* 2016;3(1):2053951715622512.

47. Char DS, Shah NH, Magnus D. Implementing machine learning in health care: addressing ethical challenges. *N Engl J Med.* 2018;378(11):981-983.

48. Wartman S, Combs CD. Reimagining medical education in the age of AI. *AMA J Ethics.* 2019;21(2):E146-E152.

49. Nelson J. Arizona high court reestablishes the "learned intermediary" doctrine. Practice Points. Vol 2019. American Bar Association, 2016. Accessed October 7, 2020. https://www.americanbar.org/groups/litigation/committees/mass-torts/practice/2016/learned-intermediary-doctrine/.

50. Brown SH, Miller RA. Legal and regulatory issues related to the use of clinical software in health care delivery. In: Greenes RA, ed. *Clinical Decision Support.* 2nd ed. Academic Press; 2014:711-740.

51. Price WN. Artificial intelligence in health care: applications and legal issues. University of Michigan Public Law Research Paper No 599. 2017;14(10). Accessed October 7, 2020. https://repository.law.umich.edu/cgi/viewcontent.cgi?article=2932&context=articles.

52. Froomkin AM, Kerr IR, Pineau J. When AIs outperform doctors: confronting the challenges of a tort-induced over-reliance on machine learning. University of Miami Legal Studies Research Paper No 18-3. 2019;61(33). Accessed October 7, 2020. https://papers.ssrn.com/sol3/papers.cfm?abstract_id=3114347.

53. O'Sullivan S, Nevejans N, Allen C, et al. Legal, regulatory, and ethical frameworks for development of standards in artificial intelligence (AI) and autonomous robotic surgery. *Int J Med Robot Comput Assist Surg.* 2019;15(1):e1968.

54. Malangoni MA, Shiffer CD. The American Board of Surgery maintenance of certification program: the first 10 years. Accessed October 7, 2020. https://bulletin.facs.org/2015/07/the-american-board-of-surgery-maintenance-of-certification-program-the-first-10-years/#:~:text=The%20American%20Board%20of%20Surgery%20Maintenance%20of%20Certification,and%20discusses%20possible%20future%20directions%20for%20the%20program.

55. Lu J. Will medical technology deskill doctors? *Int Educ Studies.* 2016;9:7.

56. Ebbatson M, Harris D, Huddlestone J, Sears R. The relationship between manual handling performance and recent flying experience in air transport pilots. *Ergonomics.* 2010;53(2):268-277.

57. Casner SM, Schooler JW. Thoughts in flight: automation use and pilots' task-related and task-unrelated thought. *Hum Factors.* 2013;56(3):433-442.

58. Edmond CV Jr. Impact of the endoscopic sinus surgical simulator on operating room performance. *Laryngoscope.* 2002;112(7 Pt 1):1148-1158.

59. Hamilton EC, Scott DJ, Kapoor A, et al. Improving operative performance using a laparoscopic hernia simulator. *Am J Surg.* 2001;182(6):725-728.

60. Stefanidis D, Sevdalis N, Paige J, et al. Simulation in surgery: what's needed next? *Ann Surg.* 2015;261(5):846-853.

PRACTICAL CONSIDERATIONS IN UTILIZATION OF COMPUTER VISION

16

Thomas Ward

HIGHLIGHTS

- Adherence to and compliance with local laws and regulations in data capture, storage, and use are just as important as compliance with accepted ethical guidelines around research.
- True anonymization and full deidentification of data are difficult to achieve. Appropriate measures must be in place to ensure optimal protection of patient privacy.
- To obtain a reliable result in your research, establishing a well-planned database structure for storage and access to data is as important as your machine learning model and analysis.

INTRODUCTION

Computer vision is a young field. Its current era started in 2012 with Krizhevsky's application of deep convolutional neural networks,[1] and this "deep learning revolution" made accurate image and video classification a reality with a resultant explosion in computer vision research (nearly 30,000 publications in 2017). The medical community, though, has underperformed in contributions, with less than 1000 annual publications in artificial intelligence.[2] Computer vision medical research, particularly that focused on surgery, is therefore an even smaller slice of the pie.

With a paucity of research groups, there is no definitive roadmap to creating an effective medical computer vision group. New labs will inevitably encounter hurdles and unforeseen complications. Our group, the Surgical Artificial Intelligence and Innovation Laboratory (SAIIL) at the Massachusetts General Hospital (MGH), is one of just a handful of groups that focus on computer vision and surgery. Using our laboratory's experience, this chapter will provide a roadmap to navigating these poorly charted waters.

Overview

Key Point

Chapters 6, 7, 8, and 10 in particular touch on various research questions that have been tackled in the field of surgical computer vision.

Prior to embarking on a computer vision study in surgery, a researcher must first determine a question to address. This question will be unique to each group's interests, with common computer vision problems including operative temporal segmentation, phase recognition, tool recognition, operative skill assessment, and clinical decision support. Once there is a question, one must then identify the appropriate technical expertise in answering the question.

As with any research, the selection of appropriate methodology is critical. Thus, the first recommendation for anyone looking to engage in computer vision research is to partner with an expert in, at least, the technical aspects of the field. Guidance from a PhD-trained expert will help you refine your question to be specific, measurable, and achievable while also preventing you from falling into common traps regarding data set selection and model evaluation.

Although the specifics for any particular research project will vary, the remaining chapter will review the 3 major considerations when conducting research in surgical computer vision:

1. Data acquisition and preparation
2. Data annotation
3. Modeling

▌ DATA ACQUISITION AND PREPARATION

Machine learning and computer vision models live or die on their data inputs. For these image and video data to be useful for modeling, they must go through a multistep pipeline. First, researchers must acquire data, either from a publicly available data set or from data captured de novo. Second, the data must be processed to a standardized format for use with the modeling tools. Finally, the data need proper labels for supervised model training. Although this pipeline seems straightforward, it actually presents numerous challenges. Without consideration of the various minutiae, a research group will ultimately lose months and years in data preparation, which for such a fast-moving field as machine learning translates to numerous research discoveries lost to other groups.

Existing Data Sets

As a relatively nascent field bound by numerous health privacy regulations, few publicly available medical data sets for computer vision in surgery exist. Most readily available medical data sets consist of radiographic images or clinical still images. For example, the KiTS19 Challenge Data has computed tomography (CT) images and clinical outcomes for 300 patients with kidney tumors.[3] Other data sets include the ChestX-ray8 (>100,000 chest x-rays for 32,000 patients), Messidor (1200 eye fundus images for diabetic retinopathy), and HAM10000 (10,000 dermatoscopic images).[4-6] Many more examples are centrally located on the Cancer Imaging Archive (TCIA).[7]

Although there are several medical image data sets, few have data that can answer surgical questions. Ophthalmology groups have generated some useful data sets from their procedures. These procedures lend themselves to recording because they occur in a nonmoving field under a microscope. The CATARACTS data set holds 15 cataract operations with included surgical tool labels.[8] Zisimopoulos et al[9] built upon this data set by adding labels for the surgical phases. The same group then, over a select 200 frames per video, performed highly granular labeling of tools and anatomy for the CATARACTS data set.[10]

Laparoscopic and robotic-assisted surgery similarly lends itself to video recording given the camera stability and continuous video feed inherent to minimally invasive operations. One group published a small data set of 9 partial nephrectomies that included surgical phase annotations.[11] The 2017 Robotic Instrument Segmentation Challenge also published nephrectomy videos, although their data set contained robotic instrument data for 10 sequences of porcine abdominal operations.[12] Another robotic instrument data set comes from the JIGSAWS study, with videos of a robotic surgery system performing surgical tasks on a model. Their data set includes annotations for instrument kinematics, surgical gestures, and operator skill.[13]

Multiple groups have also published data sets for laparoscopic cholecystectomies. The Computational Analysis and Modeling of Medical Activities (CAMMA) group in Strasbourg, France, has released a series of successively larger data sets, and their most recent publicly available data set contains 80 surgeries with annotations for both surgical phases and tools.[14] Technische Universität München (TUM) released another data set, the TUM LapChole, which has 20 surgeries with annotated surgical phases.[15]

These examples are, for the time being, a nearly comprehensive list of surgical video data sets. Unfortunately, the vast majority of surgical computer vision questions cannot be answered with this little data. Therefore, most computer vision groups will need to pursue de novo data acquisition, which brings its own unique set of challenges.

New Data Set Creation

Medical media acquisition is a process fraught with hurdles and challenges. This section presents an overview map with acquisition of surgical video as a case example to help with navigation of this difficult process, starting from steps that precede even data acquisition and ending with labeled data suitable for computer vision modeling.

First, prior to media acquisition, one must obtain patient and institutional consent. These processes are specific to the institution's policies and its country's laws. Some institutions have media recording consent included in all procedure consents, whereas others require specific consent forms or addenda to allow for video recording of an operation. This may vary based on each individual institution's culture regarding use of video for quality improvement, education, and research purposes. For the time being, US regulations are simpler to comply with than data regulation laws in Europe, especially General Data Protection Regulation (GDPR). Because regulations are apt to change year to year, all researchers should use the available resources of their institution to maintain compliance at all times. It is the responsibility of the investigator to ensure that all data are captured in an ethical manner that preserves patient autonomy and privacy.

Once a patient grants permission to capture media, there are then many ways to actually capture the raw data. Early standardization of the capturing process will yield the most useful data without needing to discard ultimately inutile captures. All data should be captured at the highest quality and resolution possible. Capturing devices (eg, cameras, video recorders) save the visual data in various file formats. File formats are either "lossless" or "lossy." Lossy formats, to save disk space, compress similar data together (eg, various shades of blue will save to the disk as just one type of blue). There are many common examples for both images (JPEG, WMP) and videos (MPEG-4, Quicktime).[16,17] Using a lossy format may save an image that appears to the human eye identical to the original photo. To computer vision models, though, which analyze at the pixel level, this compression may negatively hamper analysis and model performance. Astronomy, with its massive petabyte level of data input, has dealt with this trade-off extensively and still argues for highest-resolution input.[18]

The importance of capture process standardization cannot be emphasized enough. Capture devices should ideally be identical or at least of similar capabilities. In the early stages of our data acquisition, we had disparate video capture devices that ultimately led to significant downstream headaches with differences in file formats, captured metadata, and video quality. Even for simple photo acquisition, there are numerous variables to consider for standardization (eg, image orientation, ambient light, flash vs no flash). Although images can be processed after acquisition through normalization techniques, *a priori* consideration of the needs of a project will allow for more robust data capture.

Even the most perfect capture plan falls short if it fails to capture a sufficient quantity of data. Although the process of hitting a record button seems to be an easy task, asking already busy nurses and physicians to add an additional step to only certain procedures will inevitably lead to poor initial data capture. Institutions may have a "culture of capture," where video recording becomes the default rather than the exception—primarily for purposes of patient safety and quality improvement. The work performed with the OR Black Box (see Chapter 10) is an excellent example of how a culture of capture can assist in improving acquisition of surgical video data.

All personnel in the operating room should ideally be trained to use the data capture devices so that recording video does not become dependent on one individual (eg, most often the circulating nurse). For institutions that do not already routinely record surgical video, there may be significant inertia to changing workflows to accommodate video recording, even when the change in workflow involves just pressing the "record" button on a preexisting device. Communicating clearly the value of the recordings in potentially improving patient care can help with acceptance. For example, the research video database could be used not only for computer vision projects but also as a repository for surgeons to compare their techniques to other surgeons, review cases during morbidity and mortality conferences, and instruct residents. Do not be discouraged with initially low video yields; as more and more people record and the culture changes, increasing media capture will happen.

Once surgical media is captured reliably, the data must be centralized and processed. Ideally, capture systems, such as operative video recorders, will connect to the hospital's network and allow for easy transfer of data to a central, secure repository. If not, regular weekly data pulls should occur to prevent buildup of data and possible lost footage. Having various media files scattered across different laptops, flash drives, and computers can lead to data loss and risk patient privacy. Rapid centralization prevents inadvertent data loss and also increases the informational security of the group. This centralized data storage must also undergo regular secure backups. The American Society of Media Photographers proposes the 3-2-1 rule: all files have 3 copies, on 2 different types of media (hard drives or tapes), with at least 1 copy off-site.[19] Although the 3-2-1 rule seems cumbersome, data redundancy ensures no data loss.

Be cognizant that media take up significant disk space, especially surgical videos; 1 minute of high-definition surgical video has 25 times the amount of data in a high-resolution CT scan.[20] Data storage costs are expensive, so these must factor into a laboratory's budget. For example, storing 500 operative videos will take nearly half a terabyte of storage, which translates to a minimum of $1000 annually for the cheapest of offline backups (as of end of 2019).[21]

Once the data are centrally located and reliably backed up, local (and possibly remote) researchers will need access. Multiple factors will affect data access. First, decide where the data should reside: either on the local network or at a remote off-site server. A local network will guarantee higher data transfer speeds and data security, whereas remote servers will make collaborations easier (collaborators will not need to do the training and accreditation necessary to access the local hospital or university network). Compliance with local and institutional requirements will likely determine the ultimate storage location. Second, there needs to be guaranteed data availability. Many remote storage options provide a website to browse files, but any file manipulation and modeling then requires the user to download the files locally, which with hundreds of videos, can quickly outstrip any local hardware's storage capabilities. We prefer solutions that allow researchers to browse files on their computer like regular folders, which requires using systems such as Samba or the Network File System.[22,23] This allows for easy, user-transparent file browsing and data manipulation over remote links. Finally, consider the network speed link. Many networks still use slower speeds (100 megabits per second [Mbps]) rather than 1000 Mbps. This 10-fold speed difference significantly affects workload times. For example, transferring 100 surgical videos of a 45-minute procedure across the network would take an estimated 9 hours with the 100-Mbps link, whereas the faster link allows the files to transfer in under an hour.

At this point in our example process, video data are now centrally located, replicated, and quickly accessible. Next, the data must undergo meticulous tracking in a database. You should evaluate all the variables you are recording for each patient. An example initial database structure for operative videos could store records for file name, medical record number (or other identifier), and type of operation. Depending on the research question, you may also want to track other associated data, such as the surgeon's prior experience or presence of assistants. Be flexible and open to changing the database structure early on as you start to scale. Additionally, you may wish to plan for the unknown future and consider tracking more information than may initially seem necessary (if approved by your institutional review board). Collecting data prospectively will always be more accurate than retrospectively filling in missing data variables.

There are various programs suited to database creation. Using a spreadsheet (eg, Microsoft Excel), is an easy initial choice with a low barrier to entry. We have found, though, that with a burgeoning data set size, spreadsheets rapidly become messy and are prone to errors. We suggest using a formal database system (eg, PostgreSQL) due to its considerable benefits.[24] Formal databases allow for concurrent editing and for setting information sanity checks to ensure clean data. For example, our data enterers can only input certain surgeons' names and certain procedures rather than having free text input fields. The database also checks that valid times are entered (eg, procedure start times must be numbers that occur before the recorded end times). These simple sanity checks can bolster confidence in the data quality during informal assessments of the captured data. Although deploying a formal database seems daunting, check your institution's resources. You may find that your institution can offer you these services for free or at a low cost. For example, we leveraged an institutional database server to offload the mundane, though highly important, tasks of database administration such as backups, tuning, and security, giving us the benefits of a formal information database without the administrative headaches.

Once the data are appropriately captured and stored, they must undergo processing from their raw state to a state amenable to analysis and modeling. Bennett et al[25] present a framework for optimal workflow for radiology data sets that shares many similarities with our own pipeline (Figure 16-1).[25] Think of data processing as a series of finer and finer filters; each filter removes extraneous details and standardizes the data until they reach a usable final state. In the case of videos, videos for one operation often span multiple smaller video files that will need to be combined, trimmed to contain only operative footage, stripped of audio (if necessary), deidentified, and finally, converted to an appropriate format for long-term storage and model creation. Performing each step by hand would take hours per video, and quickly, the captured data volume (once a culture of capture has been established at your institution!) will consume the lab member's time and prevent actual research from occurring. Fortunately, for videos and images, there is FFmpeg and ImageMagick, both powerful open-source tools that can perform all this manipulation and more in an automated fashion.[26,27]

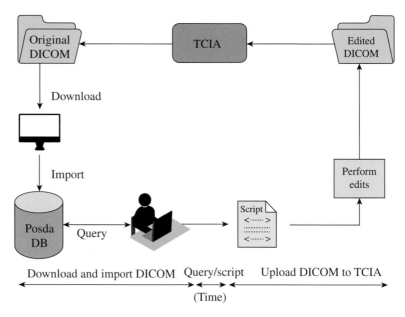

Figure 16-1 • Optimal workflow for radiology data sets. DICOM, Digital Imaging and Communications in Medicine; TCIA, the Cancer Imaging Archive. (Reproduced, with permission, from Bennett W, Smith K, Jarosz Q, Nolan T, Bosch W. Reengineering workflow for curation of DICOM datasets. *J Digit Imaging.* 2018;31(6):783-791.)

Our group created a program to expedite our data pipeline, and now all videos are rapidly processed, uploaded to the central server, and cataloged in the database, with just a single command, freeing up members for more important tasks. Thus, automating as much of the capture, processing, and storage of the database as possible will be important to preserve your research team's time for actual research tasks. However, we stress that the initial, appropriate capture and catalog of data is just as critical a step as the modeling and analysis.

Data Security and Anonymity

A comprehensive guide on data security and safe protected health information (PHI) handling is beyond the scope of this chapter. We do, however, want to underline the importance of data safety and anonymity. You should create, for each research project, a thoughtful data security plan.

Data security occurs at 3 phases: rest, motion, and in use. Data at rest refers to stored data on a computer, server, or portable hard drive. Storage, especially if the data travel off the main research campus, must be encrypted. Similarly, during data transfer between remote storage and data-processing servers, all communication should be encrypted.

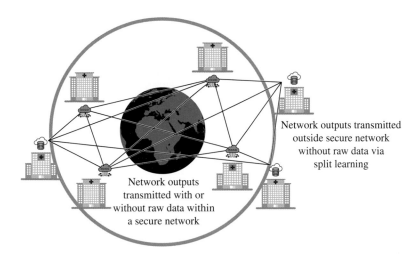

Figure 16-2 • Distributed learning can be performed within a secure network of both large and small hospitals. For hospitals that do not wish to share raw patient data, split learning allows participation in large-scale machine learning projects by sharing network outputs only.

Encryption while the data are actively in use is a yet-unsolved problem; in order for the data to make sense to any program using them, they have to be decrypted. Raskar's group at the Massachusetts Institute of Technology (MIT) have proposed an interesting workaround: split learning.[28] Split learning allows neural networks to train across multiple data sources so that data never need to leave a local facility and risk compromise (Figure 16-2). There is no large-scale application of this technology as of yet, but implementations may become more common as data privacy laws such as the GDPR continue to be enacted.

The hassle that comes with encryption and enhanced data safety may seem unnecessary, especially if surgical media was deidentified. True deidentification, however, is a goal that is increasingly more difficult, if not impossible, to achieve. Sweeney,[29] an expert in the "reidentification" field, could exactly identify health records for almost 50% of people who had newspaper stories written on their hospital visits from "deidentified" health record databases. Similarly, researchers showed that with increasing number of demographic attributes in a database, the likelihood of reidentification increases. With just 15 attributes, 99.98% of deidentified patients could be reidentified.[30] Therefore, because all data are essentially PHI, they should be treated as such.

Efforts should still be made to minimize the amount of PHI contained in the data, as each variable removed makes the cost function of reidentification more expensive. As an example, when the laparoscope is extracorporeal for intermittent lens cleaning during an operation, the camera often incidentally captures images from the operating room itself, such as the clock on the side of the wall or a whiteboard on which the date and surgeon are written. As an example of how reidentification can occur, we have actually been able to use this information leakage to help identify videos to particular surgeries when a glitch in the video recorder stopped it from recording medical record numbers. To eliminate this information leakage, we use FFmpeg, the software previously mentioned, which has a filter to blur images during certain time intervals. There are few published guides to systematic media deidentification, although one excellent example came from the TCIA group who describe thorough procedures for deidentification of radiology images.[31] Ultimately, applying extra effort during initial media processing will help keep videos more secure, prevent regulatory punishment in the future, and more importantly, keep patient information safe.

▍DATA ANNOTATION

The arduous journey toward usable data has one last peak to overcome: data annotation (also referred to as labeling). Much of the work thus far in surgical computer vision has used supervised learning, where models train on human-labeled data. Sadly, there is a scarcity of preexisting labeled data. These prelabeled data usually are of little utility for more than a narrow question. For example, even though a data set may have extensive labeling of surgical tools, if the model hopes to identify correct phases, each video will need to be rewatched and relabeled, similar to what Zisimopoulos's group did for their DeepPhase paper.[9] A key component of productive computer vision research is minimization of data preparation costs, so we will describe one workflow to maximize annotation efficiency.

Many tools exist for data annotation. Unfortunately, the majority of them focus on data labeling for a particular problem, such as tool tracking, gesture tracking, or labeling of objects in a video frame.[32] When searching for a suitable software, ensure that it is easy to use, works on all operating systems in the lab, can do the labeling needed for the project, and can output to a file format that your modeling tools can read. In the past, we have used 2 programs: Anvil and VIA. Anvil is an annotation tool originally meant for labeling dialogue and gestures but has convenient ways to label phases of an operation. It also outputs the labels into a file format that is easy to process (XML).[33] We also use VIA, an annotation software that runs straight in the browser and allows for similar temporal segmentation in addition to direct labeling and outlining of objects in the video. It also outputs to easily readable plain text formats (JSON and CSV).[34] These are

	Table 16-1		ANNOTATION TOOLS		
Tool	Temporal Labeling	Spatial Labeling	Open Source	Web-Based	Export Data Format
Anvil	Yes	No	No	No	XML
VIA	Yes	Yes	Yes	Yes	JSON, CSV, Pascal VOC
VOTT	No	Yes	Yes	Yes	JSON, CSV
CVAT	No	Yes	Yes	Yes	XML, Pascal VOC, YOLO, MS COCO, TFRecord, MOT, LabelMe
Eva	No	Yes	Yes	Yes	YOLO, Pascal VOC
MuViLab	Yes	No	Yes	No	JSON
Ultimate Labeling	No	Yes	No	No	CSV
VITBAT	No	Yes	No	No	Custom
IVAT	No	Yes	No	No	XML
Vatic	No	Yes	Yes	No	XML, JSON, LabelMe, Pascal VOC
VIPER-GT	No	Yes	Yes	No	XML

not the only available annotation tools, and Table 16-1 contains a (far from comprehensive) list of known annotation tools that are available.

Now with the tools to label data, an annotation consensus and standard must be reached. No community-wide surgical standard for media annotation exists at this point, so each group will need to create their own annotation consensus. Take, as an example, phase segmentation of operation videos. The group must agree upon the phases to label, their exact start and stop times, and whether or not they can repeat. Truly drill down to a granularity that will prevent disagreement between multiple annotators. With an initial draft, then annotate a select few media with multiple annotators. Afterward, compare the annotators' notes and closely review their areas of disagreement to then create a revised annotation guide.

You will likely be surprised by how many unplanned variations occur in the annotations. Take dissection of a structure: Does the phase start when the instrument is in view or when it touches the tissue? Does it end every time it leaves the tissue or just when the next phase start? What should happen when the laparoscope leaves the body? This refinement process will take time and is nicely encapsulated by the Japanese word *kaizen*, which represents an iterative testing and refinement process.[35]

Put in the time up front because inconsistent labeling will only lead to poor modeling performance. The model is only as good as its data inputs. Poor model performance from inconsistent annotations will lead to a serious time sink that a little up-front effort will avoid.

Understandably, manually labeling large numbers of images and videos is quite costly from a time perspective, particularly because it requires highly educated labelers (for many labels, only trained surgeons will suffice). Research groups must plan for an annotation budget to help accrue multiple annotators. Additionally, a training program for data annotation should be created (ie, to train new annotators). Lastly, annotators should cultivate a continued *kaizen* culture with regular annotator audits and retraining to ensure high-quality data labeling.

Recent studies have tried to reduce the labor-intensive labeling process. If computer vision models will need hundreds of videos to train, then the data-labeling task will rapidly outpace the ability of surgeons to annotate. Some groups have looked at pretraining models on unlabeled data to then reduce the amount of actual labeled data needed to perform accurate predictions.[36] Others have trained a neural network on a small proportion of labeled videos and then used this trained network to generate annotations on other videos. Using both synthetically generated annotations and a small number of human-generated annotations, Yu et al[37] could almost halve the prediction accuracy gap between a model trained solely on 20 annotations versus a model trained on 80 annotations. With continued advances, models will one day generate their own annotations and only require a trained-human input for those on which the model is uncertain (ie, semi- or weakly supervised learning). Until then, we will continue to have to dedicate large amounts of time to annotations.

MODELING

With good data, now the modeling and predictions can begin. Just like data collection, modeling requires a broad toolset. First, the lab will need to pick a programming language in which to design the models. The most commonly used languages include Python, C++, Julia, and R. We use Python given its readability, ease to learn, and extensive machine learning package availability. In fact, the top 10 packages used for machine learning on GitHub are only compatible with Python programs.[38] Next a deep learning framework should be selected for easy neural network development and to optimize model training at any scale. Our lab uses PyTorch, although there are other popular alternatives, including TensorFlow.[39,40]

Once a model is programmed, it will need appropriate hardware for training and testing. Machine learning and computer vision are quite computer resource intensive. Typically, models leverage computer graphical processing units (GPUs) to perform the myriad calculations required. These GPUs were developed originally for computer graphical tasks, such as video games, but were found to be well-suited to machine learning computations with orders of magnitude improvements over traditional computer processing units (CPUs).[41] Machine learning–specific chips also have been created, such as the Tensor Processing Unit (TPU) from Google, which runs with improved speed and energy costs.[42] GPUs can be accessed either locally using a computer or server within your institution or through third-party services such as those offered by Amazon, Microsoft, and Google.

Training and running models are costly endeavors with both resource and expertise-requiring challenges. The monetary cost of model development at first seems reasonable: one model averages 120 hours to train with a cloud compute cost of around $100. However, effective models will need parameter tuning to each data set, which estimates to nearly 2880 training hours with cloud compute costs of up to $4000. Beyond training hours and direct cost for cloud computing power, these models generate large carbon dioxide emissions. Training one model, including tuning, generates almost 80,000 pounds of carbon dioxide, which is over double that produced by an American citizen each year.[43]

Gaining the expertise to appropriately select a neural network and optimize its parameters also presents a significant challenge. It is not a field quickly learned: small changes to a model's hyperparameters can lead to an inability to train on a data set. Even modifying the random seed for a model with otherwise identical network and hyperparameters can lead to learning curves with zero overlap of distribution.[44] Machine learning and computer vision additionally are rapidly evolving fields. Few medical practitioners will have the expertise for thoughtful and productive work machine learning analysis. Typically, medical groups will overcome the knowledge gap through partnerships with groups that have the necessary computer vision expertise, as we did with MIT's Computer Science and Artificial Intelligence Laboratory. Their collaboration was critical for our success at tackling surgical computer vision problems.

If resources such as a world-leading institution are not available, there is an alternative: automated machine learning (AutoML). AutoML seeks to provide off-the-shelf solutions to nonexperts without requiring machine learning knowledge. AutoML solutions will select a model, optimize hyperparameters, interpret the results, and analyze data.[45] Currently available options include the Google Cloud AutoML and Microsoft AzureML.[46,47] Faes et al[48] performed a proof-of-concept study where they had 2 physicians with no previous programming or deep learning experience use AutoML to create models for image classification on public medical data sets. They then compared the AutoML models' predictions against the previously published human-designed models and found nearly comparable performance on smaller data sets.[48]

This AutoML approach, however, still has shortcomings. The environmental cost is significant: AutoML uses a method called neural architecture search to automatically select networks and hyperparameters.[49] Training a neural architecture search can increase the carbon dioxide emissions of a model over 3000-fold. This increase translates to a carbon emission that 5 cars would produce over their lifetime.[43] Despite this drastic increase in resource usage, AutoML unacceptably does not reach performance parity with hand-designed models. In the physician proof-of-concept paper from Faes et al,[48] AutoML performed similar to traditional models only in binary classification (abnormal vs normal) with poor performance on labeling images. For example, it classified a melanoma as a nevus 28.6% of the time. When the AutoML models were used on an external test data set, their near-perfect accuracy then dropped to less than 50%.[48] Clearly, further development is necessary before any medical practitioner can become a "machine learning" researcher in a day with an AutoML approach. Rather than replacing machine learning experts, AutoML's future may involve model development facilitation through initial guidance on hyperparameter choices and neural architecture design that then trained machine learning experts can build upon to improve performance.[50]

▌CONCLUSION

Although it is a young field, computer vision and its applications in the medical arena promise an exciting future. Computer vision work first starts with a defined question. Second, it requires meticulous data acquisition and processing. Third, experts label the data following a reproducible annotation consensus. Lastly, with the prepared data, researchers can train deep learning models to answer their question, whatever it may be. This chapter presented the MGH SAIL experience and provided a roadmap to avoid the numerous hurdles any researcher is destined to hit when using computer vision. An AI-augmented future is exciting, and we cannot wait to experience it with you.

REFERENCES

1. Krizhevsky A, Sutskever I, Hinton GE. Imagenet classification with deep convolutional neural networks. *Advances in Neural Information Processing Systems.* 2012:1097-1105. Accessed October 6, 2020. https://papers.nips.cc/paper/4824-imagenet-classification-with-deep-convolutional-neural-networks.pdf.

2. Shoham Y, Perrault R, Brynjolfsson E, et al. 2018 Annual Report. Artificial Intelligence Index. Accessed September 13, 2019. https://aiindex.org.

3. Heller N, Sathianathen N, Kalapara A, et al. The KiTS19 Challenge Data: 300 kidney tumor cases with clinical context, CT semantic segmentations, and surgical outcomes. Accessed September 11, 2019. http://arxiv.org/abs/1904.00445.

4. Wang X, Peng Y, Lu L, Lu Z, Bagheri M, Summers RM. ChestX-ray8: hospital-scale chest x-ray database and benchmarks on weakly-supervised classification and localization of common thorax diseases. Accessed September 11, 2019. http://openaccess.thecvf.com/content_cvpr_2017/html/Wang_ChestX-ray8_Hospital-Scale_Chest_CVPR_2017_paper.html.

5. Decencière E, Zhang X, Cazuguel G, et al. Feedback on a publicly distributed image database: the Messidor database. *Image Anal Stereol.* 2014;33(3): 231-234.

6. Tschandl P, Rosendahl C, Kittler H. The HAM10000 dataset, a large collection of multi-source dermatoscopic images of common pigmented skin lesions. *Sci Data.* 2018;5:180161.

7. Prior FW, Clark K, Commean P, et al. TCIA: an information resource to enable open science. In: *2013 35th Annual International Conference of the IEEE Engineering in Medicine and Biology Society (EMBC)*; 2013:1282-1285.

8. Al Hajj H, Lamard M, Conze P-H, et al. CATARACTS: challenge on automatic tool annotation for cataRACT surgery. *Med Image Anal.* 2019;52:24-41.

9. Zisimopoulos O, Flouty E, Luengo I, et al. DeepPhase: surgical phase recognition in CATARACTS videos. arXiv:180710565. July 2018. Accessed September 14, 2019. http://arxiv.org/abs/1807.10565.

10. Flouty E, Kadkhodamohammadi A, Luengo I, et al. CaDIS: Cataract Dataset for Image Segmentation. arXiv:190611586. June 2019. Accessed September 11, 2019. http://arxiv.org/abs/1906.11586.

11. Nakawala H. Nephrec9. November 2017. Accessed October 6, 2020. https://zenodo.org/record/1066831#.X3z312hKjIU.

12. Allan M, Shvets A, Kurmann T, et al. 2017 Robotic Instrument Segmentation Challenge. arXiv:190206426. February 2019. Accessed September 14, 2019. http://arxiv.org/abs/1902.06426.

13. Ahmidi N, Tao L, Sefati S, et al. A dataset and benchmarks for segmentation and recognition of gestures in robotic surgery. *IEEE Trans Biomed Eng.* 2017;64(9): 2025-2041.

14. Twinanda AP, Shehata S, Mutter D, Marescaux J, de Mathelin M, Padoy N. EndoNet: a deep architecture for recognition tasks on laparoscopic videos. arXiv:160203012. February 2016. Accessed September 11, 2019. http://arxiv.org/abs/1602.03012.

15. Stauder R, Ostler D, Kranzfelder M, Koller S, Feußner H, Navab N. The TUM LapChole dataset for the M2CAI 2016 workflow challenge. arXiv:161009278. October 2016. Accessed September 11, 2019. http://arxiv.org/abs/1610.09278.

16. Format descriptions for still image. Library of Congress. Accessed September 12, 2019. https://www.loc.gov/preservation/digital/formats/fdd/still_fdd.shtml.

17. Format descriptions for moving images. Library of Congress. Accessed September 12, 2019. https://www.loc.gov/preservation/digital/formats/fdd/video_fdd.shtml.

18. Vohl D, Fluke CJ, Vernardos G. Data compression in the petascale astronomy era: a GERLUMPH case study. *Astron Comput*. 2015;12:200-211.

19. Backup overview. dpBestflow. Accessed September 12, 2019. https://dpbestflow.org/node/262.

20. Natarajan P, Frenzel JC, Smaltz DH. *Demystifying Big Data and Machine Learning for Healthcare*. CRC Press, Taylor & Francis Group; 2017.

21. Cloud storage pricing comparison: Amazon S3 vs Azure vs B2. Accessed September 15, 2019. https://www.backblaze.com/b2/cloud-storage-pricing.html.

22. Samba—opening windows to a wider world. Accessed September 12, 2019. https://www.samba.org/.

23. Staubach P, Pawlowski B, Callaghan B. NFS version 3 protocol specification. Accessed September 12, 2019. https://tools.ietf.org/html/rfc1813.

24. PostgreSQL: The world's most advanced open source database. Accessed September 15, 2019. https://www.postgresql.org/.

25. Bennett W, Smith K, Jarosz Q, Nolan T, Bosch W. Reengineering workflow for curation of DICOM datasets. *J Digit Imaging*. 2018;31(6):783-791.

26. FFmpeg. Accessed September 12, 2019. https://www.ffmpeg.org/.

27. ImageMagick Studio LLC. ImageMagick. Accessed September 17, 2019. https://imagemagick.org/.

28. Gupta O, Raskar R. Distributed learning of deep neural network over multiple agents. arXiv:181006060. October 2018. Accessed September 17, 2019. http://arxiv.org/abs/1810.06060.

29. Sweeney L. Only you, your doctor, and many others may know. *Technol Sci*. September 2015. Accessed September 12, 2019. https://techscience.org/a/2015092903/.

30. Rocher L, Hendrickx JM, Montjoye Y-A de. Estimating the success of re-identifications in incomplete datasets using generative models. *Nat Commun*. 2019;10(1):1-9.

31. Freymann JB, Kirby JS, Perry JH, Clunie DA, Jaffe CC. Image data sharing for biomedical research—meeting HIPAA requirements for de-identification. *J Digit Imaging*. 2012;25(1):14-24.

32. Gaur E, Saxena V, Singh SK. Video annotation tools: a review. In: *2018 International Conference on Advances in Computing, Communication Control and Networking (ICACCCN)*. 2018:911-914. Accessed October 6, 2020. https://ieeexplore.ieee.org/document/8748669.

33. Kipp M. ANVIL: a generic annotation tool for multimodal dialogue. Accessed October 6, 2020. http://michaelkipp.de/publication/Kipp2001_ANVIL.pdf.

34. Dutta A, Zisserman A. The VIA annotation software for images, audio and video. arXiv:190410699. April 2019. Accessed October 6, 2020. https://arxiv.org/abs/1904.10699.

35. Imai M. *Kaizen (Ky'zen): The Key to Japan's Competitive Success*. McGraw-Hill; 1986.

36. Funke I, Jenke A, Mees ST, Weitz J, Speidel S, Bodenstedt S. Temporal coherence-based self-supervised learning for laparoscopic workflow analysis. In: Stoyanov D, Taylor Z, Sarikaya D, et al, eds. *OR 2.0 Context-Aware Operating Theaters, Computer Assisted Robotic Endoscopy, Clinical Image-Based Procedures, and Skin Image Analysis*. Lecture Notes in Computer Science. Springer International Publishing; 2018:85-93.

37. Yu T, Mutter D, Marescaux J, Padoy N. Learning from a tiny dataset of manual annotations: a teacher/student approach for surgical phase recognition. arXiv:181200033. November 2018. Accessed September 18, 2019. http://arxiv.org/abs/1812.00033.

38. The state of the Octoverse: machine learning. *The GitHub Blog*. January 2019. Accessed September 4, 2019. https://github.blog/2019-01-24-the-state-of-the-octoverse-machine-learning/.

39. Abadi M, Barham P, Chen J, et al. TensorFlow: a system for large-scale machine learning. Accessed September 20, 2019. https://www.usenix.org/conference/osdi16/technical-sessions/presentation/abadi.

40. Paszke A, Gross S, Chintala S, et al. Automatic differentiation in PyTorch. October 2017. Accessed September 20, 2019. https://openreview.net/forum?id=BJJsrmfCZ.

41. Mittal S, Vaishay S. A survey of techniques for optimizing deep learning on GPUs. *J Syst Architect*. 2019;99:101635.

42. Jouppi N, Young C, Patil N, Patterson D. Motivation for and evaluation of the first tensor processing unit. *IEEE Micro*. 2018;38(3):10-19.

43. Strubell E, Ganesh A, McCallum A. Energy and policy considerations for deep learning in NLP. arXiv:190602243. June 2019. Accessed September 4, 2019. http://arxiv.org/abs/1906.02243.

44. Henderson P, Islam R, Bachman P, Pineau J, Precup D, Meger D. Deep reinforcement learning that matters. arXiv:170906560. September 2017. Accessed September 10, 2019. http://arxiv.org/abs/1709.06560.

45. Truong A, Walters A, Goodsitt J, Hines K, Bruss CB, Farivar R. Towards automated machine learning: evaluation and comparison of AutoML approaches and tools. arXiv:190805557. August 2019. Accessed September 12, 2019. http://arxiv.org/abs/1908.05557.

46. Cloud AutoML: Custom machine learning models AutoML. *Google Cloud*. Accessed September 20, 2019. https://cloud.google.com/automl/.

47. AutoML. Microsoft Research. Accessed September 20, 2019. https://www.microsoft.com/en-us/research/project/automl/.

48. Faes L, Wagner SK, Fu DJ, et al. Automated deep learning design for medical image classification by health-care professionals with no coding experience: a feasibility study. *Lancet Digit Health*. 2019;1(5):e232-e242.

49. Zoph B, Le QV. Neural architecture search with reinforcement learning. arXiv:161101578. November 2016. Accessed September 20, 2019. http://arxiv.org/abs/1611.01578.

50. Wang D, Weisz JD, Muller M, et al. Human-AI collaboration in data science: exploring data scientists' perceptions of automated AI. arXiv:190902309. September 2019. Accessed October 6, 2020. https://arxiv.org/pdf/1909.02309.pdf.

ASSESSMENT OF ARTIFICIAL INTELLIGENCE RESEARCH IN SURGERY

17

Daniel A. Hashimoto

HIGHLIGHTS

- Key questions to ask while evaluating the literature:
  - Was the right question asked?
  - Were the right methods used?
  - Were the right data analyzed?
  - Are the conclusions of this paper supported by the data?
  - How will this change my practice or affect my patients?

▌ INTRODUCTION

With the growing output in machine learning papers for surgical applications, it is becoming more important for surgeons and surgical researchers to have a better understanding of key principles in machine learning research. Thus, the previous chapters of this book have provided a foundation for understanding the key techniques and existing applications for techniques in artificial intelligence (AI), especially deep learning. Although it is difficult to cover all possible methodologies and applications of AI to surgery, we hope that the previous chapters have armed you with the ability to begin learning more about the field.

Although additional mathematical and computational knowledge and skills are necessary to begin engaging in AI research, reading the literature is a good way to continue one's education and expand the scope of one's appreciation for the field. While this chapter does not review individual methods of machine learning (some methods are covered in Chapters 3-6), it is intended to provide a basic strategy to reading and

Key Point

JAMA's user guide on evaluating machine learning papers provides an excellent framework for reviewing machine learning literature.[10]

assessing predominantly clinical papers that utilize machine learning (as opposed to technical papers in computer science or engineering on the development of machine learning methods). This strategy is certainly not the only way (nor is it likely the best way) to evaluate a clinical machine learning paper; however, it provides a systematic framework to support the curious clinician or surgical researcher in evaluating such work.

SUGGESTED PREREQUISITES

As was introduced in Chapters 1 and 3, AI draws from a wide range of fields. Although one does not have to be familiar with all of psychology, neuroscience, linguistics, and so on, knowledge of core mathematical and statistical principles is vital to understanding and assessing papers that use techniques in AI. Many studies in the medical literature today are based on frequentist statistics that are often taught in high school, college, and medical school. Yet, multiple studies have demonstrated that statistical literacy among clinicians (both those in training and those in practice) is poor. A survey assessing physicians' knowledge of risk and benefit of common screening tools and therapeutics demonstrated that 79% of the surveyed physicians overestimated the benefits of these tools, whereas 66% overestimated the harms. Furthermore, 67% of these physicians reported low confidence in their own awareness of the probability of risk or benefit.[1] In a large study of over 4700 obstetrics and gynecology residents, only 42% could correctly define P value on a multiple-choice examination.[2]

Therefore, the best recommendation is to brush up on statistics first and foremost. It is outside the scope of this book to review all topics in statistics; however, Table 17-1 provides a list of some of the most high-yield

Table 17-1 SUGGESTED STATISTICAL TOPICS TO REVIEW	
Suggested Statistical Topics to Review	**Examples**
Mathematical notation	Set notation, summation, integration, derivation, combinatorics, matrices
Measures of central tendency	Mean, median, mode
Distributions	Distribution density functions
Frequentist statistics	P value, confidence intervals, effect size
Bayesian statistics	Prior probability, posterior probability
Regression	Linear and logistic regression

topics in statistics to review. Although a solid understanding of statistics is important to understanding articles that deal with the more clinical applications of AI research, articles that are geared more toward describing new technical approaches to AI will require a deeper level of comfort with other mathematical fields such as linear algebra and calculus.

Many forms of machine learning use at least some elements from linear algebra, especially matrix mathematics. Reviewing the behavior and utilization of matrices will be helpful in understanding how many machine learning techniques work "under the hood," especially when reviewing technical papers. Basic matrix concepts include matrix notation, symmetry, identity, transposition, addition/subtraction/multiplication, and the algebraic properties of matrices (eg, associativity, commutativity, distributivity, transposition, inversion). In addition, knowledge of basic calculus (integrals and derivatives) is also important.

Key Point

See Khan Academy's video tutorials on matrices at https://www.khanacademy.org/math/precalculus/x9e81a4f98389efdf:matrices

SCREENING AN ARTICLE

The reality of the demands of a busy schedule forces everyone to be selective with the literature they read. Articles to review can come to the attention of a reader in a multitude of ways. In some cases, articles may come up during a focused search on a specific topic. In other cases, one may come across an interesting paper while reading through a journal's table of contents, or a colleague may send a paper of interest to you. Regardless of how the paper comes to your attention, a systematic approach to screening and subsequently evaluating the article will be important.

The title will undoubtedly be the first element of the paper you will read. As with any scientific writing, the title may provide clues on the overall topic of the paper, but the abstract will—hopefully—contain more meaningful information on the methodology used and help you determine whether the paper warrants further evaluation. Depending on the source journal (ie, clinical vs more technical journal), the level of detail in the abstract's methodology may be insufficient to give you a sense of what specific techniques may have been used. You may find that abstracts just state that "machine learning techniques" or "deep learning" were used.

Within the field, keep in mind that traditional databases of articles may not cover work that has been published in technical journals. Thus, although PubMed, Medline, Embase, and other databases remain great resources for biomedical articles, consider also searching through the IEEE Xplore (https://ieeexplore.ieee.org/) database for papers in Institute of Electrical and Electronics Engineers (IEEE) journals and conference proceedings. IEEE Xplore is where one will find peer-reviewed papers presented at the top engineering conferences such as NeurIPS (Neural Information Processing Systems), MICCAI (Medical Image Computing and Computer Assisted Intervention), IROS (International Conference on Intelligent Robots and Systems), and ICRA (International Conference on Robotics and Automation). Another source is Google Scholar, which, not surprisingly, has a robust search engine that crosses multiple databases and also provides results from patent filings and gray literature.

Because the field of surgical AI moves quickly, one may wish to also assess the non–peer-reviewed literature, particularly pre-prints. arXiv.org (https://www.arxiv.org) hosted by Cornell University is the largest and most popular preprint repository, featuring over 1.5 million scholarly articles in physics, mathematics, computer science, electrical engineering, and other fields.

▊ EVALUATING AN ARTICLE

Each scientist has a different strategy for reviewing a paper. Some prefer to review the figures first, before reading any of the paper's text, to see if the figures present enough data from which to draw a conclusion. Others start with the conclusion and then move to the figures to see if the authors' conclusions about the work match their own. Often, multiple read throughs of an article are required to truly grasp the content.[3] Regardless of your approach, each section of the paper should generate a set of questions to help you evaluate the quality of the research approach and the conclusions drawn from the data.[4]

Keshav's "How to Read a Paper" suggests considering the "Five C's" of a paper after a first-pass read through[3]:

1. Category: What type of paper are you reading?
2. Context: To what other papers is this paper related, and what theoretical framework does it use?
3. Correctness: Are the assumptions on which the work is done valid?
4. Contributions: What are the contributions to the literature made by the work?
5. Clarity: How well written is the paper?

Introduction

The introduction of the article should provide a rationale for the work that the authors are proposing to conduct. Although the background exposition will frame the problem, it is important to focus specifically on the question or problem and the hypothesis being tested. Questions to ask oneself include the following:

1. Is the problem under investigation clearly stated? The lack of a clearly defined problem may result in methodology that is unable to assess or incompletely assesses a phenomenon.
2. Is a well-defined hypothesis driving the research, or is this an exploration of data for hypothesis generation? The underlying goal of the research will influence the methodology selected.

Methods

Each aspect of the methods should be described in sufficient detail to allow independent replication of the study. In fact, you should consider mentally reconstructing the experiment as described in the paper. With a particularly critical eye to detail, consider whether the methodology used is appropriate for the question presented in the introduction, whether sufficient detail is presented in the manuscript or references to be able to reproduce the study, and whether the data are appropriate for the conclusions that are drawn in the discussion.

The Data Set

Key Point

Recall from Chapter 3 that channel effects (ie, where a model learns characteristics of the manner in which data were recorded) can affect the outcome of a study. Channel effects should be identified *a priori* where possible and controlled as covariates.

In surgical research, the data set will mostly be composed of clinical data (eg, electronic medical record data, images, videos). For studies involving images and videos, annotations will also be a key component of the data (see Chapter 16 for more details). In evaluating work, readers should consider whether the data set selected was appropriate for the problem and hypothesis stated in the introduction. In particular, data sets should contain data that are representative of the problem under investigation.

For supervised learning problems, careful attention should be paid to the method of annotation that was used for the training data set. For studies using computer vision on images or videos, annotator identity—at least at the level of experience—can be critical. As an example, are images being annotated by experienced clinicians trained in annotation or by a lay crowd that has been recruited through means such as Amazon MTurk (Amazon, Seattle, WA)?[5] Even experienced clinicians can vary in their conceptualization of clinical phenomena and annotate the same image or video differently using the same criteria.[6] Thus, depending on the specific clinical problem being investigated, different levels of annotator may be appropriate. For example, annotation of tools, such as clip appliers or graspers, could be performed by students or the lay public, while more complex phenomena, such as identification of surgical planes, likely require domain expertise from surgeons. Furthermore, consider whether there is a reference standard against which the annotation is being performed. For example, if a study is attempting to investigate whether a model can predict cirrhosis based on a laparoscopic image of the liver, one should consider whether a liver biopsy was used as the criterion for establishing the ground truth against which the model's prediction can be compared.

A reference standard is similarly important for nonimage work. When models are trained to predict clinical phenomena such as surgical site infection or sepsis, it is important to identify how such phenomena were identified and labeled. Are specific and accepted diagnostic criteria available and used or were the ground-truth labels based on claims data such as International Classification of Diseases (ICD) or Common Procedural Technology (CPT) codes? If so, as with health services research, one must remember that these codes were not designed for research and clinical care purposes but to track services for billing.

The availability of the data set should be considered. For studies that use publicly available data sets such as the MIMIC-III[7] or Cholec80[8] databases, it is much easier to independently verify results. For papers using proprietary data sets, independent verification may not be possible. The reader should consider whether use of an existing public data set could have helped to verify results. For example, as part of the methodology, authors may elect to train and validate their results on their proprietary data set and then subsequently demonstrate performance of that model on a public data set, if applicable.

The amount of data is also important. Although big data is often thought to require tens of thousands, if not millions, of data entries, the actual scale of data necessary can vary based on the problem and the approach. For regressions, simulations have suggested that anywhere from 5 to 10 events per variable are necessary depending on the tolerance for Type I error.[9] For deep learning, such as convolutional and recurrent neural networks, others have suggested more than 10,000 data points are required (see eTable 2 in Liu et al[10]). For novel data sets or applications without prior examples to suggest an appropriate sample size, "ablation" testing can demonstrate how much data might be necessary to reach an asymptote on performance. For example, Twinanda et al[8] demonstrated improving performance in identification of phases with the addition of 10 videos from 65.9% accuracy with 20 videos to 75.2% accuracy with 40 videos and ultimately 91% accuracy with 80 videos. Such findings suggest that for a single-institution data set, thousands of videos may not be necessary; however, such conclusions cannot be made about whether models trained on similarly sized data sets generalize to data sets from other institutions or contexts.

Key Point

It is important to recognize the underlying research question and to think carefully about whether the selected data contain a population that is appropriate for answering the question and has been labeled to an acceptable standard.

Preprocessing of data is common in machine learning studies and can help mitigate against data issues such as incompleteness, inconsistency, or inaccuracy. In any data processing, the typical stages are (1) cleaning, (2) integration, (3) reduction, and (4) transformation.[11] For studies of large data sets of electronic medical record information, preprocessing may involve removal of missing, incorrect, or implausible data; generation of new variables (eg, clinical ratios of existing data such as mean arterial pressure from systolic and diastolic pressure); or transformation of time series data (eg, Fourier transforms, regression adjustments).[12] For computer vision studies, transformation may involve resizing (especially common in deep-learning studies), reorienting, or flipping and inverting images. For any preprocessing methods, readers should carefully consider whether the preprocessing was explicitly stated, how it was applied to the different data sets (if multiple data sets or across both training and testing sets), and whether the preprocessing steps taken were appropriate for the research question under investigation. Table 17-2 demonstrates examples of data processing steps and considerations for each.

Modeling

As described in Chapters 3 through 6, there are a number of methodologic considerations in various applications of AI techniques. Selection of the appropriate model should be reviewed and considered based on the study's objective. Although it is outside the scope of this chapter to dive specifically into the appropriate or preferred uses of one model over another, it is helpful to approach the modeling with some broad considerations. Key again is that there should be sufficient detail either in the manuscript or in references to replicate the study independently, assuming access to the same data.

Did the authors select a supervised, unsupervised, semi-supervised, or reinforcement method? As detailed in Chapter 3, supervised learning approaches are appropriate when the input data for training have labels and the goal is to assign labels to new data. Unsupervised learning approaches are most often used when one has unlabeled data for which an underlying structure or relationship between data points is being sought. Semi-supervised approaches are a combination of supervised and unsupervised learning wherein a fraction of data is labeled for training and the remainder of the data can be assessed in an unsupervised fashion. Reinforcement learning approaches seek to optimize a function through a series of experiments that rewards or punishes the model.

How interpretable is the model that the authors selected? Approaches such as decision trees provide a high degree of interpretability, whereas

Table 17-2	STAGES OF DATA PREPROCESSING AND EXAMPLE METHODS AND PITFALLS[11]	
Data Preprocessing Stages	Preprocessing Method	Notes
Cleaning data	Drop patients with missing data	Can imbalance data set, affect representation, and remove other potentially valuable features associated with the patient
	Replace missing data with measure of central tendency	Can reflect data set but need to assume minimal missing data
	Replace missing data with predicted value	Replacement data are limited by assumption of the predictive model used, so may bias the data
Integrating data	Consolidate data	Can be achieved through relational databases or condensing into one database
Reducing data	Principal component analysis	Reduce correlated data into principal components; may introduce bias from assumptions
	Filter data	Compare correlations of normalized data to remove highly covariant data; may introduce bias from assumptions
Transforming data	Smooth data	Filter statistical noise
	Normalize data	Rescale data into a normalized range for more consistent comparisons
	Construct/aggregate features from data	Combine existing variables into new variables reflective of clinical phenomena; incorrect assumptions may lead to inappropriate aggregation of data points that introduce researcher bias into the data

neural networks offer lower interpretability. However, decision trees work best with tabular data, while neural networks have greater flexibility to allow application to data as disparate as tabular data, images, and audio. That being said, there are approaches to make traditionally black box algorithms more interpretable.[13] For example, automated detection of nodules on a pulmonary computed tomography scan with deep learning may be able to provide reference examples from the training set of images with similar features that influenced the prediction of a node on the output scan. Understanding the interpretability of a model can help the reader assess its potential impact or utility in clinical practice because models with greater interpretability are more likely to have rapid clinical adoption.[14]

Optimization (also known as tuning) of hyperparameters plays an important role in the performance of a model (see Chapter 3). In many of the machine learning papers in the surgical literature, a model is first pretrained on an existing (and often unrelated) set of data such as ImageNet, which is a data set of over 1 million images of common objects.[15] The model is then fine-tuned on more applicable data that specifically relate to the surgical task at hand. For example, Hashimoto et al[6] fine-tuned a residual neural network that was originally trained on ImageNet by training the model to identify phases of laparoscopic sleeve gastrectomy. Cross-validation, described later, can also be used to tune the hyperparameters of a model. For studies that do not report on tuning of hyperparameters, readers should carefully assess whether the "test" set was, in fact, inadvertently used to tune hyperparameters. Such a step can make the reported metrics of performance of the model unreliable, with likely overestimation of performance.

If the authors selected a deep-learning approach, they should have reported on the construction of the deep neural network. The specific type of network (eg, convolutional neural network, recurrent neural network) and any pretrained architecture (eg, AlexNet, Resnet16, Mask R-CNN) should be reported. Any tuning of hyperparameters and the data on which it was tuned should also be reported. Finally, any regularization and optimization techniques (see Chapters 3 and 4) used in the study should be explicit to help the reader understand the exact methodology that was used.

Validation

Validation in the clinical sense differs from validation in many machine learning studies, where a single set of data may be divided into separate training and testing sets, and the test set is intended to "validate" the model's performance on unseen data. Division of a single set of data (even with data sourced from multiple institutions) leads to internal validation but does not necessarily mean that results will generalize to a population independent from those included in the training and testing sets. Furthermore, in some papers, you may find that "validation set" refers to a subsample of the data on which the model is fine-tuned (ie, has hyperparameters adjusted as mentioned earlier). External validation, particularly when considering clinical impact, requires an independent data set. This ensures that results obtained from training and testing generalize to previously unseen populations. Most importantly, does the model generalize to a patient population that matches the objective of the study set forth in the introduction? When assessing the methodology used in the study, careful attention should be paid to whether or not data from the training set was allowed to also enter the test or validation set. As detailed in Chapter 3, contamination of the test set with data from the training set allows the model to "cheat" on its predictions.

Cross-validation in machine learning, broadly, refers to partitioning the data into subsamples to preserve an "unseen" subsample. Two common methods of cross-validation are K-fold cross-validation and leave-p-out cross-validation. In K-fold cross-validation, a sample of data is divided into k-sized segments, and one subsample is held out as a test set. This is then repeated across the different k-sized segments until mean error of the model can be estimated (Figure 17-1). In leave-p-out cross-validation, a p number of observations is selected from the data sample as a test set with the remaining data used for training (Figure 17-2). The model is then

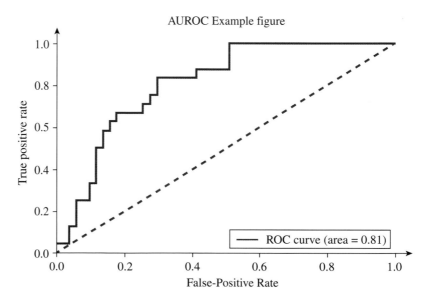

Figure 17-1 • Example of a receiver operating curve (ROC) with an area under the curve (AUROC) of 0.81.

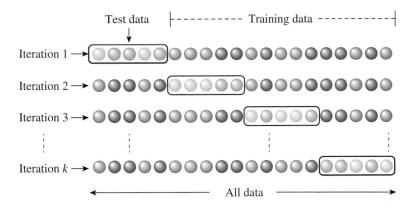

Figure 17-2 • Example of k-fold cross-validation.

repeated in all possible ways such that all data have, at one point, been part of subsample p. Leave-p-out cross-validation is considered a form of exhaustive cross-validation in which all possible ways of dividing the data are explored; however, for large data sets, exhaustive cross-validation is computationally infeasible due to the time and computational power needed. Therefore, many studies favor K-fold cross-validation or other nonexhaustive techniques, and this is a well-accepted methodology.

Validation is an important step to assess for issues such as overfitting. When overfitting occurs, the model too tightly approximates the current data set by describing the random error in the data and not the phenomenon in question. It is unable to subsequently generalize to data outside those in the current study because outside data may not have the same kind of random error. Thus, although performance may seem good with high accuracy, it is applicable only to the data in question and cannot be considered a model that has good performance on other representative data. Although not always the case, one possible clue that a model is overfit to data is when a study using a small sample size demonstrates markedly higher accuracy on the training set than on the test set. Therefore, validation (either on external data, if possible, or on repeated subsamples) is critical.

Perhaps most importantly when considering the validity of a study, one should consider whether the circumstances under which a set of analyses were performed were representative of real-world scenarios. Immaculate, clean data sets in machine learning research are, in some ways, similar to the tightly controlled settings in which we see randomized controlled trials for new drugs—unrealistic and unachievable in real clinical practice. Thus, if a paper claims to use machine learning that can disrupt clinical practice, the validation set should not only be based on a generalizable population but should also be on real-world data that mimic or at least

Table 17-3   TABLE OF DEFINITIONS OF METRICS OF PERFORMANCE IN CLASSIFICATION TASKS

Metric	Mathematical Definition
Accuracy	(TP + FP)/(TP + FP + TN + FN)
Precision	(TP)/(TP + FP)
Recall	(TP)/(TP + FN)
F1 score	$2 \times \dfrac{\text{precision} \times \text{recall}}{\text{precision} + \text{recall}}$

FN, false negative; FP, false positive; TN, true negative; TP, true positive.

approximate the type of data on which it would be asked to perform if launched clinically.

Results

Do the results of the validation lead to support or rejection of the null hypothesis? A vital component of evaluating the performance of machine learning models is to consider which metrics are used to assess the performance (see Chapter 3).

For classification problems, common metrics of performance include accuracy, precision, recall, and the F1 score (Tables 17-3 and 17-4). Although accuracy can potentially be variably defined according to the study at hand, it is commonly considered to be defined as the proportion of true positives and true negatives divided by the total set. To compare to more traditional terms in medicine, recall is analogous to sensitivity,

Table 17-4   HOW DIFFERENT METHODOLOGIC STEPS MAY INFLUENCE PERFORMANCE CLASSIFICATION METRICS

Metric	Increase Number of Training Examples	Improve Representative Training Examples	Improve Annotation of Data	Improve Annotation Consistency
Precision				Increase
Recall	Increase	Increase	Increase	Increase
F1	Increase	Increase	Increase	Increase

Adapted from IBM Watson Knowledge Studio.[16]

whereas precision is analogous to positive predictive value. The F1 score refers to the harmonic or weighted mean of precision and recall, where, as with the other metrics, 1 is best performance and 0 is worst. The receiver operating characteristic (ROC) curve shows performance of a model by plotting true positive on the *y*-axis over false positive on the *x*-axis. Depending on the methodology, studies may choose to maximize one performance metric over another or balance across different metrics by adjusting the classification threshold of their model(s).

By calculating the area under the ROC curve (AUC, AUROC, or c-statistic), one can evaluate the aggregate performance of the model under the different classification thresholds—again, with area of 1 reflecting best performance and 0 reflecting worst (Figure 17-3). The AUC is often reported because it provides a measure of performance of the model that can be used to compare ROC curves at different classification thresholds.

When considering the choice of metrics, think first about the problem at hand and whether, as the reader, you are evaluating the mathematical implications of the results or the clinical implications. For studies attempting to improve prediction of highly lethal or morbid diagnoses, recall may be the most appropriate metric to assess, as the cost of low precision may be offset by the benefit of high recall. In such situations, looking specifically at recall would be a better metric than looking at AUC, which may be low due to low precision of the model, whereas the intended purpose of the model would be unaffected due to its high recall.

In another example of considering the best metric of performance, consider a study analyzing the performance of a computer vision model in identifying anatomic structures such as the cystic duct (Figure 17-4).

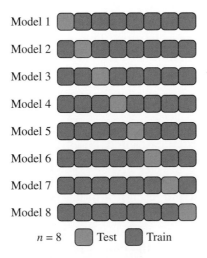

Figure 17-3 • Example of leave-p-out cross-validation.

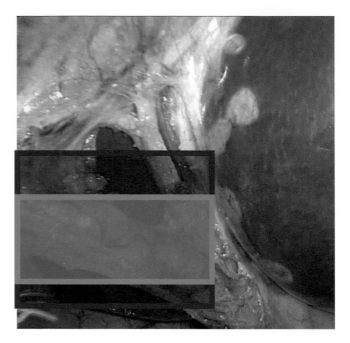

Figure 17-4 • Image of Calot's triangle during cholecystectomy with green box representing ground-truth annotation and red box representing machine prediction. Shaded green represents true positive; shaded red represents false positive.

The ground-truth bounding box and the predicted bounding box may not exactly overlap, leading to low precision; however, the clinical goal of assisting a physician in identifying the cystic duct could likely be accomplished.

Careful evaluation of the reported distribution of events in the data set is critical. For many surgical topics, the event of interest (eg, complication, mortality) may be rare. This predisposes a data set to class imbalance, where the number of event cases (eg, complications) is far outnumbered by nonevent cases. This imbalance can affect the interpretation of results for classification problems in several ways. First, for severely imbalanced data sets, a model's performance can achieve high "accuracy" by simply opting to predict the higher incidence label. For example, if a data set has 99% normal cases and 1% of cases with a bile duct injury, the model will perform at high accuracy by predicting "normal" for every input. Being wrong about 1% of cases would still result in high accuracy performance. Second, even if a model is attempting to classify low-incidence events, poor performance can be masked by good performance on high incidence events. Take Table 17-5 as an example from a study on automated identification of the phases of per oral endoscopic myotomy. The prevalence of the "submucosal injection" phase is less than 1% of all

Table 17-5 DIFFERENCE IN PERFORMANCE METRICS POEM				
	Precision	Recall	F1 score	Prevalence
Submucosal Injection	0.667	0.361	0.468	0.006
Mucosotomy	0.837	0.602	0.700	0.044
Submucosal Tunnel	0.955	0.840	0.894	0.513
Myotomy	0.791	0.945	0.861	0.278
Mucosotomy Closure	0.848	0.971	0.906	0.159
Overall (Unweighted)	0.820	0.744	0.766	
Overall (Weighted)	**0.885**	**0.876**	**0.875**	

Ward TM, Hashimoto DA, Ban Y, Rattner DW, Inoue H, Lillemoe KD, Rus DL, Rosman G, Meireles OR. Automated operative phase identification in peroral endoscopic myotomy. Surg Endosc. 2020 Jul 27. doi: 10.1007/s00464-020-07833-9. PMID: 32720177.

available frames. The overall weighted F1 score for identifying phases was 0.875; however, the performance on "submucosal injection" was 0.468.

For studies investigating risk (or conversely, benefit) prediction, one must also consider how well a model may discriminate across risk categories first,[17] including performance of the model not just overall but also between subgroups (if intended). In these models, classification metrics are most often reported (eg, c-statistic) with the threshold determined by the aims of the study. A higher c-statistic suggests greater discriminative ability of the model. For studies with poor discriminative ability between low- and high-risk patients, there is little utility to the model.

Discrimination alone, however, is not the only necessary trait of a predictive model. For risk prediction, the model should also be appropriately calibrated to offer absolute risk. In an example from Alba et al[17] in *JAMA*, a model that discriminates between patients at a predicted 1%, 2%, and 3% risk has little utility if the absolute risk is actually 10%, 20%, and 30%, respectively. Thus, the model's calibration should be assessed by checking its performance on one's population of interest to ensure that events of interest such as morbidity and mortality are not being under- or overestimated (Figure 17-5).

In assessing the clinical utility of a risk prediction model, perhaps the most important evidence to consider is whether the model has undergone prospective validation on a sample distinct from the sample on which it was developed. Many of the current models that use machine learning techniques have been developed on retrospective databases with split samples rather than prospectively collected data with independent validation. These models should be used cautiously because generalizability may be limited.

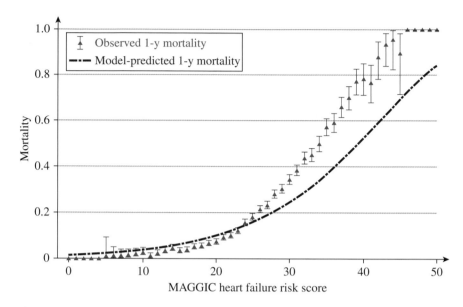

Figure 17-5 • Underestimation of predicted 1-year mortality by the MAGGIC score in heart failure patients. (Reproduced from Alba AC, Agoritsas T, Walsh M, et al. Discrimination and calibration of clinical prediction models: users' guides to the medical literature. *JAMA.* 2017;318:1377-1384.)

When comparing the performance of 2 models on the same data, it can be tempting to simply compare metrics such as c-statistic and assume that the higher c-statistic must point to the better model. However, such a comparison does not provide any insight into how well a model actually predicts the observed risk.[17,18] Net reclassification improvement (NRI) is a technique that is meant to quantify a model's ability to accurately reclassify patients into affected (ie, event) and not affected (ie, nonevent) categories as compared to another model. However, NRI can be limited by miscalibration of models, lack of access to underlying data on which to determine the true rate of events and nonevents, and some underlying lack of applicability to noncategorical predictions.[19] Comparison of the performance of 2 models is not a straightforward task. Researchers should strongly consider statistical consultation when reviewing manuscripts for publication and especially if comparison of models is part of the proposed methodology for an upcoming research project.

Author Interpretations of Results

As with any academic publication, the discussion provides the authors' interpretation of the data and their perceived impact on the field. It is important to first review the methodology and results apart from the authors' discussion to allow one to come to his or her own conclusions from the data. The discussion can then be reviewed to assess whether the authors' interpretations are congruent with your own. Reporting of the limitations of the study is the section of the discussion to evaluate. Consider the data set, the modeling, and validation, and determine whether the authors appropriately identified the limitations of their work and interpreted their results in the context of those limitations. Furthermore, in light of the limitations, consider whether any claims of clinical applicability are merited. Ultimately, a thorough evaluation of the earlier parts of the article should allow you to either agree or disagree with the conclusions of the authors.

CONCLUSION

For additional resources on critically evaluating medical literature, *JAMA: The Journal of the American Medical Association* has, since 1993, been publishing a series entitled "Users' Guide to the Medical Literature" that provides an excellent overview to evaluating different types of papers.[20] For papers that use AI techniques, the questions to ask in assessing the papers remain the same as when reading any other clinical investigation: (1) Was the right question asked? (2) Were the right methods used? (3) Were the right data analyzed? (4) Are the conclusions of this paper supported by the data? (5) How will this change my practice or affect my patients?

At the time of this writing, efforts have been underway to develop a Consolidated Standards of Reporting Trials (CONSORT) guideline for AI as well as a Standard Protocol Items: Recommendations for Interventional Trials (SPIRIT) statement for AI.[21,22] These guidelines will hopefully improve the design and reporting of trials involving AI techniques, and we highly recommend that readers keep an eye out for the publication of these statements to further guide evaluation of the literature.

REFERENCES

1. Krouss M, Croft L, Morgan DJ. Physician understanding and ability to communicate harms and benefits of common medical treatments. *JAMA Intern Med.* 2016;176:1565-1567.
2. Anderson BL, Williams S, Schulkin J. Statistical literacy of obstetrics-gynecology residents. *J Grad Med Educ.* 2013;5:272–275.
3. Keshav S. How to read a paper. *ACM SIGCOMM Comput Commun Rev.* 2007;37:83-84.
4. Cormode G. How NOT to review a paper. *ACM SIGMOD Record.* 2009;37:100-104.

5. Deal SB, Stefanidis D, Telem D, et al. Evaluation of crowd-sourced assessment of the critical view of safety in laparoscopic cholecystectomy. *Surg Endosc.* 2017;31:5094-5100.

6. Hashimoto DA, Rosman G, Witkowski ER, et al. Computer vision analysis of intraoperative video: automated recognition of operative steps in laparoscopic sleeve gastrectomy. *Ann Surg.* 2019;270:414-421.

7. Celi LA, Citi L, Ghassemi M, Pollard TJ. The PLOS ONE collection on machine learning in health and biomedicine: towards open code and open data. *PLoS One.* 2019;14:e0210232.

8. Twinanda AP, Shehata S, Mutter D, et al. EndoNet: a deep architecture for recognition tasks on laparoscopic videos. *IEEE Trans Med Imaging.* 2017;36:86-97.

9. Vittinghoff E, McCulloch CE. Relaxing the rule of ten events per variable in logistic and Cox regression. *Am J Epidemiol.* 2007;165:710-718.

10. Liu Y, Chen P-HC, Krause J, Peng L. How to read articles that use machine learning: users' guides to the medical literature. *JAMA.* 2019;322:1806-1816.

11. Data preprocessing in detail. IBM Developer. Accessed October 7, 2020. https://developer.ibm.com/technologies/data-science/articles/data-preprocessing-in-detail/.

12. Roimi M, Neuberger A, Shrot A, et al. Early diagnosis of bloodstream infections in the intensive care unit using machine-learning algorithms. *Intensive Care Med.* 2020;46:454-462.

13. Gordon L, Grantcharov T, Rudzicz F. Explainable artificial intelligence for safe intraoperative decision support. *JAMA Surg.* 2019;154:1064-1065.

14. Bertsimas D, Dunn J, Velmahos GC, Kaafarani HMA. Surgical risk is not linear: derivation and validation of a novel, user-friendly, and machine-learning-based Predictive OpTimal Trees in Emergency Surgery Risk (POTTER) Calculator. *Ann Surg.* 2018;268:574-583.

15. Russakovsky O, Deng J, Su H, et al. ImageNet large scale visual recognition challenge. *Int J Comput Vision.* 2015;115:211-252.

16. Analyzing machine-learning model performance. IBM. https://cloud.ibm.com/docs/services/knowledge-studio?topic=knowledge-studio-evaluate-ml.

17. Alba AC, Agoritsas T, Walsh M, et al. Discrimination and calibration of clinical prediction models: users' guides to the medical literature. *JAMA.* 2017;318:1377-1384.

18. Han K, Song K, Choi BW. How to develop, validate, and compare clinical prediction models involving radiological parameters: study design and statistical methods. *Korean J Radiol.* 2016;17:339-350.

19. Leening MJG, Vedder MM, Witteman JCM, Pencina MJ, Steyerberg EW. Net reclassification improvement: computation, interpretation, and controversies. *Ann Intern Med.* 2014;160:122-131.

20. Oxman AD. Users' guides to the medical literature. I. How to get started. The Evidence-Based Medicine Working Group. *JAMA.* 1993;270:2093-2095.

21. Schulz KF, Altman DG, Moher D. CONSORT 2010 statement: updated guidelines for reporting parallel group randomised trials. *BMJ.* 2010;340:c332.

22. Chan A-W, Tetzlaff JM, Altman DG, et al. SPIRIT 2013 statement: defining standard protocol items for clinical trials. *Ann Intern Med.* 2013;158:200-207.

AUTOMATION AND THE FUTURE OF SURGERY

18

Ozanan R. Meireles, Daniela Rus, and Daniel A. Hashimoto

HIGHLIGHTS

- Adoption of new technologies in surgery is appropriately slow to allow for the accumulation of evidence to support the use of such technology.
- In the automotive industry, cars are defined by 6 levels of automation ranging from no automation to full automation, and automation for surgical robots can similarly be considered on 6 levels.
- Important considerations for the implementation of autonomous surgical robots include patient safety, cost, surgical education, and surgical credentialing.
- A large-scale effort at sharing quantitative operative data, known as the collective surgical consciousness, will likely be needed to enable research that can lead to generalizable results in artificial intelligence–enabled surgery.

INTRODUCTION

Prior chapters introduced and explored the current state of artificial intelligence (AI) in surgery and opined on specific areas under development in surgical AI. We have seen how various machine learning techniques are having impact on risk prediction and patient selection (Chapters 3 and 9); how natural language processing is alleviating documentation burden and catalyzing clinical workflows (Chapters 5 and 13); and how computer vision has been augmenting intraoperative data streams to allow for more quantitative analysis of surgical events (Chapter 6). Deep learning has had a significant impact across many subfields in AI and has sped the application of AI to surgical environments (Chapters 4, 7, and 11). Robotics, despite significant advances in technology and availability for nearly 2 decades as a surgical tool, is still relatively early in terms of its maturity in many surgical specialties (Chapter 12). The pace of adoption of surgical technology such as robotics and AI has been variable.

Surgery is certainly a conservative profession. Given the stakes at hand (ie, patient lives), adoption of new technologies is appropriately slow to allow for the accumulation of evidence to support the use of such technology. It is therefore not surprising that automation has not entered surgery, where highly complex, unique physiologic and pathophysiologic conditions are treated by humans who, after training for a decade or more, must perform at the peak of their technical skill, critical assessment, and judgment. Surgeons are tasked with demonstrating exceptional coordination between their eyes and hands to deliver the finest and most precise movements, to the point that the phrase "surgical precision" epitomizes the pinnacle of precision in other professions and industries. Furthermore, surgeons have a duty to ensure that any technology is introduced with the goal of improving patient care and preventing patient harm (Chapter 14).

However, as described in Chapter 12, advances in digital technologies have catalyzed conversations and inspired dreams of what an autonomous operation might entail. Furthermore, advances in automated identification of operative steps, instruments, and events through deep learning (Chapters 4, 6, 10, and 11) raise the possibility that clinical decision support from AI could give way to automation of, at least, aspects of surgical care. Although predicting the future can never be certain, we present one possible path through which surgery may see increased adoption of AI and robotics, particularly as it relates to clinical decision making and automation.

▌ CURRENT LANDSCAPE OF AUTOMATION IN SURGERY

The industrial revolution served as a breakthrough, with machine automation beginning to be widely used in manufacturing, farming, and other industries. As technology advanced, automation became incorporated into more advanced and refined fields such as aviation, space exploration, textiles, communication, and others; however, despite significant advances in surgical device technology, automation seen at the scale of these other fields has not been incorporated into surgery. Some barriers are technologic, whereas others are cultural, as described earlier.

Over the course of the past 20 years, surgical robots have entered the operating room, providing assistance to surgeons through increased stability and robotic positioning of the camera, enhanced dexterity, elimination of tremors, 3-dimensional visualization, improved ergonomics for surgeons, and decreased barriers to entry to perform advanced minimally invasive surgery. However, such advances have been costly, and increased capital investments in robotic systems have not yielded evidence of improved clinical outcomes.[1]

The current generation of approved surgical robots is not intelligent. As reviewed in Chapter 12, the algorithms used on their operating systems are largely deprived of AI in the sense that these machines are constrained to specific tasks and operate either as leader-follower devices or as devices designed to function within a preregistered operative environment. Soft tissue surgical robotic systems (ie, robots designed for use in the abdomen) currently available for clinical use are deprived of autonomous capabilities. These robots are fully dependent on a human operator. Some "hard tissue" robotic systems are capable of performing low-level tasks to alert and assist the surgeon in placement of objects such as screws, catheters, or electrodes, similar to cars equipped with intelligent cruise control and lane assist.

At the research level, there has been some work done on low-level automation of straightforward soft tissue surgical subtasks and primitive actions, such as steering a needle, grasping, suturing,[2] and cutting.[3] For example, Shademan et al[4] successfully demonstrated the feasibility of supervised autonomous anastomosis with near-infrared fluorescent imaging to track tissue motion by designing the Smart Tissue Autonomous Robot (STAR) system, built with a 7-degree-of-freedom (DOF) Kuka LWR 4+ industrial arm and a 1-DOF Endo360 suturing tool. This system was able to outperform human surgeons in leak pressure and suture spacing, although the conditions under which these anastomoses were performed were quite artificial.[4]

Additionally, ongoing work on improving the understanding of kinematics (ie, the motion of the robotic arms) and their impact on clinical outcomes and surgeon experience may lead to advances in decision support related to appropriate use of robotic positioning and arm motion. For example, Andrew Hung's team at the University of Southern California has published numerous studies demonstrating that certain metrics gleaned from the da Vinci Surgical System (Intuitive Surgical, Sunnyvale, CA) correlate with differences in both outcomes of patients[5] and surgical expertise.[6] Such work suggests that, as the field evolves, automated clinical decision support in robotic systems could base suggestions on data related to patient outcome and potentially offer targeted intervention through automated delivery of robotic arm motion.[6,7]

In clinical use, some solid tissue surgical robots used in orthopedic surgery already support some low levels of automation, such as the ROBODOC system (Think Surgical, Fremont, CA), which generates motion plans that the surgeon verifies and supervises during the execution of knee arthroplasty. Another example of low-level automation in orthopedic surgery is the Mako-Stryker Surgical System (Stryker, Kalamazoo, MI), in which the robot applies constraints to the surgeon's actions when approaching the boundaries of a previously determined safe region for knee arthroplasty.

A PATH TOWARD AUTOMATION IN SURGERY

For some, the ultimate goal is to enable surgical robots with the necessary technology to become fully autonomous and to perform surgery independent of a human surgeon, with the hope that the technology may allow robotic systems to surpass human capabilities. Given the rapid advancements seen in AI on high-level cognitive tasks such as complex gaming and autonomous driving, it may be tempting to think that fully autonomous surgical robots are on the horizon. However, AI and robotics researchers have described what is known as Moravec's paradox, which is the observation that, contrary to common assumptions, cognitive reasoning (a high-level function in humans) requires less computation than sensorimotor functions (considered a relatively low-level function in humans), which require enormous computational resources.[8] Thus, although a fully autonomous robot performing surgery is far from achievable with the current technology (and difficult to predict when it will happen), the automation of small surgical tasks and subtasks is likely to be seen in the more proximate future.

Surgical procedures are divided into steps, where, within a given period of time, tasks (eg, mobilize the stomach) are performed by the operator to accomplish predetermined goals (eg, perform a gastrectomy). The tasks can then be deconstructed into subtasks (eg, free the greater curvature), which then can be broken down into actions (eg, apply bipolar current to the omentum and cut the coagulated tissue). Therefore, we predict that the natural progression to a semi-autonomous surgical robot will be to first automate actions that are universal and can be adopted in different tasks before ultimately scaling to specific steps of operations. Similar to other industries, the adoption framework will likely be based on the gradual introduction of different levels of autonomy, although over a much longer period of time.

It is important to remember that automating surgical robots, especially those operating on soft tissue, is very different than automating robots that function in factories or self-driving cars, which may be designed for regulated, if not chaotic, constrained environments (eg, assembly lines or highways). Autonomous surgical robots will have to function in the complex environment of the human body, dealing with deformable structures with a wide variety of unique tissue characteristics that can be difficult to model.

Human Driver Monitors Environment			System Monitors Environment		
0 No Automation Solely reliant on human control and guidance.	1 Driver Assistance Human control; systems to assist navigation or speed.	2 Partial Automation Automated assistance, eg, cruise control, lane keeping.	3 Conditional Automation Automated navigation and monitoring, human backup.	4 High Automation Fully automated, human backup only in limited circumstances.	5 Full Automation Fully automated "smart vehicle" capable of operating in any circumstance.

Human vs Robot Surgeons					
0 No Automation Traditional surgery: Human surgeon performs all tasks.	1 Some Assistance eg, intraoperative image guidance; human still physically performs all surgery.	2 Partial Automation eg, ROBODOC hip arthroplasty robot: reduced level of human input required but range of procedures.	3 Conditional Automation eg, CyberKnife, automated pre-operative planning and radiosurgery (but not technically "surgery").	4 High Automation eg, Robot capable of performing most, if not all parts of a complex procedure. Negligible human input required.	5 Full Automation eg, Robot for deep space exploration? Fully autonomous, versatile; no human assistance needed.

Figure 18-1 • A comparison of levels of autonomy in self-driving cars (top) and robotic surgical systems (bottom).[9]

Despite differences between surgery and driving, the autonomous vehicle industry provides an excellent framework with which to consider the levels of autonomy that can be attained. In the automotive industry, cars are defined by 6 levels of automation, as demonstrated in Figure 18-1.[9] An analogous framework to consider has been presented by Yip and Das[10] with a gradient from direct control to full autonomy (Figure 18-2).

As is already evident in our currently available robotic surgical systems, development and implementation of surgical autonomy will be incremental. Even when considering the examples provided in Figure 18-2,

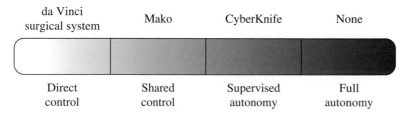

Figure 18-2 • A growing gradient of autonomy in robotic systems ranging from direct human control to full autonomy.[10]

the CyberKnife system (Accuray, Sunnyvale, CA), considered a supervised autonomous system, is a radiotherapy device rather than a true surgical robotic system. Although work such as the STAR provides hope that surgical tasks like suturing, which is complex for even novice humans to learn, can be achieved by robotic systems, the same work demonstrates the significant constraints that must be present to allow such systems to function autonomously at near-human levels of skill.[4] Such constraints are not realistic for operating room environments. Furthermore, one must consider the speed with which surgical tasks can be achieved by autonomous systems. Research performed on a modified da Vinci Surgical System designed to perform autonomous tasks such as pattern cutting (a skill from the Fundamentals of Laparoscopic Surgery certification program[11]) demonstrated that the success rate of the system in cutting a circle was 70% and that the mean time to perform the task was 284 seconds, well above the expert proficiency cutoff of 162 seconds.[3]

It will be critical to develop robotic capabilities that are not only precise but also efficient. Automated functions must be performed in a manner that leads to significant improvement in patient outcome, either at the individual level or at a population level. For example, a robot designed to perform automated suturing of bowel anastomoses should yield results that are superior to human hand-sewn or stapled anastomoses to justify an increase in the cost of performing the operation through utilization of a robotic system. This does not necessarily have to be for any and every anastomosis; rather, it may be in select situations such as deep in the pelvis or high above the diaphragmatic hiatus through an abdominal approach. Alternatively, if results are equivalent, the robot should enable other benefits such as reduced operative time or an increase in access to minimally invasive surgery for patients.

The advancement of automation in surgical robotics will likely mirror advances we have seen in self-driving vehicles. Consider that many vehicles now offer some form of automated assistance even with base-level packages (eg, lane detection, adaptive cruise control, automated headlights). Others still offer more advanced automated features such as automated parking (Smart Park by Hyundai) or even some autonomous driving (Tesla). These capabilities can be set up to merely warn drivers, as with lane detection; to selectively assist drivers in specific tasks, as with adaptive cruise control; or to provide targeted conditional automation, such as with Tesla's self-driving feature.

We anticipate that AI systems, such as those reviewed throughout this book, will first provide clinical decision support through warnings (both in robotic and nonrobotic surgery) that augment surgeons' abilities to make informed operative decisions in all phases of care from pre- to postoperative care. As we have already seen with orthopedic and neurosurgical robotics, robotic assistance is already present in select cases, providing surgeons with operative versions of "lane assist." As research in computer vision and robotics advances, we anticipate conditional automation of surgical tasks will be demonstrated in research environments. However, as stated earlier, ultimate translation into clinical practice will have to be rolled out with consideration of the benefits that will be afforded to patients, surgeons, and the health system overall.

THE COLLECTIVE SURGICAL CONSCIOUSNESS

Although many efforts have been made to gather high-quality surgical data (see Chapter 2), collection of intraoperative data that can be used to assist in the development and ultimate deployment of AI-based clinical decision support and autonomous surgical robotics is not widespread. Many of these databases are from single institutions or proprietary to the medical device companies that are currently working in the field. In fact, data to enable further development of many AI technologies for surgery, especially those related to computer vision, are also limited in scope and scale. Operative video is largely held by individual hospitals, companies, or surgical societies. Studies in computer vision and robotic surgery kinematics are largely limited to single-institution databases.[5,12,13] Such databases are important for the foundational work necessary to establish the feasibility of AI and autonomous robotics but are of limited utility when investigating clinical application outside of limited use cases.

Therefore, we strongly advocate for the establishment of a shared database of objective, quantitative surgical data. Medical device manufacturers should implement data collection capabilities in all "smart" devices, cameras, robots, and other technology (including technology for the protection of patient privacy) to allow intraoperative data to be collected, analyzed, and shared in real time across multiple surgeons. Importantly, the data collection should be conducted in a standardized manner that enables interoperability and comparison of data across devices from different manufacturers.

Ultimately, the data must be shared across institutions in a collaborative manner. Isolating the data within specific groups defeats the purpose of democratizing surgical data and knowledge. This does not mean that all data must be centralized. Advances in cloud computing and new techniques such as federated learning allow for data to be accessed and shared for machine learning purposes without revealing the actual raw data.[14,15]

A worldwide database of operative videos, kinematics, outcomes, and other health data could bring together the collective experience of hundreds

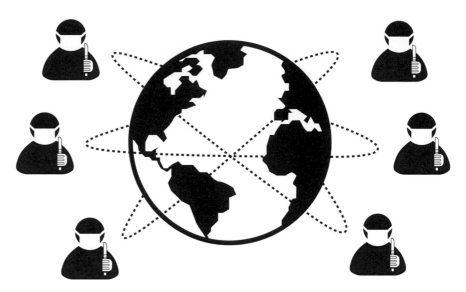

Figure 18-3 • The collective surgical consciousness has the potential to bring together the expertise of surgeons from around the world through comprehensive, quantitative data.

of surgeons—a "collective surgical consciousness" that pools the experience of a multitude of surgeons (Figure 18-3). Although current regulations in data sharing make such an effort difficult, efforts across surgical organizations, data privacy groups, patient advocacy groups, device companies, and technology foundations are ongoing to determine how best to proceed with the dream of democratizing surgical data with the hope of improving access to high-quality surgical care for the global patient population.

CONSIDERATIONS FOR CLINICAL IMPLEMENTATION OF AUTONOMOUS SYSTEMS

Let us assume that ongoing advances in technology will drive down the capital investment necessary to secure increasingly autonomous machines in the operating room with a concomitant increase in the overall adoption of robotic surgery. It is important to consider how to introduce semiautonomous robots into the clinical workflow, how to supervise them, and how to prevent deskilling of human surgeons as risk mitigation if the machine fails.

Automating surgical tasks has the potential to increase efficiency in the operating room by decreasing human involvement in tedious tasks and enabling multiple operations to be supervised by a single surgeon simultaneously (eg, similar to how anesthesiologists might supervise multiple nurse anesthetists). We would hope that automation of some tasks would diminish fatigue and allow surgeons to concentrate on more important tasks and clinical decision making. Furthermore, it could improve access to advanced surgical skills to a broader base of surgeons across different geographic locations and practice settings.

Early models of training in robotic surgery involved short bursts of training through 1- to 2-day courses followed by a handful of proctored operations. There is concern that such a training model may have contributed to a higher level of complications in robotic surgery than might otherwise have been expected.[1] The increased adoption of robotic surgery across the world has resulted in earlier and more prolonged exposure to robotic training through the surgical residency system. However, the introduction of even partially autonomous robotic systems could upend current models of training and supervision as surgeons would have to rapidly determine their personal comfort level in supervising a machine.

It will be critically important for regulatory bodies such as the US Food and Drug Administration to require very specific guidance on the data that must be collected to establish safety profiles for the use of these systems. Specific use cases should be outlined by the manufacturers, and extensive stress testing of the system should ensure that any circumstance in which failure of the robotic system could lead to a complication could be easily corrected by a human surgeon.

Inherent to the introduction of an autonomous system is the downstream effect of deskilling of surgeons. If robots are used to perform all anastomoses, how will human surgeons learn to perform them or maintain their skill in performing them? Surgical training and maintenance of certification will have to adapt appropriately to ensure that basic competencies are met and that new competencies in digital surgery are also gained.

Additionally, financial implications of acquiring and maintaining these systems should be considered in the context of the local health care system along with the implications of likely needing a specialized workforce to maintain and adjust such systems. Of course, there are significant legal ramifications regarding liability in case of a complication. If an autonomous system were to cause harm to a patient, would the surgeon, the health system, or the manufacturer be held responsible? The answer will likely depend on the extent of autonomy used and the circumstances under which the system was deployed.

Ultimately, the future for surgery is an exciting one. Although we have focused predominantly on traditional robotic systems that mimic the manner in which human surgeons intervene on surgical disease, it is

Key Point

For a video demonstration of "origami" robots, see https://www.youtube.com/watch?v=3Waj08gk7v8

important to note that many creative innovations may bypass our traditional notions of surgery. For example, self-folding, ingestible "origami" robots could one day serve as a tool to achieve foreign body neutralization and extraction, perforation repair, or anastomosis.[16] Clinicians, researchers, patients, regulators, and many others will need to work together to bring about a data-enabled world of surgery that truly changes the way we operate.

REFERENCES

1. Sheetz KH, Dimick JB. Is it time for safeguards in the adoption of robotic surgery? *JAMA*. 2019;321:1971-1972.
2. Sen S, Garg A, Gealy DV, et al. Automating multi-throw multilateral surgical suturing with a mechanical needle guide and sequential convex optimization. 2016 IEEE International Conference on Robotics and Automation (ICRA). Accessed October 7, 2020. https://goldberg.berkeley.edu/pubs/icra2016-final-suturing.pdf.
3. Murali A, Sen S, Kehoe B, et al. Learning by observation for surgical subtasks: multilateral cutting of 3D viscoelastic and 2D orthotropic tissue phantoms. 2015 IEEE International Conference on Robotics and Automation (ICRA). Accessed October 7, 2020. https://ieeexplore.ieee.org/document/7139344.
4. Shademan A, Decker RS, Opfermann JD, et al. Supervised autonomous robotic soft tissue surgery. *Sci Trans Med.* 2016;8:337ra64.
5. Chen A, Ghodoussipour S, Titus MB, et al. Comparison of clinical outcomes and automated performance metrics in robot-assisted radical prostatectomy with and without trainee involvement. *World J Urol.* 2019;38(7):1615-1621.
6. Nguyen JH, Chen J, Marshall SP, et al. Using objective robotic automated performance metrics and task-evoked pupillary response to distinguish surgeon expertise. *World J Urol.* 2020;38(7):1599-1605.
7. Hung AJ, Chen J, Ghodoussipour S, et al. A deep-learning model using automated performance metrics and clinical features to predict urinary continence recovery after robot-assisted radical prostatectomy. *BJU Int.* 2019;124:487-495.
8. Falco J, Van Wyk K, Liu S, Carpin S. Grasping the performance: facilitating replicable performance measures via benchmarking and standardized methodologies. *IEEE Robot Automation Mag.* 2015;22:125-136.
9. Panesar S, Cagle Y, Chander D, et al. Artificial intelligence and the future of surgical robotics. *Ann Surg.* 2019;270:223-226.
10. Yip M, Das N. Robot autonomy for surgery. *Encyclop Med Robot.* 2018;281-313.
11. Marks JM. Fundamentals of laparoscopic surgery (FLS) and of endoscopic surgery (FES). In: Soper N, Scott-Conner C, eds. *The SAGES Manual*. Springer; 2012.
12. Twinanda AP, Shehata S, Mutter D, et al. EndoNet: a deep architecture for recognition tasks on laparoscopic videos. *IEEE Trans Med Imaging.* 2017;36:86-97.
13. Hashimoto DA, Rosman G, Witkowski ER, et al. Computer vision analysis of intraoperative video: automated recognition of operative steps in laparoscopic sleeve gastrectomy. *Ann Surg.* 2019;270:414-421.

14. Wu Q, He K, Chen X. Personalized federated learning for intelligent IoT applications: a cloud-edge based framework. *IEEE Comput Graph Appl.* 2020. doi:10.1109/OJCS.2020.2993259.
15. Ilias C, Georgios S. Machine learning for all: a more robust federated learning framework. Proceedings of the 5th International Conference on Information Systems Security and Privacy. Accessed October 7, 2020. https://www.scitepress.org/Link.aspx?doi=10.5220/0007571705440551.
16. Miyashita S, Guitron S, Yoshida K, et al. Ingestible, controllable, and degradable origami robot for patching stomach wounds. 2016 IEEE International Conference on Robotics and Automation (ICRA). Accessed October 7, 2020. https://ppm.csail.mit.edu/sites/default/files/publications/201605ICRA_MiyashitaEtAl_Preprint.pdf.

GLOSSARY Appendix

1

Accuracy The total correct predictions (true positives and true negatives) divided by the total set of predictions; see Table 17-3 for mathematical description.

Adaptive histogram equalization Histogram equalization that occurs at the "local" level, wherein distinct sections of an image are equalized across a histogram of light intensity; it can enhance edges in each region of an image.

Artificial intelligence A field of study that focuses on the study of algorithms that give machines the ability to reason and perform cognitive functions.

Aspect ratio Ratio of an image's or video's width to height; the traditional aspect ratio is 4:3, whereas the more modern or widescreen aspect ratio is 16:9.

Automatic speech recognition (ASR) See computerized voice recognition.

Autonomy With regard to ethical principles in medicine, refers to the respect for the decisions of adults who have decision-making capacity.

Back-end speech recognition (BESR) A human-hybrid production approach that applies computerized voice recognition to prepare a draft transcript of human-dictated speech, which is then passed to human transcriptionists for final review and editing.

Backpropagation An algorithm to adjust weights within a neural network from final layer back to input layer based on each weight's contribution to error during forward propagation.

Beneficence The moral obligation to act for the benefit of others.

Biomedical informatics Branch of health informatics that uses data to help clinicians, researchers, and scientists improve human health and provide health care.

Channel effect An effect wherein a model may learn characteristics of the manner in which data were recorded, in addition to the nature of the data themselves.

Classification decision trees A hierarchical structure to achieve classification of data in an iterative fashion such that the final structure represents a "tree." Each tree is composed of a node, which reflects the test or question on which the data is divided; a branch, which is the outcome of a test performed at the preceding node; and leaf nodes, which represent the final node that yields an outcome. The data are split iteratively into partitions until each partition is sufficiently homogenous to yield an acceptable results based on predefined stopping criteria.

Computer vision   Machine understanding of visual data (ie, images and videos).

Computerized voice recognition   An extension of signal processing to include recognition of speech utterances, application of language and speech models, and computational machine learning (assisted by neural networks and cloud computing) to enable machine awareness and understanding of spoken human speech.

Conditional random field   A statistical modeling method that is used for structured predictions and takes context into account. For example, in natural language processing, sequential data about surrounding words can be taken into account, or in computer vision, data about nearby structures can be used to help predictions.

Contextual bias   Bias that may occur if one ignores what may appear to be trivial caveats (eg, whether the operating surgeon is right- or left-handed) or if one presumes that the same level of resources is available across operating rooms and hospitals.

Convolutional neural network   A type of neural network that uses convolution operations and pooling to generate an output; it is constructed, at minimum, of a convolutional layer, a pooling layer, and a fully connected layer.

Cost function   See loss function.

Current Procedural Terminology (CPT)   A medical code set that is used to report medical, surgical, and diagnostic procedures and services to entities such as physicians, health insurance companies, and accreditation organizations.

Cyber-physical systems   Systems with both computational (software) and physical (hardware) components.

Data augmentation   Increasing the size of the training subset by adding additional data generated using modifications of the available training data set.

Deep learning   A machine learning method that is equivalent to neural networks but with greater than 3 layers; deep learning utilizes automatic feature extraction to generate a prediction.

Diagnosis-related group (DRG)   A patient classification system that standardizes prospective payment to hospitals and encourages cost containment initiatives.

Electronic health record (EHR)   A digital version of a patient's paper chart. EHRs are real-time, patient-centered records that make information available instantly and securely to authorized users.

F1 score   The harmonic or weighted mean of precision and recall; see Table 17-3 for mathematical description.

Filter   Mathematical operations to adjust images at the local level, with adjustments made to a pixel based on surrounding pixel information.

Focus bias   Bias arising from the differential usage of information in training artificial intelligence systems (ie, more heavily weighting the impact of one source of data over another); this bias may be exploited to account for causal mechanisms or interaction effects with other variables.

Forward propagation   The transmission of data "forward" within a neural network from the input layer through hidden layers to the final output layer. The input is modified by a hidden weight and passed through an activation function, the result of which is then forward propagated to the next layer.

Generative adversarial networks (GANs)   A model is trained to synthesize images resembling examples from a given training data set using 2 neural networks. The first network, or generator, tries to synthesize an output resembling the training data, whereas a second network, or discriminator, competes to identify whether the generated example was a fake. During training, as the discriminator gets better at discerning fake examples, the generator becomes more efficient at generating realistic fakes.

Global Objective Assessment of Laparoscopic Skills (GOALS)   Like the Objective Structured Assessment of Technical Skills, a Likert scale questionnaire to measure performance but specifically for laparoscopic tasks. It was first described in Vassiliou MC, Feldman LS, Andrew CG, et al. A global assessment tool for evaluation of intraoperative laparoscopic skills. *Am J Surg.* 2005;190(1):107-113.

Gradient boosted decision trees A machine learning technique where decision trees are built in a stepwise fashion, with each subsequent tree measuring and correcting the error of the tree that preceded it. It is an ensemble method that utilizes the output of several weaker models.

Gradient descent An optimization algorithm whereby the loss function is minimized by moving iteratively toward the direction of steepest descent (ie, down a negative gradient) to find the local or global minimum of a function, depending on the context.

Graphical processing unit (GPU) Computer chips originally designed for graphical tasks but that were found to be well suited to machine learning computations and other parallel processing tasks.

Ground truth Refers to underlying truth on which an algorithm's accuracy is judged for supervised learning techniques.

Hidden Markov Model (HMM) A statistical model that considers a series of events that are observable yet influenced by factors that are not directly observable (hidden states). The hidden states are first-order Markovian; that is, the probability of entering the next state depends on only the current state and that probability is fixed.

Hierarchical condition categories (HCCs) Used by third-party payers for scoring risk-adjusted patient panels and justifying increased payments under value-based contracts.

Histogram equalization A technique for adjusting contrast in an image by modifying the intensity distribution across a histogram of an entire image.

Human factors research The study of how people interact psychologically and physically with their working environment.

Hyperparameters The numeric hand-tunable configurations of a machine learning algorithm (eg, learning rate, number of neurons in a neural network).

Image classification An algorithmic task to label a set of images with a particular category.

Instance detection An algorithmic task to detect and label each instance of an object within an image that fits a particular category.

Instance segmentation An algorithmic task to detect all objects within an image while providing pixel-wise segmentation of each instance.

International Classification of Diseases (ICD) The diagnostic classification standard for all clinical and research purposes. ICD defines the universe of diseases, disorders, injuries, and other related health conditions, listed in a comprehensive, hierarchical fashion.

Interpretation bias Bias arising from the misinterpretation of an algorithm's output by either a human user or by the broader system within which the algorithm functions.

JHU–ISI Gesture and Skill Assessment Working Set (JIGSAWS) A data set of robotic surgical data that contains kinematic data such as Cartesian positions, orientations, velocities, angular velocities, and gripper angles along with the stereo videos captured during the operation and is manually assessed with different expertise levels.

K-fold cross-validation A nonexhaustive form of cross-validation; a sample of data is divided into k-sized segments, and one subsample is held out as a test set. This is then repeated across the different k-sized segments until mean error of the model can be estimated.

Kaizen cycle A continuous improvement process of observing a situation, identifying problems, and implementing solutions with the cycle repeating continuously to yield better and better processes with each iteration.

Kernel Small n × n matrix of pixels that represents a specific localized portion of the image and their associated weights; an algorithm can use a kernel to run a mathematical function for every matrix of pixels in that particular image, producing a single output for each matrix to create a modified view of the data.

Latent space A "hidden" world of structure and dimension within the data, but one that we cannot observe.

Leader-follower system A machine system with a leader that generates commands to a second unit, the follower, that executes tasks as commanded by the leader; this type of system does not function autonomously; rather, a human (surgeon) controls the leader unit to generate action by the follower.

Learning rate The amount to change in the components of a model from iteration to iteration.

Least absolute shrinkage and selection operator (lasso) penalized logistic regression A feature selection algorithm that is an extension of the ordinary least squares regression algorithm; it minimizes the residual sum of squares (RSS) and adds a penalty to the RSS based on the absolute value of the coefficients in the regression.

Leave-one-out cross-validation   A form of leave-p-out cross-validation; one observation is selected from the data sample as a test set with the remaining data used for training.

Leave-p-out cross-validation   A form of exhaustive cross-validation; a p number of observations is selected from the data sample as a test set with the remaining data used for training. The model is then repeated in all possible ways such that all data have, at one point, been part of subsample p.

Long short-term memory (LSTM)   Specific type of recurrent neural network that allows for "memory" of data to persist within a neural network so that it can be used in other layers of a neural network.

Loss function (also known as cost function)   A function of the modeling process that maps observations or outcomes onto a real number that we wish to minimize.

Lossless compression   Type of compression that results in a file in which the original file can be reconstructed perfectly from the compressed file.

Machine learning   The study of computer algorithms that seek to improve performance automatically through experience.

Markov assumption   An assumption that an observation at time t depends not on the entire history of observations that preceded it, but is approximately estimated by only the recent past.

Medical Language Extraction and Encoding (MedLEE)   A natural language processing algorithm with the goal to extract, structure, and encode clinical information in textual patient reports so that the data can be used by subsequent automated processes.

MySurgeryRisk   An analytics platform developed by the University of Florida; it pulls raw data continuously from a patient's electronic health record and calculates risk of morbidity and mortality related to procedures.

Named-entity recognition (NER)   A subtask of information extraction that seeks out and categorizes specified entities in a body or bodies of text.

Natural language inference (NLI) The task of classifying the relationship between 2 sentences—a premise and a hypothesis—as entailment, neutral, or contradiction.

Natural language processing (NLP) A collection of tools and computer algorithmic techniques that aim to help humans automatically "structure" and model relationships between words to gain an in-depth, contextual understanding of free text information; a subfield of artificial intelligence and machine learning that concentrates on the capture, interpretation, and manipulation of human-generated spoken or written data.

Natural language text A human language. For example, English, French, and Chinese are natural languages. Computer languages, such as FORTRAN and C, are not.

Near miss Potential adverse event that did not reach the patient due to random chance or recovery from other processes.

Neural network An algorithmic technique composed of a collection of computational units (called neurons) that are interconnected in layers in a manner that loosely mimics neurons in a biological brain. At minimum, a neural network is composed of an input layer, a hidden layer, and an output layer. Features can be automatically extracted to generate a prediction.

Nonmaleficence The moral obligation to not inflict harm on others.

Normalization Preprocessing strategy where the input data are scaled down to a smaller range of values such as between 0 and 1.

Objective Structured Assessment of Technical Skills (OSATS) Validated global rating scale consisting of 7 domains graded on a Likert scale from 1 to 5: respect for tissue, time and motion, instrument handling, knowledge of instruments, the flow of operation, use of assistants, and knowledge of the specific procedure. It was first described in Martin JA, Regehr G, Reznick R, et al. Objective Structured Assessment of Technical Skill (OSATS) for surgical residents. *Br J Surg*. 1997;84(2):273-278.

Optimal classification tree (OCT) A type of classification decision tree that creates the entire decision tree at once instead of iteratively; this approach attempts to overcome the limitation of traditional decision trees that create node partitions at local optima rather than considering the overall optimization problem.

Overfitting A model that is tightly fitted to the training data and has low bias but high variance and will not generalize well to unseen data.

Perceptron   A computational model of a neuron that takes the weighted sum of inputs and outputs a "1" if the sum exceeds a given threshold, a process analogous to neurons firing an action potential if a certain threshold potential is reached. The perceptron's internal parameters update much like neurons' connections strengthen or weaken with learning.

Point operation   Image transformation in which the output of a pixel's value is dependent only on that pixel's input value.

Precision   Positive predictive value; true positives divided by the sum of true positives and false positives; see Table 17-3 for mathematical description.

Preprocessing   Suitably altering the data set before passing it to the network can greatly improve the learning process in terms of stability, preventing overfitting and time to converge to a good minimum corresponding to a sufficiently low loss.

Prior knowledge inference (PKI)   Probabilistic method that, when used to analyze video, takes the probability of the previous frames as input and updates the predictions according to the previously known ordering of phases.

Processing bias   Algorithmic bias introduced from the use of statistically biased estimators, which may reduce the variance of the model.

Random forest   An ensemble method where multiple decision trees (called estimators) are constructed by randomly sampling the data with replacement and aggregating the predictions of the estimators to yield an overall prediction.

Recall sensitivity   True positives divided by the sum of true positives and false negatives; see Table 17-3 for mathematical description.

Recurrent neural networks   A type of neural network that is particularly adept at modeling data in a sequence because it can use prior outputs as inputs.

Regularization   Process of providing additional constraints to a model to reduce overfitting.

Reinforcement learning   A form of learning that is goal directed, wherein a machine learns, through a series of trial-and-error decisions that are either rewarded or punished, to achieve a goal; analogous to operant conditioning in biological organisms.

Robot   A machine equipped with sensors to observe the physical world and actuators to physically affect the world with computation involved between the sensor and actuator to generate action.

Rule-based expert systems (also known as production systems or expert systems)   These are the simplest form of artificial intelligence. A rule-based system uses rules as the knowledge representation for knowledge coded into the system.

Semantic segmentation   The task of classifying every pixel of an image target into a particular category (see Figure 4-8C).

Sequence-to-sequence (seq2seq) architecture   A model that consists of an encoder for processing a variable-length sequence as input and a decoder for generating the output sequence (usually variable-length too) in an autoregression fashion.

Sobel filter   A 3 × 3 kernel designed to detect either horizontal or vertical edges.

Supervised learning   A form of learning where human labelers may apply their insights or expertise to provide the targets of a presumed function over the features of the data.

Support vector machine   A supervised machine learning algorithm that maps data and attempts to maximize the distance between any 2 classes to optimize performance.

Surgemes   The shortest surgical motion units with semantic sense.

Surgical coaching   Partnering with surgeons in a process that inspires them to maximize their personal and professional potential, often through video review.

Surgical phase recognition   Field of research concerned with classifying frames of a video into an operation's component phases or steps.

Total project life cycle approach   A Food and Drug Administration regulation strategy centered around 4 key steps: validation of manufacturer reputation, review of safety and efficacy through testing, establishment of a protocol for changes to the device/software, and extensive real-world monitoring of performance after release.

Transfer learning   Pretrain the network on an alternate but similar task and/or data set and then optimize or fine-tune a subset of the network's parameters on the target data set.

Transfer of context bias   Bias introduced when an algorithm or trained model is employed outside the context of its training. An unwarranted application or extension of an artificial intelligence system outside of its intended contexts will not necessarily perform according to appropriate statistical, moral, or legal standards.

Underfitting   A model that does not appropriately describe the data and whose output shows high bias and low variance.

Unified Medical Language System (UMLS)   Set of files and software that brings hierarchies, definitions, and other relationships and attributes from health and biomedical vocabularies and standards to enable and improve interoperability between electronic health systems.

Unsupervised learning   A form of learning that involves automatically recognizing patterns emergent from the data, such as latent or hidden structures, without any guidance whatsoever.

Unsupervised Learning   A type of machine learning algorithm used to draw inferences from data sets consisting of input data without labeled responses.

Virtual coach (VC)   A digital replacement or augmentation of a surgical coach that can provide feedback to a surgeon on performance.

Virtual scribes   Application of computerized voice recognition to generate clinical documentation from monitoring the ambient discussion in the exam room or operating room.

Voice assistants   Application of computerized voice recognition that can execute human orders, including requests for information, clinical orders, and computational instructions.

Word2vec   A 2-layer neural net that processes text. Its input is a text corpus (a collection of written texts), and its output is a set of vectors (ie, feature vectors for words in the corpus). Word2vec can be applied for parsing sentences, genes, code, likes, playlists, social media graphs, and other verbal or symbolic series in which patterns can be recognized.

RESOURCES FOR ADDITIONAL EDUCATION IN ARTIFICIAL INTELLIGENCE

Although this textbook was meant to provide an understanding of the nontechnical fundamentals to artificial intelligence (AI) in surgery, we hope that your journey through this book has inspired you to pursue additional education in AI. As such, we have curated a list of resources ranging from textbooks to online courses and code repositories. For online courses, all resources listed are free with, in some cases, an option to purchase a certificate for those interested.

▎TEXTBOOKS

Artificial Intelligence

Russell S, Norvig P. *Artificial Intelligence: A Modern Approach*. Pearson; 2009. (One of the definitive textbooks for AI. A comprehensive textbook on the theory and application of AI that is often used for both undergraduate and graduate courses in AI.)

James G, Witten D, Hastie T, Tibshirani R. *An Introduction to Statistical Learning With Applications in R*. Springer; 2013. (A textbook that provides an accessible introduction to concepts in statistical learning. Each chapter contains a tutorial on implementing the analyses and methods presented in R.)

Gopal M. *Applied Machine Learning*. McGraw-Hill Education; 2018. (For readers with a solid grasp of calculus and linear algebra, this textbook provides an overview of concepts within AI, many of which are covered in the current book you are reading, but with more mathematical explanation and intuition.)

Deisenroth MP, Faisal AA, Ong CS. *Mathematics for Machine Learning*. Cambridge University Press; 2020. (This book provides a concise review of the key mathematical concepts necessary to understand machine learning for those wishing to conduct a deeper dive into understanding or building algorithms and networks.

It provides a particular emphasis on how these key mathematical concepts apply to machine learning problems.)

Programming

Wickham H, Grolemund G. *R for Data Science: Import, Tidy, Transform, Visualize, and Model Data*. O'Reilly Media; 2016.
Free online copy from the authors at https://r4ds.had.co.nz/index.html.
An easy to comprehend book that walks through the use of R programming language specifically for applications in data science.

Wickham H. *Advanced R*. CRC Press; 2019.
Free online copy from the author at https://adv-r.hadley.nz/.
For those interested in expanding their understanding of the R language, this book delves into more specific and advanced concepts.

▌ ONLINE COURSES

Mathematics Helpful for AI

Khan Academy
Linear algebra: https://www.khanacademy.org/math/linear-algebra
Calculus 1: https://www.khanacademy.org/math/calculus-1
Calculus 2: https://www.khanacademy.org/math/calculus-2
Multivariable Calculus: https://www.khanacademy.org/math/multivariable-calculus
Khan Academy's visual approach to teaching has been popular with students in middle and high school. However, they also provide valuable lessons at the college level, which is more than sufficient to help you regain a fundamental understanding of the most common mathematical approaches used in machine learning.

Mathematics for Machine Learning Specialization
Coursera: https://www.coursera.org/specializations/mathematics-machine-learning
This specialization is comprised of a series of courses to develop a deeper understanding of the mathematics used for machine learning.

Machine Learning

Machine Learning by Andrew Ng
Coursera: https://www.coursera.org/learn/machine-learning
Perhaps one of the most popular machine learning courses online. This provides a walk-through of basic concepts in linear algebra before progressing to more advanced topics such as neural networks, providing an overview of how these algorithms work "under the hood."

Neural Networks and Deep Learning by Andrew Ng
Coursera: https://www.coursera.org/learn/neural-networks-deep-learning
A follow-up to his popular Machine Learning course, this online course extends knowledge gained in the Machine Learning course and provides further training in the design and construction of deep neural networks.

fast.AI
https://course.fast.ai/
A massive open online course (MOOC) for people who have at least an introductory level of experience in coding in Python. This course provides a walk-through for training machine learning models using fastai and PyTorch.

Programming

Introduction to Computer Science and Programming Using Python by John Guttag
MIT EdX: https://www.edx.org/course/introduction-to-computer-science-and -programming-7
This course covers fundamental concepts in computer science using Python 3.5 as the programming language of choice.

Python for Everybody Specialization by Charles Severance
Coursera: https://www.coursera.org/specializations/python
This series of online courses covers the basics of Python 3.5 for individuals with no prior programming experience. It serves as an accessible yet solid introduction to programming in Python for complete novices.

R Programming by Dr. Roger Peng
Coursera: https://www.coursera.org/learn/r-programming
This course provides an introduction to using R, a popular statistical analysis software. It serves as an accessible yet solid introduction to programming in R.

▌ ONLINE VIDEOS

Stanford Engineering Lecture Collections
YouTube: https://www.youtube.com/c/stanfordengineering
The Stanford Engineering department provides several lecture collections featuring videos of their courses that include computer vision and natural language processing.

▌ CODING RESOURCES

Research Group CAMMA Chapter 4 Tutorial on Neural Networks and Deep Learning
https://github.com/CAMMA-public/ai4surgery

This short tutorial is designed to offer hands-on experience with artificial neural networks to surgeons with little to no coding experience and is specifically created for readers of this textbook.

The coding resources below refer specifically to various libraries and their specific tutorials. Background experience in programming is highly recommended if not required to engage more fully in these tutorials.

NumPy Beginner's Tutorial
NumPy: https://numpy.org/doc/stable/user/absolute_beginners.html
NumPy is a Python library for handling numerical data, including arrays and matrices.

Pandas Tutorial
Pandas: https://pandas.pydata.org/docs/user_guide/index.html
Pandas is a Python library for data loading and manipulation.

Scikit-learn Tutorial
Scikit-learn: https://scikit-learn.org/stable/tutorial/index.html
Scikit-learn is a Python library for conducting machine learning such as regression, classification, and clustering.

PyTorch Tutorials
PyTorch: https://pytorch.org/tutorials/
PyTorch is an open source machine learning library with applications in computer vision and natural language processing. This library was primarily developed by Facebook's AI Research group.

TensorFlow Tutorials
TensorFlow: https://www.tensorflow.org/tutorials
TensorFlow is an open source machine learning library with particular utility in deep learning, including for applications in computer vision. This library was developed by the Google Brain team.

▍SOFTWARE

Anaconda
https://www.anaconda.com/products/individual
Open source distribution platform for Python.

R
https://cran.r-project.org/
Offers precompiled binaries of the R environment.

Index

Note: Page numbers followed by "*f*" indicate figures and "*t*" indicate tables in the text.